Managing Chronic Pain: A Clinical Guide

Managing Chronic Pain: A Clinical Guide

Editor: Emerson Haynes

MURPHY & MOORE
www.murphy-moorepublishing.com

www.murphy-moorepublishing.com

MURPHY & MOORE

Cataloging-in-Publication Data

Managing chronic pain : a clinical guide / edited by Emerson Haynes.
p. cm.
Includes bibliographical references and index.
ISBN 978-1-63987-803-1
1. Chronic pain. 2. Chronic pain--Treatment. 3. Chronic pain--Prevention.
4. Chronic pain--Patients--Drug use. I. Haynes, Emerson.
RB127 .M363 2023
616.047 2--dc23

Murphy & Moore Publishing
1 Rockefeller Plaza,
New York City,
NY 10020, USA

ISBN 978-1-63987-803-1 (Hardback)

Contents

Preface

Pain refers to a signal in the nervous system that indicates something is wrong. There are two types of pain, namely, acute pain and chronic pain. Acute pain is short lived and intense, and activates the body's fight response. Chronic pain usually lasts longer than six months and can be either mild or severe. It is associated with complications such as arthritis, cancer, nerve pain, back pain and fibromyalgia. It causes stress in the body, which creates physical conditions, such as tense muscles, low energy, decreased ability to move, and change in appetite. The management of chronic pain involves a range of non-drug therapies including acupuncture, nerve blocks, psychotherapy, surgery, biofeedback, relaxation therapies, physical therapy, and physical manipulation. Rhizotomy, decompression, and electrical deep brain and spinal cord stimulation procedures are various types of surgeries for managing chronic pain. This book outlines the methods of chronic pain management in detail. It will serve as an invaluable source of reference for students and researchers interested in the field of chronic pain management.

When I was approached with the idea of this book and the proposal to edit it, I was overwhelmed. It gave me an opportunity to reach out to all those who share a common interest with me in this field. I had 3 main parameters for editing this text:

1. Accuracy - The data and information provided in this book should be up-to-date and valuable to the readers.

2. Structure - The data must be presented in a structured format for easy understanding and better grasping of the readers.

3. Universal Approach - This book not only targets students but also experts and innovators in the field, thus my aim was to present topics which are of use to all.

Thus, it took me a couple of months to finish the editing of this book.

I would like to make a special mention of my publisher who considered me worthy of this opportunity and also supported me throughout the editing process. I would also like to thank the editing team at the back-end who extended their help whenever required.

Editor

1

Psychometric Properties of the Polish Version of the 36-Item WHODAS 2.0 in Patients with Low Back Pain

Agnieszka Ćwirlej-Sozańska [1,*], Agnieszka Bejer [1], Agnieszka Wiśniowska-Szurlej [1], Anna Wilmowska-Pietruszyńska [2], Alessandro de Sire [3,4], Renata Spalek [4,5] and Bernard Sozański [1]

1. Institute of Health Sciences, College of Medical Sciences of the University of Rzeszow, University of Rzeszow, Rejtana16C, 35-959 Rzeszow, Poland; agnbej@wp.pl (A.B.); wisniowska@vp.pl (A.W.-S.); benieks@poczta.onet.pl (B.S.)
2. Faculty of Medicine, Lazarski University, Świeradowska Street 43, 02-662 Warsaw, Poland; anna.wilmowska@gmail.com
3. Physical and Rehabilitative Medicine, Department of Health Sciences, University of Eastern Piedmont, Viale Piazza D'Armi 1, 28100 Novara, Italy; alessandro.desire@gmail.com
4. Department of Geriatrics, Neurosciences, Orthopedics, Center for Geriatric Medicine (CEMI), Institute of Internal Medicine and Geriatrics, Catholic University of the Sacred Heart, L.go F.Vito 8, 00168 Rome, Italy; renata.spalek@unicatt.it or r.spalek-to@libero.it
5. Rehabilitation Unit, 'Mons. L. Novarese' Hospital, Str. Sotto Cerca, 13040 Vercelli, Italy

* Correspondence: sozanska@ur.edu.pl

Abstract: The World Health Organization Disability Assessment Schedule 2.0 (WHODAS 2.0) is considered by the World Health Organization (WHO) to be a useful tool for assessing the functioning and disability of the general population as well as the effectiveness of the applied interventions. Until this study, no data regarding the validity of the 36-item WHODAS 2.0 in chronic low back pain (LBP) in Poland have been explored. This study was conducted on 92 patients suffering from chronic LBP admitted to the rehabilitation ward. The Polish version of the 36-item WHODAS 2.0, the Sf-36 Health Survey (SF-36), the Oswestry Disability Index (ODI), the Hospital Anxiety and Depression Scale (HADS) and the Visual Analogue Scale (VAS) questionnaires were applied to assess patients. The scale score reliability of the entire tool for the study population was very high. The Cronbach's alpha test result for the entire scale was 0.92. For the overall result of the WHODAS 2.0, the Intraclass Correlation Coefficient ($ICC_{1,2}$) was 0.928, which confirmed that the scale was consistent over time. The total result and the vast majority of domains of the 36-item WHODAS 2.0 correlated negatively with domains of the SF-36 questionnaire; thus, a higher WHODAS 2.0 score was associated with a lower score on the SF-36 questionnaire. We found that the minimal clinically important difference (MCID) for the total WHODAS 2.0 score in patients after rehabilitation for LBP was 4.87. Overall, the results indicated that the Polish version of the 36-item WHODAS is suitable for assessing health and disability status in patients with LBP.

Keywords: ICF; disability; low back pain; rehabilitation; validity; reliability

---

1. Introduction

Currently, low back pain (LBP) is the most common health problem [1], affecting an estimated 70% to 85% of the population [2,3]. The frequency of LBP problems is still increasing [4]. LBP puts significant limitations on the functioning of individuals [5]. Chronic LBP is a serious burden on health, social, and work systems [6,7]. LBP is a major contributor to disability worldwide [8] and is in sixth place in terms of overall disease burden [9].

The World Health Organization (WHO) defines disability as a difficulty in the functioning at the level of the body, activity, or participation in social life, as experienced by a person experiencing a health problem in interaction with contextual factors [10]. The biopsychosocial conceptual model has been described in WHO's International Classification of Functioning, Disability, and Health (ICF) [11]. In this context, the ICF might be considered to be the ideal conceptual framework to adequately describe and measure the impairments, activity limitations, and participation restrictions in people affected by LBP [12]. Indeed, a recent Italian multicenter cross-sectional study reported that back pain was the most common disease (9.6%) and the sensation of pain (ICF b280) was the most common alerted ICF item (76.3%) in a cohort of 864 patients [13].

The most common tools that have been used to measure disability in patients affected by LBP are the Oswestry Disability Index (ODI) and the Roland–Morris Disability Questionnaire [14]. However, neither of them was developed with the ICF biopsychosocial conceptual model [15]. In order to get a broader perspective of the problems experienced by people with LBP, the use of the World Health Organization Disability Assessment Schedule 2.0 (WHODAS 2.0) instrument based on the ICF may be of value [16]. A comprehensive disability assessment is important for identifying problems and needs for planning health care and rehabilitation services and for assessing the results and effectiveness of interventions [17,18].

The 36-item WHODAS 2.0 has been validated in some populations where some psychological and physical disease states occur [19]. Previous studies investigated the psychometric properties of the WHODAS 2.0, including arthritis [20], stroke [21], systemic sclerosis [22], psychotic disorders [23] or depression, and back pain [24]. Lee et al. suggested that WHODAS 2.0 may be a useful measure for patients with LBP [25]. The scale was translated and validated among patients with musculoskeletal problems in various countries, including Portugal [26], Finland [27] and Turkey [28]. The WHODAS 2.0 might be among the best measures for assessing LBP disability, being the most supportive of the biopsychosocial disability model [29]. Moreover, the Measuring Health and Disability in Europe: Supporting policy development - MHADIE, an observational, longitudinal, multicentric study conducted in seven European centers (Czech Republic, Germany, Italy, Slovenia and Spain) indicated that WHODAS 2.0 conformed good metric properties in clinical and rehabilitation samples in patients with chronic diseases including LBP [30]. Results from the World Health Organization (WHO) study on global ageing and adult health (SAGE) suggested that comparable evidence on back pain and its impact on disability is needed and internationally important so that governments can invest in rehabilitation to reduce the growing economic and social burden resulting from disability [31].

However, there are no data regarding the validity of the 36-item WHODAS 2.0 in chronic low back pain in Poland. Therefore, the present study aimed to investigate the psychometric properties of the Polish version of the 36-item WHODAS 2.0 in patients with chronic LBP.

2. Materials and Methods

2.1. Study Design and Data Collection

This study was conducted on patients with chronic LBP admitted to the rehabilitation ward of the Holy Family Specialist Hospital, Rudna Mała, Poland.

Inclusion criteria were admission to the rehabilitation ward for LBP during the study period; suffering from LBP for at least 12 weeks; aged ≥50 years. The exclusion criteria were severe neurological disorders of the central nervous system (stroke and traumatic brain injury), unstable cardiovascular diseases, active cancer, amputations and lack of consent by the patient.

All consecutively admitted patients with chronic LBP from June 2019 to March 2020 meeting the inclusion criteria were qualified for the study. The study was conducted by properly prepared and trained physiotherapists in the rehabilitation ward. The investigation was performed using a direct interview implementing a pen and paper interview method. The examination was carried out three times: study I—in the first day after hospital admission using the following tools: the 36-item

WHODAS 2.0, the SF-36 Health Survey (SF-36), ODI, the Hospital Anxiety and Depression Scale (HADS), the Visual Analogue Scale (VAS), and sociodemographic data were also collected; study II—mainly two days after the study I (using the WHODAS 2.0) and study III–1 month after the completion of rehabilitation in the hospital (to assess responsiveness, the WHODAS 2.0 and VAS were used) (Figure 1).

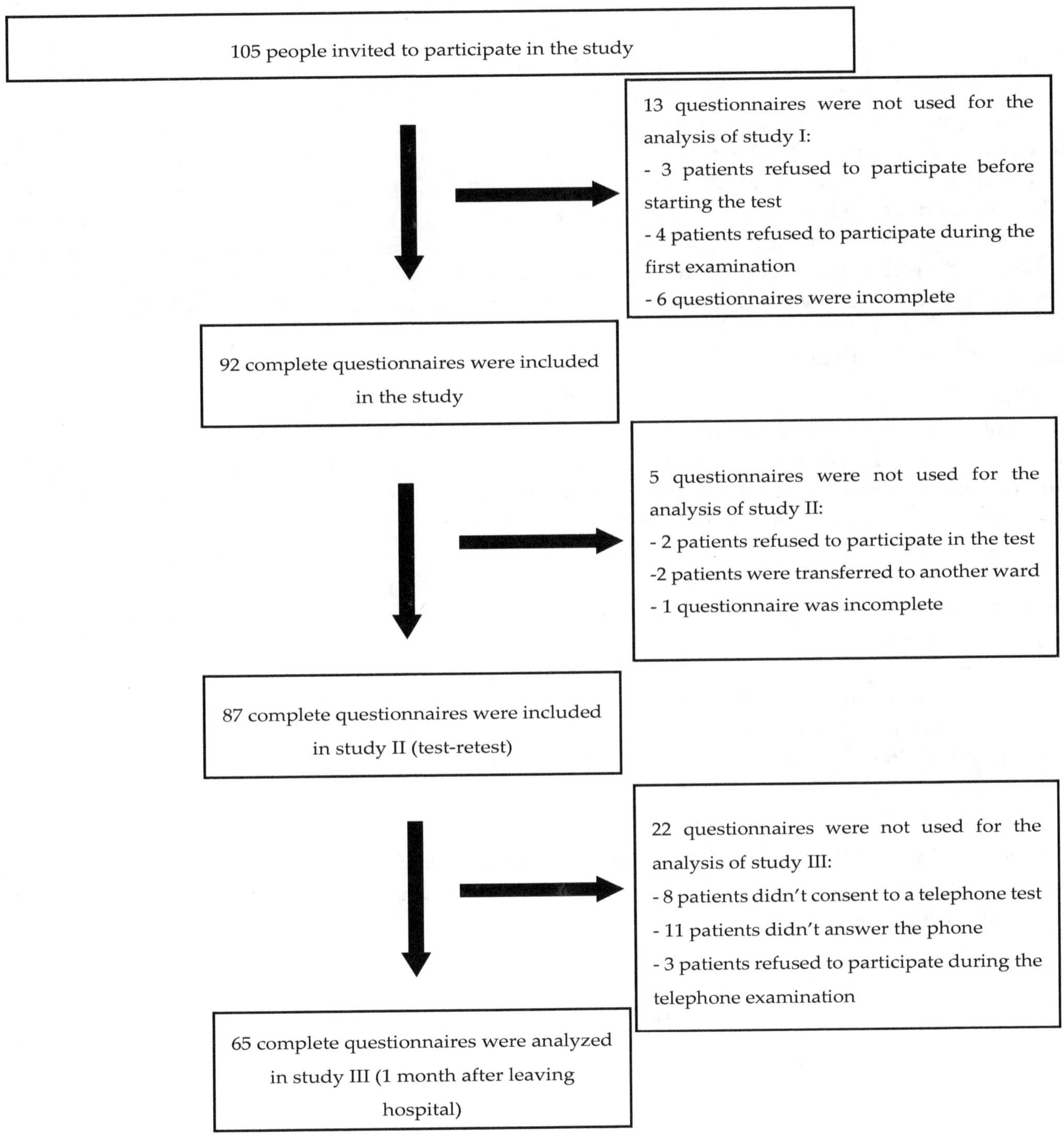

Figure 1. Flow diagram of the study.

2.2. *Ethics Approval*

This study was approved by the Bioethics Committee of the University of Rzeszów (Resolution No. 33/05/2019). All participants were instructed on the purpose and course of the study. They also received information that they could withdraw from participation at any time without any consequences. Moreover, they were asked to sign informed consent in order to take part in the research.

2.3. Measurements

2.3.1. The 36-item WHODAS 2.0

In accordance with the WHO rules, the 36-item WHODAS 2.0 was translated and culturally adapted by the ICF Council at the Poland Health Protection IT Systems, led by Professor Anna Wilmowska-Pietruszyńska, based on the agreement with the WHO [32].

The 36-item WHODAS 2.0 is used to measure general disability and disability in six domains: Do1 Cognition (6 items), Do2 Mobility (5 items), Do3 Self-care (4 items), Do4 Getting along (5 items), Do5 Life activities (8 items), and Do6 Participation (8 items). During the interview, the response refers to the last 30 days. Answers to the questions are rated on a 5-point scale identifying the level of difficulty or problem (1 = none; 2 = mild; 3 = moderate; 4 = severe; 5 = extreme or cannot to do). The obtained results are converted on the scale from 0 to 100 [33]. The psychometric properties of the 36-item WHODAS 2.0 have been examined in a cross-sectional study of older people in Poland [34].

2.3.2. The SF-36 Health Survey (SF-36)

The SF-36 version 2.0 is a general tool for measuring the health-related quality of life. The questionnaire contains 36 items used to measure eight domains: Physical functioning (10 items), Role limitations due to physical health (4 items), Bodily pain (2 items), General health perceptions (5 items), Vitality (4 items), Social functioning (2 items), Role limitations due to emotional problems (3 items), Mental health (5 items), Reported health transition (1 item).

Additionally, changes in general health over the preceding year are recorded. The remaining items in the questionnaire concern the experiences from the preceding month. In addition, the first four domains form the Physical component scale (PCS), whereas the next four ones create the Mental component scale (MCS).

The answers given by the participants are normalized so that the quality of life measures calculated on this basis are in the range of 0–100 points, where the value 0 is always the worst and the value 100 points relates to the best quality of life [35,36]. License agreement number QM030224 was obtained for using the SF-36 v. 2.0 questionnaire for the research.

2.3.3. The Oswestry Disability Index (ODI)

The modified ODI is a tool assessing the functional disability of a patient with LBP. It includes 10 items referring to pain and activities of daily living, each scored from 0 to 5. The total score is calculated through multiplying the sum, giving a range of 0 to 50 [37,38].

2.3.4. The Hospital Anxiety and Depression Scale (HADS)

The HADS is a tool commonly used for self-assessment detecting non-physical symptoms of anxiety and depression. It includes 14 items, i.e., seven items refer to the anxiety subscale (HADS anxiety) and seven other items refer to the depression subscale (HADS depression) [39]. Each item is rated on a 4-point scale ranging from 3 to 0. After adjusting for six items that are scored reversely, the sum of all responses is used to calculate the two subscales [40,41].

2.3.5. The Visual Analogue Scale (VAS)

The VAS is used to assess the intensity of pain using a visual scale, where 0 represents the total absence of pain, and 10 indicates unbearable pain.

2.3.6. Sociodemographic Data

Sociodemographic data were collected to provide basic information concerning sex, age, place of residence and education.

2.4. *Statistical Analyzes*

In order to receive the results, it is necessary to perform statistical analyses. The obtained data were analyzed using the R software, version 3.6.1. For the initial data analysis, the researchers used descriptive statistics measures.

2.4.1. Reliability Analysis

Internal Consistency

In order to assess the internal consistency, the Cronbach's alpha-coefficient was used. Cronbach's alpha values between 0.70 and <0.95 indicated the adequate internal consistency reliability of the scale [42,43].

Test–Retest Reliability and Measurement Error

The reliability of the 36-item WHODAS 2.0 was assessed using the test–retest method. The time between the two measurements made by different interviewers amounted to 2 days on average. During this period there should have not been significant changes in the phenomenon under study. The Intraclass Correlation Coefficient ($ICC_{2,1}$), with a 95% confidence interval (CI), was used to measure the relative reliability [42,44]. It is the ability of a questionnaire to capture similar scores on 2 separate occasions of test administration, given when the patient's condition has not changed [45]. The relative reliability indicates the degree of consistency and agreement between two measures [46]. The standard error of measurement (SEM) quantifies what was assessed to measure the absolute reliability. The determination of the absolute reliability of measures is critical to ensure repeated measurements with satisfactory stability and sensitivity to real changes over time [45]. The absolute reliability indicates how much dispersion and error this measurement contains [46]. As for the discussed study, the SEM was calculated as follows: $SEM = SD \sqrt{(1 - ICC_{2,1})}$ [44,47–49]. In addition, the minimal detectable change at the level 95% (MDC_{95}) was calculated. The MDC estimates the minimal amount of change in the score that confirms that the change is truly eliminating measurement error. In this case, the MDC was obtained using the formula: $MDC = SEM \times 1.96 \times \sqrt{2}$, where 1.96 was derived from the 0.95% CI of no change, and $\sqrt{2}$ showed two measurements assessing the change [44,47,50].

Internal Structure

The internal structure of the 36-item WHODAS 2.0 was also assessed by analyzing the correlations between the items in a given domain and the domain itself, as well as correlations appearing between the items and the overall result. Pearson's correlation coefficient was used.

2.4.2. Floor and Ceiling Effects

To detect the floor and ceiling effects, they were established by determining the percentage of subjects who scored the lowest or highest results with reference to the 36-item WHODAS 2.0. Floor or ceiling effects was observed if there were more than 15% of participants providing the lowest or highest possible score, respectively [51].

2.4.3. Validity

Convergent Validity

The convergent validity was assessed by correlating the results of the 36-item WHODAS 2.0 and the SF-36 questionnaire, the HADS and the ODI. The analysis was performed by examining Pearson's correlation coefficient. Adults with a lower quality of life and lower mood should have a higher level of disability [52]. We also assumed that the disability assessment using the ODI questionnaire would correlate with the assessment using the 36-item WHODAS 2.0. The greater the disability in the assessment of the ODI questionnaire, the higher the disability in the 36-item WHODAS 2.0.

Known Group Validity

The known group validity was assessed to test whether the 36-item WHODAS 2.0 distinguished two groups which should have different levels of construct. We took into account the simplicity in assessing these problems and the possibility of assigning function problems to the ICF framework. The occurrence of pain (ICF b280, a sensation of pain) was considered a health problem affecting the disability. The pain level was assessed using the VAS scale. For the purposes of the analysis, a dichotomous variable was created to divide the studied population into groups based on the following cutoffs: VAS ≤ 5 and VAS ≥ 6. Adults with higher levels of pain should be characterized by a higher level of disability [53,54]. The comparison of the 36-item WHODAS 2.0 results in the two groups was performed using the Student's *t*-test.

2.4.4. Responsiveness

The responsiveness refers to the ability of an instrument to distinguish clinically important changes as the result of an intervention. In order to assess the responsiveness, standard effect size (ES) and standardized response mean were calculated (SRM). ES is defined as a change in the mean score of the 36-item WHODAS 2.0 (between test 1 and 3) divided by the SD of the baseline score. Paired-samples *t*-test was used to examine the mean change between test 1 and test 3. SRM was calculated by dividing the mean score change by the SD of that score change. Absolute values of 0.20 or less, 0.21–0.79, and 0.80 or greater represent small, moderate, and large responsiveness, respectively, for ES and SRM [55].

To access responsiveness, the minimal clinically important difference (MCID) with its standard error (SE) was assessed [56]. The MCID was calculated on the basis of linear regression analysis, where the dependent variable was the change between 1st and the 3rd study in the 36-item WHODAS 2.0 (separately for each domain), and independent variable—change by 1 point on the VAS.

3. Results

3.1. Socio-Demographic Characteristics

In the studied adult population, 61.96% were women. The average age was 66.0 (SD = 11.6) years. Slightly more of the respondents lived in the countryside (52.17%). Most of the respondents had secondary education (48.91%). The average level of pain on the VAS scale in the studied population was 5.77 points. According to the 36-item WHODAS 2.0, the average disability score for the study group was 41.53 ± 13.84. The highest average level of disability was observed in Do2 Mobility (65.08 ± 20.49) and Do5 Life activities (60.43 ± 21.83). Regarding the quality of life, the respondents rated the worst functioning in the domains: Physical functioning, Role physical and body pain, respectively:

35.11 ± 20.91; 36.07 ± 19.87; 35.16 ± 17.06. According the ODI, the average degree of disability caused by lower back pain was 29.57 ± 6.40. The average HADS subscales anxiety and depression were 7.67 ± 3.63 and 5.51 ± 3.14 (Table 1), respectively.

Table 1. General socio-demographic characteristics of the study population (n = 92).

Variables	Mean ± SD n (%)
1. Gender	
Female	57 (61.96)
Male	35 (38.04)
2. Age (years)	66.0 ± 11.6
3. Place of residence	
City	44 (47.82)
Countryside	48 (52.17)
4. Education	
Primary education	18 (19.57)
Vocational education	17 (18.48)
Secondary education	45 (48.91)
Higher education	12 (13.04)
5. Pain (VAS)	5.77 ± 1.31
6. 36-item WHODAS 2.0	41.53 ± 13.84
Do1 Cognition	15.98 ± 20.78
Do2 Mobility	65.08 ± 20.49
Do3 Self-care	34.13 ± 21.80
Do4 Getting along	23.37 ± 18.00
Do5 Life activities	60.43 ± 21.83
Do6 Participation	51.4 ± 18.17
7. SF-36	
Physical functioning	35.11 ± 20.91
Role physical	36.07 ± 19.87
Body pain	35.16 ± 17.06
General health	42.83 ± 14.92
Vitality	48.70 ± 15.37
Social functioning	57.34 ± 25.15
Role emotional	62.14 ± 28.26
Mental health	56.48 ± 13.89
PCS	37.14 ± 14.84
MCS	55.59 ± 14.55
8. ODI	29.57 ± 6.40
9. HADS	
Anxiety	7.67 ± 3.63
Depression	5.51 ± 3.14

3.2. *Reliability Analysis*

3.2.1. Internal Consistency

The scale score reliability of the 36-item WHODAS 2.0 for the study population was very high. The Cronbach's alpha test result for the entire scale was 0.921. As for the Cronbach's alpha for the individual domains, it ranged from 0.786 (Do4 Getting along) to 0.904 (Do5 Life activities) (Table 2).

Table 2. Reliability of the 36-item WHODAS 2.0 for patients with LBP.

WHODAS 2.0	Floor Score	Ceiling Score	Cronbach's α	$ICC_{2,1}$ (95% CI)	SEM	MDC_{95}
Do1 Cognition	35.87%	0.00%	0.896	0.899 (0.859–0.928)	6.48	17.96
Do2 Mobility	0.00%	7.61%	0.823	0.950 (0.93–0.965)	4.44	12.31
Do3 Self-care	8.70%	2.17%	0.815	0.805 (0.733–0.859)	10.06	27.88
Do4 Getting along	15.22%	0.00%	0.786	0.936 (0.910–0.955)	4.51	12.50
Do5 Life activities	0.00%	7.61%	0.904	0.759 (0.673–0.825)	11.01	30.52
Do6 Participation	0.00%	0.00%	0.830	0.897 (0.857–0.927)	5.61	15.55
Total score	0.00%	0.00%	0.921	0.928 (0.898–0.949)	3.77	10.45

3.2.2. Test–Retest Reliability and Measurement Error

The value of the $ICC_{2,1}$ ranged from very high (for Do4, $ICC_{2,1}$ was 0.936) to high (for Do5, $ICC_{2,1}$ was 0.759). For the overall result of the WHODAS 2.0, the $ICC_{2,1}$ was 0.928, which confirmed that the scale was consistent over an approximate 2 day period (Table 2). The total score WHODAS 2.0 result was characterized by a low measurement error (SEM = 3.77). The smallest SEM was found in the Do4 Getting along domain (SEM = 4.44), and the largest in Do5 Life activities (SEM = 11.01). The SEM for the overall result and all WHODAS 2.0 domains were less than 50% of the respective standard deviation values, except for Do3 Self-care and Do5 Life activities, where the measurement error was recorded at the limit of 50% of the standard deviation values for these domains. The MDC was the best (the smallest) for the total result (MDC_{95} = 10.45), indicating that 10.45 was the minimal amount of change in the score of an instrument that must occur for an individual in order to be sure that the change in the score is not simply attributable to measurement error (Table 2).

3.2.3. Internal Structure

All subscales for WHODAS 2.0 were moderately strongly or strongly correlated with the total result (r ranged from 0.482 to 0.762) (Table 3).

Table 3. Internal Structure of the 36-item WHODAS 2.0 for patients with LBP.

WHODAS 2.0 Domains	WHODAS 2.0 Total Score Pearson's Correlation Coefficient
Do1 Cognition	r = 0.663, $p < 0.001$
Do2 Mobility	r = 0.762, $p < 0.001$
Do3 Self-care	r = 0.688, $p < 0.001$
Do4 Getting along	r = 0.482, $p < 0.001$
Do5 Life activities	r = 0.751, $p < 0.001$
Do6 Participation	r = 0.758, $p < 0.001$

3.3. *Floor and Ceiling Effects*

No floor or ceiling effects for the overall result the 36-item WHODAS 2.0 were found. However, over 15% of respondents reported the lowest possible score for WHODAS 2.0 Do1 cognition and Do4 getting along, indicating possible floor effects for these two domains (Table 2).

3.4. *Validity*

3.4.1. Convergent Validity

The convergent validity was tested by correlating the results obtained with the 36-item WHODAS 2.0, the results of the SF-36, the HADS and the ODI questionnaires.

The total result and the vast majority of domains of the 36-item WHODAS 2.0 were negatively correlated with domains of the SF-36 questionnaire; thus, a higher score on the WHODAS (higher disability) was associated with a lower score on the SF-36 questionnaire (lower quality of life). The weakest correlation was found with Do3 Self-care and Do4 Getting along.

The total result and all the domains of the 36-item WHODAS 2.0 were positively correlated with each domain of the HADS questionnaire; thus, a higher score on the 36-item WHODAS 2.0 (higher disability) was associated with a higher score on the HADS questionnaire (anxiety and depression). These findings confirm that adults with higher anxiety and depression are characterized by a higher level of disability (Table 4).

Table 4. Convergent validity of the 36-item WHODAS 2.0 for patients with LBP.

WHODAS 2.0		Do1 Cognition	Do2 Mobility	Do3 Self-Care	Do4 Getting Alone	Do5 Life Activities	Do6 Participation	Total Score
SF-36	Physical functioning	r = −0.388, $p < 0.001$	r = −0.784, $p < 0.001$	r = −0.502, $p < 0.001$	r = −0.312, $p = 0.002$	r = −0.647, $p < 0.001$	r = −0.666, $p < 0.001$	r = −0.810, $p < 0.001$
	Role physical	r = −0.125, $p = 0.276$	r = −0.554, $p < 0.001$	r = −0.362, $p < 0.001$	r = −0.133, $p = 0.207$	r = −0.540, $p < 0.001$	r = −0.551, $p < 0.001$	r = −0.539, $p < 0.001$
	Body pain	r = −0.466, $p < 0.001$	r = −0.784, $p < 0.001$	r = −0.525, $p < 0.001$	r = −0.389, $p < 0.001$	r = −0672, $p < 0.001$	r = −0.724, $p < 0.001$	r = −0.873, $p < 0.001$
	General health	r = −0.232, $p = 0.026$	r = −0.223, $p = 0.033$	r = −0.099, $p = 0.350$	r = −0.354, $p < 0.001$	r = −0.248, $p = 0.017$	r = −0.280, $p = 0.007$	r = −0.349, $p = 0.001$
	Vitality	r = −0.271, $p = 0.009$	r = −0.381, $p < 0.001$	r = −0.185, $p = 0.078$	r = −0.229, $p = 0.028$	r = −0.257, $p = 0.014$	r = −0.327, $p = 0.001$	r = −0.413, $p < 0.001$
	Social functioning	r = −0.260, $p = 0.012$	r = −0.477, $p < 0.001$	r = −0.075, $p = 0.478$	r = −0.010, $p = 0.921$	r = −0.325, $p = 0.002$	r = −0.579, $p < 0.001$	r = −0.476, $p < 0.001$
	Role emotional	r = −0.312, $p = 0.003$	r = −0.270, $p = 0.009$	r = −0.119, $p = 0.257$	r = −0.166, $p = 0.113$	r = −0.197, $p = 0.059$	r = −0.545, $p < 0.001$	r = −0.440, $p < 0.001$
	Mental health	r = −0.362, $p < 0.001$	r = −0.231, $p = 0.027$	r = −0.16, $p = 0.126$	r = −0.224, $p = 0.032$	r = −0.341, $p = 0.001$	r = −0.339, $p = 0.001$	r = −0.417, $p < 0.001$
	PCS	r = −0.395, $p < 0.001$	r = −0.781, $p < 0.001$	r = −0.495, $p < 0.001$	r = −0.361, $p < 0.001$	r = −0.681, $p < 0.001$	r = −0.705, $p < 0.001$	r = −0.834, $p < 0.001$
	MCS	r = −0.391, $p < 0.001$	r = −0.421, $p < 0.001$	r = −0.177, $p = 0.091$	r = −0.214, $p = 0.041$	r = −0.356, $p < 0.001$	r = −0.562, $p < 0.001$	r = −0.556, $p < 0.001$
HADS	Anxiety	r = 0.448, $p < 0.001$	r = 0.2, $p = 0.046$	r = 0.310, $p = 0.003$	r = 0.297, $p = 0.004$	r = 0.305, $p = 0.003$	r = 0.296, $p = 0.004$	r = 0.455, $p < 0.001$
	Depression	r = 0.294, $p = 0.004$	r = 0.358, $p < 0.001$	r = 0.319, $p = 0.002$	r = 0.360, $p < 0.001$	r = 0.398, $p < 0.001$	r = 0.342, $p = 0.001$	r = 0.489, $p < 0.001$
ODI		r = 0.585, $p < 0.001$	r = 0.667, $p < 0.001$	r = 0.526, $p < 0.001$	r = 0.345, $p = 0.001$	r = 0.645, $p < 0.001$	r = 0.716, $p < 0.001$	r = 0.867, $p < 0.001$

r from the Pearson's correlation coefficient.

The total result of the 36-item WHODAS 2.0 and all the domains were correlated with the ODI questionnaire. These findings confirming that adults with a higher physical disability measured by the ODI have a higher level of disability by the 36-item WHODAS 2.0 (Table 4).

3.4.2. Known Group Validity

We found significant differences among the selected subgroups of pain. With the possible exception of Do4 Getting along, we found differences between the selected subgroups and the total score of the 36-item WHODAS 2.0. These findings indicate that adults with higher levels of pain are likely characterized by a higher level of disability (Table 5).

3.5. Responsiveness

The statistical evidence indicates that all WHODAS 2.0 domains decreased between the first and third study (i.e., from test 1 to test 3). Nearly all domains showed a moderate to large degree of responsiveness, respectively, as signified by the ES and SRM values. The largest MCID was found in the case of Do2 Mobility (7.93 ± 0.70), and the smallest in the case of Do1 Cognition (1.71 ± 0.34) (Table 6).

Table 5. Known group validity of the 36-item WHODAS 2.0.

WHODAS 2.0		Pain (VAS Scale) 0 to 4	Pain (VAS Scale) 5 to 10	p-Value
Do1 Cognition	M ± SD	6.05 ± 9.51	18.56 ± 22.15	$p = 0.018$
	Median	0.00	10.00	
	Quartiles	0.00–10.00	0.00–30.00	
Do2 Mobility	M ± SD	44.74 ± 9.38	70.38 ± 19.26	$p < 0.001$
	Median	43.75	75.00	
	Quartiles	37.50–50.00	56.25–81.25	
Do3 Self-care	M ± SD	24.21 ± 16.10	36.71 ± 22.43	$p = 0.004$
	Median	20.00	30.00	
	Quartiles	20.00–30.00	20.00–50.00	
Do4 Getting along	M ± SD	18.42 ± 11.31	24.66 ± 19.22	$p = 0.284$
	Median	16.67	25.00	
	Quartiles	8.33–25.00	8.33–33.33	
Do5 Life activities	M ± SD	46.32 ± 10.65	64.11 ± 22.54	$p = 0.001$
	Median	40.00	60.00	
	Quartiles	40.00–50.00	50.00–90.00	
Do6 Participation	M ± SD	30.26 ± 9.81	56.91 ± 15.64	$p < 0.001$
	Median	29.17	56.25	
	Quartiles	25.00–37.50	45.83–66.67	
Total score	M ± SD	27.06 ± 6.85	45.29 ± 12.68	$p < 0.001$
	Median	25.00	43.48	
	Quartiles	23.91–28.26	35.87–52.17	

p-values from Student's *t*-test.

Table 6. Responsiveness of the 36-item WHODAS 2.0.

WHODAS 2.0	Change between 1st and 3rd Study: Mean	Median	SD	p-Value	SRM	ES	MCID	SE
Do1 Cognition	−3.69	0.00	8.49	$p = 0.001$	−0.43	−0.18	1.71	0.34
Do2 Mobility	−20.29	−18.75	18.75	$p < 0.001$	−1.08	−0.99	7.93	0.70
Do3 Self-care	−13.85	−10.00	14.76	$p < 0.001$	−0.94	−0.64	5.67	0.54
Do4 Getting along	−12.82	−8.33	15.46	$p < 0.001$	−0.83	−0.71	4.85	0.64
Do5 Life activities	−14.31	−10.00	17.76	$p < 0.001$	−0.81	−0.66	6.07	0.65
Do6 Participation	−11.15	−8.33	12.72	$p < 0.001$	−0.88	−0.61	4.62	0.47
Total score	−11.97	−11.96	8.86	$p < 0.001$	−1.35	−0.86	4.87	0.24

p-values from paired Student's *t*-test.

4. Discussion

To the best of our knowledge, this is the first study in which the researchers have evaluated the psychometric properties and validation of the Polish version of the 36-item WHODAS 2.0 engaging the patients with chronic LBP. This study is important due to the need for the implementation of valuable and reliable clinical tools for assessing the functioning and disability of patients with musculoskeletal pathology and for assessing rehabilitation progress. The 36-item WHODAS 2.0 implementation in Poland is associated with the simultaneous implementation of ICF. Indeed, in the recent past, the LBP Core Set Self-Report Checklist (LBP-CS-SRC) has been recently developed to facilitate people in self-rating activity limitations and participation restrictions [57]. Albeit LBP-CS-SRC is useful to understand the patients' perspectives [58], the 36-item WHODAS 2.0 has been defined as an instrumental tool for the clinical assessment of disability and the ability to function in patients with LBP by the latest WHO resolution for the International Classification of Diseases 11th Revision (ICD-11) [59].

The results of our research have shown that the Polish version of the 36-item WHODAS 2.0 presents good psychometric properties and can be useful for the clinical examination of adult patients with LBP in Poland.

We found a very good scale score reliability of the entire Polish version of the 36-item WHODAS 2.0. In our case, the Cronbach's alpha test value for the whole scale was 0.92. The Cronbach's alpha value for individual domains ranged from 0.79 to 0.90. The tool is reliable and not "redundant" i.e., it does not contain too many questions still exploring the same subject. The tool meets Nunnally's criteria, according to which for a good Cronbach's alpha scale it must be >0.70 [43]. Similar reliability of the WHODAS 2.0 test was received by Silva et al. while validating the Portuguese version of the 36-item WHODAS among 204 patients with musculoskeletal pain [26]. The authors of this article have confirmed the reliability of the WHODAS 2.0 by also examining 60–70 year-olds living in Poland, establishing Cronbach's alpha for the whole scale on the level 0.89 and for individual domains it ranged from 0.85 to 0.86 [34]. Moreover, the reliability of the WHODAS 2.0 test was correspondingly obtained by Moen et al., where the Cronbach's alpha was 0.93 for the whole score and for individual domains it ranged from 0.75 to 0.94 [60]. It is worth mentioning that other authors also obtained high WHODAS 2.0 reliability scores [61–63].

We confirmed the good repeatability of the 36-item Polish WHODAS 2.0. For the overall result the 36-item WHODAS 2.0, the $ICC_{2,1}$ was 0.93 and for domains it ranged from 0.76 to 0.94. Kutlay et al. examined patients with osteoarthritis who received the ICC retest–test value for the overall score of 0.97, and for individual domains in the range of 0.87–097 [64]. As for the Chinese version of the WHODAS 2.0, the ICC values for the total score was 0.80 and for domains it ranged 0.83–0.89 [65]. Moen et al., examining patients referred for somatic rehabilitation, found an acceptable ICC reproducibility of the total score and the different domains except for self-care [60].

In our study, the SEM for the overall score and the WHODAS 2.0 domains were less than 50% of the respective standard deviation values. The exceptions were the domains of Do3 self-care and Do5 life ctivities, for which the measurement error was found to be at the level of 50% of the standard deviation value. For the overall result of the 36-item WHODAS 2.0, the SEM was 3.77, while the MCD_{95} was 10.45. In the studies of Serrano-Dueñas et al., the SEM for the WHODAS overall result slightly exceeded 50% of the measurement error (SEM = 51.7%) [66]. Silva et al., in their research, received the relatively small deviations of the SEM (2.94) and the MDC (8.15) indicated the good reliability of the 36-item WHODAS 2.0 summary score [26].

No floor effect and ceiling for the overall result of the 36-item WHODAS 2.0 was found. However, the Do1 Cognition and Do4 Getting along domains showed floor effects over 15%. The result for Do4 was actually on the border of the adopted norm. In contrast, due to the attributable proportion of patients with no cognitive problems, a high floor result was expected in the cognition domain. The low percentage of ceiling and floor scores obtained in the summary score and in the other domains could support the use of these scores in rehabilitation assessment in patients with LBP. Serrano-Dueñas et al., assessing patients with Parkinson's disease, found floor effects in the Do1 Cognition domain, and the Do5 Life activities domain of the WHODAS 2.0 scale receiving 17.2% and 22.9%, respectively [66].

We found a positive correlation between the six domains of the Polish version of the 36-item WHODAS 2.0 ($p < 0.001$). A good correlation coefficient was identified between the total score and each domain (r = 0.482–0.762), demonstrating a good internal structure. Similarly, the total score had a good correlation with the six domains of the 36-item WHODAS 2.0 in the case of the traditional Chinese version ($p < 0.05$; r = 0.7–0.76) [67].

We also tested the convergent validity of the 36-item WHODAS 2.0. The overall result and the vast majority of domains of the 36-item WHODAS 2.0 were negatively correlated with domains of the SF-36 questionnaire; hence, a higher score on the WHODAS (higher disability) was associated with a lower score on the SF-36 questionnaire (i.e., lower quality of life). All WHODAS 2.0 domains were correlated with SF-36 domains like physical functioning, body pain, PCS and MCS. The weakest correlation was found between Do3 Self-care and Do4 Getting along of the WHODAS 2.0 questionnaire, and other SF-36 domains. Baron et al. demonstrated the strong correlation of WHODAS 2.0's total score with the SF-36 PCS ($\tau = -0.51$, $p < 0.001$) and moderate correlation with the SF-36 MCS ($\tau = -0.43$, $p < 0.001$). The WHODAS 2.0 domains, likewise, were all moderately to strongly correlated with the subscale domains and total scores of the SF-36 [20]. Other authors also obtained correlations between the 36-item WHODAS 2.0 and the SF-36 from weak to high [22,24,68]. These findings confirm that adults with a lower quality of life have a higher level of disability.

The total result and entire domains of the 36-item WHODAS 2.0 were statistically positively correlated with each domain of the HADS questionnaire; thus, a higher score on the 36-item WHODAS (higher disability) was associated with a higher score on the HADS questionnaire (anxiety and depression). These findings confirm that adults with higher anxiety and depression are characterized by a higher level of disability. We did not find any other studies in which the HADS scale was used for convergent validity for the 36-item WHODAS 2.0. However, studies using other scales assessing the occurrence of depression confirm the significant relationship between a higher level of depression and a higher level of disability. For instance, Rotarou et al. noticed a strong association of functional disability with increased depression in patients [69], whereas Sjonnesen indicated that the WHODAS 2.0 was sensitive in case of assessing the impact of depression [70].

The total result and all domains of the 36-item WHODAS 2.0 were significantly correlated with the ODI questionnaire. These findings confirm the hypothesis that adults with a higher physical disability measured by the ODI have a higher level of disability measured by the WHODAS 2.0. Saltychev et al. showed that the total scores of the WHODAS and the ODI were strongly correlated. Authors also suggested that the assessment of disability in the case of the population with LBP might be better estimated by the WHODAS 2.0 unlike the ODI [27]. According to Varjonen, both the WHODAS 2.0 and the ODI assessed the level of functioning of people experiencing LBP equivalently [28].

We confirmed that the 36-item WHODAS 2.0 had satisfactory validity for people with a different health status. In our study, the results of the WHODAS differed between people experiencing less and more pain. Similar situations were in all domains, except Do4 Getting along. These findings confirm our hypothesis that adults with higher levels of pain are characterized by a higher level of disability. With reference to the research performed by Baron et al., the patients with early arthritis were divided into two subgroups according to the results of the Center for Epidemiological Studies Depression Scale. These researchers noticed that the 36-item WHODAS 2.0 was able to distinguish patients with low and high depression symptoms [20]. Additionally, Garin et al. pointed out that as for most of the WHODAS 2.0 domains there were statistically significant, differences regarding groups with various clinical severity as for their medical condition and between professionally active and inactive due to poor health ($p < 0.001$) [30]. Serrano-Dueñas et al. revealed that in respect of the WHODAS 2.0, the getting along domain and the life activities domain were not significantly different in terms of staging according to the Hoehn and Yahrfor scale, whereas other domains and the total scale indicated differences [66].

The values of all WHODAS 2.0 domains changed between the first and third study. Results in all domains decreased significantly, i.e., the disability decreased. Almost all domains showed a moderate to large degree of responsiveness, respectively, for ES and SRM. The WHODAS 2.0 responsiveness scores for the total results were −1.35 (SRM) and −0.86 (ES) at 4 weeks after discharge. Meesters et al. found the WHODAS 2.0 responsiveness scores −0.35 (SRM), −0.34 (ES) at 6 weeks after discharge [71]. Moreover, in the research performed by Garin et al., analyzing the group of patients whose health condition had improved, they indicated small to moderate responsiveness coefficients (ES = 0.3–0.7), but higher than in the group of the SF-36 [30]. Additionally, Chwastiak et al. showed that the WHODAS 2.0 was well responsive (ES = 0.65) while assessing the treatment results [24].

Federici et al. emphasized that the 36-item WHODAS 2.0 is adequate for assessing disability and health status. Although it is an important issue for rehabilitation, MCID score for the WHODAS 2.0 should be established [19]. We found that the minimal clinically important difference in case of the total WHODAS 2.0 score in patients after rehabilitation for low back pain was 4.87. The largest

MCID was found for Do2 Mobility (7.93 ± 0.70), and the smallest for Do1 Cognition (1.71 ± 0.347). The 36-item WHODAS can accurately capture changes in disability after rehabilitation in patients with LBP and thus can be used as a valid primary endpoint for clinical trials [72].

A weakness of our analysis is that our sample size prevented the use of a more robust test of the internal factor structure of the WHODAS 2.0 such as confirmatory factor analysis (CFA) [73]. The study's strengths include the use of standardized methods for the assessment of psychometric properties. It is the first study in Poland and one of the few in the world to analyze the usefulness of the WHODAS 2.0 questionnaire in assessing the disability of patients with chronic back pain. The scientific foundation of this issue is particularly important in the context of the implementation of the ICF and the WHODAS 2.0 questionnaire in Poland for general use in rehabilitation departments and other physiotherapy units.

5. Conclusions

These findings show that the 36-item WHODAS is suitable for evaluating health status and disability, and that it is a reliable and valid tool for assessing patients with chronic LBP according to its psychometric properties. Because it can capture changes in disability after rehabilitation in patients with LBP, the 36-item WHODAS 2.0 can thus be used as a valid primary endpoint for clinical trials. Regarding that the 36-item WHODAS 2.0 is an easy-to-use, generic instrument, based on the principles of ICF, with high feasibility, it could be considered as a first-choice tool in the rehabilitation field that might implement the management of people with disability due to LBP.

Author Contributions: Conceptualization, A.Ć.-S.; methodology, A.Ć.-S., A.B.; software, B.S.; validation, A.Ć.-S., A.B., formal analysis, A.Ć.-S., B.S.; investigation, A.Ć.-S., A.B., A.W.-S.; writing—original draft preparation, A.Ć.-S.; writing—review and editing, A.Ć.-S., A.B., B.S., A.W.-S., A.W.-P.; visualization, A.Ć.-S., R.S., A.d.S.; supervision, A.W.-P., R.S., A.d.S.; project administration and coordination A.Ć.-S.; cooperation and support in the clinical field of ICF in the project, R.S., A.d.S. All authors have read and agreed to the published version of the manuscript.

References

1. Rapoport, J.; Jacobs, P.; Bell, N.R.; Klarenbach, S. Refining the measurement of the economic burden of chronic diseases in Canada. *Chronic. Dis. Can.* **2004**, *25*, 13–21. [PubMed]
2. Andersson, G.B. Epidemiological features of chronic low-back pain. *Lancet* **1999**, *354*, 581–585. [CrossRef]
3. Rubin, D.I. Epidemiology and risk factors for spine pain. *Neurol. Clin.* **2007**, *25*, 353–371. [CrossRef] [PubMed]
4. Freburger, J.K.; Holmes, G.M.; Agans, R.P.; Jackman, A.M.; Darter, J.D.; Wallace, A.S.; Castel, L.D.; Kalsbeek, W.D.; Carey, T.S. The rising prevalence of chronic low back pain. *Arch. Intern. Med.* **2009**, *169*, 251–258. [CrossRef]
5. Palazzo, C.; Ravaud, J.F.; Papelard, A.; Ravaud, P.; Poiraudeau, S. The burden ofmusculoskeletal conditions. *PLoS ONE* **2014**, *9*, e90633. [CrossRef]
6. Palazzo, C.; Ravaud, J.F.; Trinquart, L.; Dalichampt, M.; Ravaud, P.; Poiraudeau, S. Respective contribution of chronic conditions to disability in France: Results fromthe national Disability-Health Survey. *PLoS ONE* **2012**, *9*, e44994. [CrossRef]
7. Boonen, A.; van den Heuvel, R.; van Tubergen, A.; Goossens, M.; Severens, J.L.; van der Heijde, D.; van der Linden, S. Large differences in cost of illness and wellbeing between patients withfibromyalgia, chronic low back pain, or ankylosing spondylitis. *Ann. Rheum. Dis.* **2005**, *3*, 396–402.
8. Vos, T.; Flaxman, A.D.; Naghavi, M.; Lozano, R.; Michaud, C.; Ezzati, M.; Shibuya, K.; Salomon, J.A.; Abdalla, S.; Aboyans, V.; et al. Years livedwith disability (YLDs) for 1160 sequelae of 289 diseases and injuries 1990–2010: A systematic analysis for the Global Burden of Disease Study 2010. *Lancet* **2012**, *380*, 2163–2196. [CrossRef]

9. Global Burden of Disease Study 2013 Collaborators. Global, regional, and national incidence, prevalence, and years lived with disability for 301 acute and chronic diseases and injuries in 188 countries, 1990–2013: A systematic analysis for the Global. Burden of Disease Study 2013. *Lancet* **2015**, *386*, 743–800. [CrossRef]
10. Leonardi, M.; Bickenbach, J.; Ustun, T.B.; Kostanjsek, N.; Chatterji, S. The definition of disability: What is in a name? *Lancet* **2006**, *368*, 1219–1221. [CrossRef]
11. World Health Organization. *International Classification of Functioning, Disability and Health*; WHO: Geneva, Switzerland, 2001.
12. Cieza, A.; Stucki, G.; Weigl, M.; Disler, P.; Jackel, W.; van der Linden, S.; Kostanjsek, N.; de Bie, R. ICF Core Sets for low back pain. *J. Rehabil. Med.* **2004**, *44*, 69–74. [CrossRef] [PubMed]
13. Gimigliano, F.; de Sire, A.; Gastaldo, M.; Maghini, I.; Paoletta, M.; Pasquini, A.; Boldrini, P.; Selb, M.; Prodinger, B.; Abbamonte, M.; et al. Use of the International Classification of Functioning, Disability and Health Generic-30 Set for the characterization of outpatients: Italian Society of Physical and Rehabilitative Medicine Residents Section Project. *Eur. J. Phys. Rehabil. Med.* **2019**, *55*, 258–264. [CrossRef] [PubMed]
14. Stevens, A.; Gillam, S. Needs assessment: From theory to practice. *BMJ.* **1998**, *316*, 1448–1452. [CrossRef] [PubMed]
15. Sigl, T.; Cieza, A.; Brockow, T.; Chatterji, S.; Kostanjsek, N.; Stucki, G. Content comparison of low back pain-specifi c measures based on the International Classifi cation of Functioning, Disability and Health (ICF). *Clin. J. Pain* **2006**, *22*, 147–153. [CrossRef] [PubMed]
16. Rehabilitation Institute of Chicago Center for Rehabilitation Outcomes Research, and Northwestern University Feinberg School of Medicine Department of Medical Social Sciences Informatics Group. Rehabilitation Measures Database. Available online: http://www.rehabmeasures.org/ (accessed on 10 May 2020).
17. World Health Organization. *WHO Global Disability Action Plan 2014–2021: Better Health for All People with Disabilities*; WHO: Geneva, Switzerland, 2015.
18. Klokkerud, M.; Dagfinrud, H.; Uhlig, T.; Dager, T.N.; Furunes, K.A.; Klokkeide, Å.; Larsen, M.; Nygård, S.; Nylenna, S.; Øie, L.; et al. Developing and testing a consensus-based core set of outcome measures for rehabilitation in musculoskeletal diseases. *Scand. J. Rheumatol.* **2018**, *47*, 225–234. [CrossRef]
19. Federici, S.; Bracalenti, M.; Meloni, F.; Luciano, J.V. World Health Organization disability assessment schedule 2.0: An international systematic review. *Disabil. Rehabil.* **2017**, *39*, 2347–2380. [CrossRef]
20. Baron, M.; Schieir, O.; Hudson, M.; Steele, R.; Kolahi, S.; Berkson, L.; Couture, F.; Fitzcharles, M.A.; Gagné, M.; Garfield, B.; et al. The clinimetric properties of the World Health. Organization Disability Assessment Schedule II in early inflammatory arthritis. *Arthritis Rheum.* **2008**, *59*, 382–390. [CrossRef]
21. Schlote, A.; Richter, M.; Wunderlich, M.T.; Poppendick, U.; Moller, C.; Wallesch, C.W. Use of the WHODAS II with stroke patients and their relatives: Reliability and inter-rater-reliability. *Rehabilitation* **2008**, *47*, 31–38. [CrossRef]
22. Hudson, M.; Steele, R.; Taillefer, S.; Baron, M. Quality of life in systemic sclerosis: Psychometric properties of the World Health Organization Disability Assessment Schedule II. *Arthritis Rheum.* **2008**, *59*, 270–278. [CrossRef]
23. Chopra, P.K.; Couper, J.W.; Herrman, H. The assessment of patients with long-term psychotic disorders: Application of the WHO Disability Assessment Schedule II. *Aust. N. Z. J. Psychiatry* **2004**, *38*, 753–759. [CrossRef]
24. Chwastiak, L.A.; Von Korff, M. Disability in depression and back pain: Evaluation of the World Health Organization Disability Assessment Schedule (WHO DAS II) in a primary care setting. *J. Clin. Epidemiol.* **2003**, *56*, 507–514. [CrossRef]
25. Lee, H.J.; Song, J.M. Analysis of the characteristics of Patients with Chronic Low Back Pain Using the ICF Concept. *J. Korean Soc. Phys. Ther.* **2013**, *25*, 282–287.
26. Silva, C.; Coleta, I.; Silva, A.G.; Amaro, A.; Alvarelhao, J.; Queiros, A.; Rocha, N. Adaptation and validation of WHODAS 2.0 in patients with musculoskeletal pain. *Rev. Saude Publica* **2013**, *47*, 752–758. [CrossRef] [PubMed]
27. Saltychev, M.; Bärlund, E.; Mattie, R.; McCormick, Z.; Paltamaa, J.; Laimi, K. A Study of the Psychometric Properties of 12-item WHODAS 2.0 in a Large Population of People with Chronic Musculoskeletal Pain. *Clin. Rehabil.* **2016**, *31*, 262–272. [CrossRef]
28. Varjonen, T.; Laimi, K.; Passoja, A.; Peltonen, J.; Silto, T.; Saltychev, M. Disability in Low Back Pain: Correlation between Oswestry Back Pain Disability Index and WHODAS 2.0. Turku ICF Study. *J. Rehabil.* **2015**, *54*, 482.

29. Igwesi-Chidobe, C.N.; Kitchen, S.; Sorinola, I.O.; Godfrey, E.L. World Health Organisation Disability Assessment Schedule (WHODAS 2.0): Development and validation of the Igbo version in patients with chronic low back pain. *BMC Musculoskelet. Disordes* **2020**. [CrossRef]
30. Garin, O.; Ayuso-Mateos, J.L.; Almansa, J.; Nieto, M.; Chatterji, S.; Vilagut, G.; Alonso, J.; Cieza, A.; Svetskova, O.; Burger, H.; et al. Validation of the "World Health Organization Disability Assessment Schedule, WHODAS-2" in patients with chronic diseases. *Health Qual. Life Outcomes* **2010**, *8*, 51. [CrossRef]
31. Stewart Williams, J.; Ng, N.; Peltzer, K.; Yawson, A.; Biritwum, R.; Maximova, T.; Wu, F.; Arokiasamy, P.; Kowal, P.; Chatterji, S. Risk Factors and Disability Associated with Low Back Pain in Older Adults in Low-and Middle-Income Countries. Results from the WHO Study on Global AGEing and Adult Health (SAGE). *PLoS ONE* **2015**, *10*, e0127880. [CrossRef]
32. *Decree No. 50/2010 of 16 April 2010 Issued by the Director of the Centre of Health Information Systems in Warsaw on the Appointment of the Council for the International Classification of Functioning, Disability and Health*; Decree No. 50/2010; Centre of Health Information Systems: Warsaw, Poland, 16 April 2010.
33. Üstün, T.B.; Kostanjsek, N.; Chatterji, S.; Rehm, J. *Measuring Health and Disability: Manual for WHO Disability Assessment Schedule (WHODAS 2.0)*; WHO: Geneva, Switzerland, 2001.
34. Ćwirlej-Sozańska, A.; Wilmowska-Pietruszyńska, A.; Sozański, B. Validation of the Polish version of the World Health Organization Disability Assessment Schedule (WHODAS 2.0) in an elderly population (60–70 years old). *Int. J. Occup. Saf. Ergon.* **2018**, *24*, 386–394. [CrossRef]
35. Ware, J.E.; Kosinski, M.; Gandek, B. *SF36® Health Survey: Manual & Interpretation Guide*; Quality Metric Incorporated: Lincoln, RI, USA, 1993.
36. Lyons, R.A.; Perry, H.M.; Littlepage, B.N. Evidence for the validity of the Short-form 36 Questionnaire (SF-36) in an elderly population. *Age Ageing* **1994**, *23*, 182–184. [CrossRef]
37. Roland, M.; Fairbank, J. The Roland-Morris Disability Questionnaire and the Oswestry Disability Questionnaire. *Spine* **2000**, *25*, 3115–3124. [CrossRef] [PubMed]
38. Fairbank, J.C.; Pynsent, P.B. The Oswestry Disability Index. *Spine* **2000**, *25*, 2940–2952. [CrossRef] [PubMed]
39. Snaith, R.P. The hospital anxiety and depression scale. *Health Qual. Life Outcomes* **2003**, *1*, 29. [CrossRef] [PubMed]
40. Zigmond, A.S.; Snaith, R.P. The hospital anxiety and depression scale. *Acta Psychiatr. Scand.* **1983**, *67*, 361–370. [CrossRef] [PubMed]
41. Herrmann, C.; Buss, U.; Lingen, R.; Kreuzer, H. The screening for anxiety anddepression in routine medical care. *Dtsch. Med. Wochenschr.* **1994**, *119*, 1283–1286. [CrossRef] [PubMed]
42. Terwee, C.B.; Bot, S.D.; de Boer, M.R.; van der Windt, D.A.; Knol, D.L.; Dekker, J.; Bouter, L.M.; de Vet, H.C. Quality criteria were proposed for measurement properties of health status questionnaires. *J. Clin. Epidemiol.* **2007**, *60*, 34–42. [CrossRef]
43. Nunnlly, J.; Bernestein, I. *Psychometric Theory*; Mackgrow Hill: New York, NY, USA, 1994.
44. Weir, J.P. Quantifying test-retest reliability using the intraclass correlation coefficient and the SEM. *J. Strength Cond. Res.* **2005**, *19*, 231–240.
45. Chuang, L.L.; Wu, C.Y.; Lin, K.C.; Hsieh, C.J. Relative and Absolute Reliability of a Vertical Numerical Pain Rating Scale Supplemented with a Faces Pain Scale after Stroke. *Phys. Ther.* **2014**, *94*, 129–138. [CrossRef]
46. Ohya, N.; Yamada, T.; Satoh, Y.; Kawamura, H. Relative and absolute reliability of ultrasound measurements for the thickness of the soft tissue around the shoulder joint of young normal subjects. *J. Phys. Ther. Sci.* **2017**, *29*, 754–759. [CrossRef]
47. Harvill, L.M. Standard Error of Measurement. *Educ. Meas.* **1991**, *2*, 33–41. [CrossRef]
48. Overend, T.; Anderson, C.; Sawant, A.; Perryman, B.; Locking-Cusolito, H. Relative and absolute reliability of physical function measures in people with end-stage renal disease. *Physiother. Can.* **2010**, *62*, 122–128. [CrossRef] [PubMed]
49. Stratford, P. Reliability: Consistency or differentiating among sub-jects? *Phys. Ther.* **1989**, *69*, 299–300. [CrossRef] [PubMed]
50. Ries, J.D.; Echternach, J.L.; Nof, L.; Gagnon Blodgett, M. Test-retest reliability and minimal detectable change scores for the timed "up & go" test, the six-minute walk test, and gait speed in people with Alzheimer disease. *Phys. Ther.* **2009**, *89*, 569–579. [PubMed]
51. McHorney, C.A.; Tarlov, A.R. Individual-patient monitoring in clinicalpractice: Are available health status surveys adequate? *Qual. Life Res.* **1995**, *4*, 293–307. [CrossRef]

52. Ünal, Ö.; Akyol, Y.; Tander, B.; Ulus, Y.; Terzi, Y.; Kuru, Ö. The relationship of illness perceptions with demographic features, pain severity, functional capacity, disability, depression, and quality of life in patients with chronic low back pain. *Turk. J. Phys. Med. Rehabil.* **2019**, *65*, 301–308. [CrossRef]
53. Hartvigsen, J.; Hancock, M.J.; Kongsted, A.; Louw, Q.; Ferreira, M.L.; Genevay, S.; Hoy, D.; Karppinen, J.; Pransky, G.; Sieper, J.; et al. What low back pain is and why we need to pay attention. *Lancet* **2018**, *391*, 2356–2367. [CrossRef]
54. Makino, K.; Lee, S.; Bae, S.; Jung, S.; Shinkai, Y.; Chiba, I.; Shimada, H. Pain characteristics and incidence of functional disability among community-dwelling older adults. *PLoS ONE* **2019**, *14*, e0215467. [CrossRef]
55. Husted, J.A.; Cook, R.J.; Farewell, V.T.; Gladman, D.D. Methods for assessing responsiveness: A critical review and recommendations. *J. Clin. Epidemiol.* **2000**, *53*, 459–468. [CrossRef]
56. Revicki, D.; Hays, R.D.; Cella, D.; Sloan, J. Recommended methods for determining responsiveness and minimally important differences for patient-reported outcomes. *J. Clin. Epidemiol.* **2008**, *61*, 102–109. [CrossRef]
57. Bagraith, K.S.; Strong, J.; Meredith, P.J.; McPhail, S.M. Rasch analysis supported the construct validity of self-report measures of activity and participation derived from patient ratings of the ICF low back pain core set. *J. Clin. Epidemiol.* **2017**, *61*, 161–172. [CrossRef]
58. Bagraith, K.S.; Strong, J.; Meredith, P.J.; McPhail, S.M. Self-reported disability according to the International Classification of Functioning, Disability and Health Low Back Pain Core Set: Test-retest agreement and reliability. *Disabil. Health J.* **2017**, *10*, 621–626. [CrossRef] [PubMed]
59. ICD-11 for Mortality and Morbidity Statistics (ICD-11 MMS) 2018 Version. Available online: https://icd.who.int/browse11/l-m/en (accessed on 8 July 2020).
60. Moen, V.P.; Drageset, J.; Eide, G.E.; Klokkerud, M.; Gjesdal, S. Validation of World Health Organization Assessment Schedule 2.0 in specialized somatic rehabilitation services in Norway. *Qual. Life Res.* **2017**, *26*, 505–514. [CrossRef] [PubMed]
61. Silveira, C.; Souza, R.T.; Costa, M.L.; Parpinelli, M.A.; Pacagnella, R.C.; Ferreira, E.C.; Mayrink, J.; Guida, J.P.; Sousa, M.H.; Say, L.; et al. Validation of the WHO Disability Assessment Schedule (WHODAS 2.0) 12-item tool against the 36-item version for measuring functioning and disability associated with pregnancy and history of severe maternal morbidity. *Int. J. Gynaecol. Obstet.* **2018**, *141* (Suppl. 1), 39–47. [CrossRef] [PubMed]
62. Wolf, A.C.; Tate, R.L.; Lannin, N.A.; Middleton, J.; Lane-Brown, A.; Cameron, I.D. The World Health Organization Disability Assessment Scale, WHODAS II: Reliability and validity in the measurement of activity and participation in a spinal cord injury population. *J. Rehabil. Med.* **2012**, *44*, 747–755. [CrossRef]
63. Tazaki, M.; Yamaguchi, T.; Yatsunami, M.; Nakane, Y. Measuring functional health among the elderly: Development of the Japanese version of the World Health Organization Disability Assessment Schedule II. *Int. J. Rehabil. Res.* **2014**, *37*, 48–53. [CrossRef]
64. Kutlay, S.; Küçükdeveci, A.A.; Elhan, A.H.; Oztuna, D.; Koç, N.; Tennant, A. Validation of the World Health Organization disability assessment schedule II (WHODAS-II) in patients with osteoarthritis. *Rheumatol. Int.* **2011**, *31*, 339–346. [CrossRef]
65. Chiu, T.Y.; Yen, C.F.; Chou, C.H.; Lin, J.D.; Hwang, A.W.; Liao, H.F.; Chi, W.C. Development of traditional Chinese version of World Health Organization disability assessment schedule 2.0 36-item (WHODAS 2.0) in Taiwan: Validity and reliability analyses. *Res. Dev. Disabil.* **2014**, *35*, 2812–2820. [CrossRef]
66. Serrano-Dueñas, M.; Serrano, M.; Mafla, D.; Martínez-Martín, P. Evaluation of the metric properties of the WHODAS 2.0, WHODAS-S, and RADS in the assessment of disability in Parkinsonian patients [published online ahead of print, 28 April 2020]. *Clin. Neurol. Neurosurg.* **2020**, *194*, 105872. [CrossRef]
67. Cheung, M.K.; Hung, A.T.; Poon, P.K.; Fong, D.Y.; Li, L.S.; Chow, E.S.; Qiu, Z.Y.; Liou, T.H. Validation of the World Health Organization Assessment Schedule II Chinese Traditional Version (WHODAS II CT) in persons with disabilities and chronic illnesses for Chinese population. *Disabil. Rehabil.* **2015**, *37*, 1902–1907. [CrossRef]
68. Posl, M.; Cieza, A.; Stucki, G. Psychometric properties of the WHODASII in rehabilitation patients. *Qual. Life Res.* **2007**, *16*, 1521–1531. [CrossRef]
69. Rotarou, E.S.; Sakellariou, D. Depressive symptoms in people with disabilities; secondary analysis of cross-sectional data from the United Kingdom and Greece. *Disabil. Health J.* **2018**, *11*, 367–373. [CrossRef] [PubMed]

70. Sjonnesen, K.; Bulloch, A.G.; Williams, J.; Lavorato, D.; Patten, S.B. Characterization of Disability in Canadians with Mental Disorders Using an Abbreviated Version of a DSM-5 Emerging Measure: The 12-Item WHO Disability Assessment Schedule (WHODAS) 2.0. *Can. J. Psychiatry* **2016**, *61*, 227–235. [CrossRef] [PubMed]
71. Meesters, J.J.; Verhoef, J.; Liem, I.S.; Putter, H.; Vliet Vlieland, T.P. Validity and responsiveness of the World Health Organization Disability Assessment Schedule II to assess disability in rheumatoid arthritis patients. *Rheumatology* **2010**, *49*, 326–333. [CrossRef] [PubMed]
72. Kalkman, C.J. Minimal Clinically Important Difference, Maximum Impact. *Anesthesiology* **2020**, *132*, 1296–1298. [CrossRef]
73. Irwing, P.; Booth, T.; Hughes, D.J. *The Wiley Handbook of Psychometric Testing: A Multidisciplinary Reference on Survey Scale, and Test Development*; Wiley Blackwell: Hoboken, NJ, USA, 2018; Volume 1, pp. 13, 113–138.

2

Prevalence of Low Back Pain among Nursing Staff in Najran, Saudi Arabia

Adel Alshahrani

Rehabilitation Sciences Department, Physical Therapy Program, Najran University, Najran 55461, Saudi Arabia; amsalshahrani@nu.edu.sa

Abstract: This study aimed to determine the various demographic and work-related professional characteristics associated with low back pain among nursing professionals in Najran, Saudi Arabia. A self-administered modified questionnaire (electronic), which included information on general subject demographics and work conditions, was sent through various electronic channels to which 187 nurses working across various health institutions in the Najran region responded. Among the included respondents, 35.3% were Saudis, 64.7% were Non-Saudis, and 88.8% were in the young to middle-age group (21–40 years). Similarly, 57.8% were females, while a majority (91%) had completed a bachelor's degree. In total, 140 respondents (74.8%) reported experiencing low back pain. Among the various work-related factors, gender, place of work, nature of work, and direct contact hours with patients per week were found to be significantly associated with low back pain. Assessment of pain characteristics found that a majority (88.2%) had mild to moderate localized back pain. A significant number of nursing professionals included herein reported to have low back pain, which appeared to be moderated by work-related characteristics, including place and nature of work. Our findings can help to establish policies and interventions aimed at reducing the risk and onset of low back pain.

Keywords: low back pain; epidemiology; nurse; prevalence; risk factors

1. Introduction

Low back pain (LBP), also known as low back ache (LBA), is a very common musculoskeletal condition that has garnered worldwide attention [1,2]. LBP has a prevalence of 84% and ranks 6th on the global burden of disease with 40–60% of individuals with acute LBP still reporting pain after a year and 5–7% having chronic pain [3,4]. Moreover, studies have observed that, on average, 45–70% of the adult population suffer from varying degrees of LBP of mechanical origin at least once during their lifetime [5]. LBP adversely affects vast populations by deterring activities of daily living (ADLs) and preventing a person from leading a physically, psychologically, economically, and socially fulfilling life [6]. LBP has been associated with a sedentary lifestyle, irrespective of gender, nationality, and a variety of other associated factors [4,6].

LBP significantly impacts society by reducing quality of life, and through its large socioeconomic influence. For instance, between 1990 and 2015, disability-adjusted life years (DALY) due to LBP increased by 54% worldwide, with a large proportion of the increase having been observed among countries in the Middle East, Africa, and Asia (low- and middle-income nations) who have inadequate resources and expertise in health and social systems needed to address this growing burden [7]. In Australia, the cost associated with LBP in 2001 exceeded AU $1 billion [8], with LBP having a lifetime prevalence of 11–84%. LBP remains one of the most frequent causes of disability worldwide, which claims around 80% of total expense [9].

In a review of 40 studies investigating the prevalence of persistent LBP in Asia, Africa, and South America (n = 80,076), Jackson found that chronic LBP was two and a half times more common among individuals with formal employment than those with non-formal employment [10]. Another study showed that lifestyle, psychological, and social factors were related to work-related LBP [10,11].

Studies have apparently shown that some professions are more likely to suffer from LBP given the nature of their work [5,6,11]. One such profession is nursing, which is physically challenging and has been associated with long working hours, prolonged standing, frequent bending, stooping, lifting, and other risk factors [12,13]. In a series of studies, including one conducted in Turkey, Karahan et al. determined that LBP onset affected as many as 77% of nurses [14]. Yet another study by Chiwaridzo et al. conducted in Zimbabwe reported that 67.9% of nurses experienced varying degrees of LBP over 12 months, while 52.7% reported that the initial episodes occurred during the first five years of working as a nurse [15].

Nurses have been the backbone of the entire health care system and remain under intense physical stress, which may consequently promote LBP. Considering the limited studies on LBP among nurses in Saudi Arabia [11,16–18], the present study aimed to primarily determine the prevalence of work-related LBP and its association with various work-related factors among nursing professionals in Najran region, Kingdom of Saudi Arabia.

2. Methods

This descriptive cross-sectional study utilized a self-administered questionnaire modified from Dionne et al. [19]. The study population consisted of nursing professionals working at hospitals and health care centers within the Najran region. A pilot study was conducted on 10 nurses with no major modifications required. The questionnaire obtained information regarding socioeconomic and demographic profiles of the nursing professionals, irrespective of their nationalities. Questions included herein were aimed at understanding LBP with respect to onset, type, nature, work settings, and impact of the nature of work on LBP.

The questionnaire was distributed electronically through various social media sites from January 2019 until June 2019. 187 nursing professionals working at clinics, hospitals, community care centers, and schools responded. Data from concerned professionals were also collected using various social media networks in order to include responses from multiple health care locations. Socioeconomic and work-related characteristics were then compared according to the prevalence of LBP irrespective of sex. Similarly, this study aimed at comparing vocational and non-vocational LBP according to gender. This study had been approved by Najran University Ethics Committee for Human Investigations, ethical number 01-10-01-2010 EC, and electronic consent was obtained from all participants.

Data were initially coded and keyed into a Microsoft Excel spreadsheet and then transferred to SPSS software for data processing. Descriptive analysis was used to summarize categorical data. The Pearson chi-square test was used as part of inferential statistics to determine the degree of association between categorical variables. A p value of <0.05 indicated significant differences between variables.

3. Results

Among the 187 respondents, 35.3% were Saudis, while 64.7% were not non-Saudis, with a maximum 88.8% of the sample population being in the young age group (21–40 years) (Table 1).

Table 1. Participant demographics.

Characteristics	Level	Number out of Total 187	Percentage %
Nationality	Saudi	66	35.3
	Non-Saudi	121	64.7
Age (in years)	21–30	83	44.4
	31–40	83	44.4
	41–50	16	8.5
	>50	5	2.7
Gender	Male	79	42.2
	Female	108	57.8
Educational qualification	Diploma	58	31
	Bachelor's degree	113	60.4
	Master's degree and higher	16	8.6
Work experience	<10	110	58.8
	10–19	58	31
	>19	19	10.2
Place of work	General hospital	111	59.4
	Private	65	34.7
	Others	11	5.9
Total		187	100

A total of 108 respondents (57.8%) were female, while approximately 91% of the participants had a diploma or a bachelor's degree in nursing. Moreover, 58.8% had a work experience of <10 years, whereas only 10.2% had a work experience of more than 19 years. After comparing various sociodemographic and work-related characteristics and determining their association with LBP, certain findings were noted (Table 2).

Table 2. Sociodemographic and work-related characteristics and their association with low back pain.

Characteristics	Level	Nurses with LBP (n = 140)	Nurses without LBP (n = 47)	p Value
Nationality	Saudi Non-Saudi	45 (68.2%) 95 (78.5%)	21 (31.8%) 26 (21.5%)	0.120
Age	21–25 26–30 31–35 36–40 41–45 46–50 >50	19 (67.9%) 41 (74.5%) 41 (82%) 25 (75.8%) 9 (69.2%) 3 (100%) 2 (40%)	9 (32.1%) 14 (25.5%) 9 (18%) 8 (24.2%) 4 (30.8%) 0 (0%) 3 (60%)	0.364
Sex	Male Female	55(69.62 %) 85(78.7%)	24 (30.38%) 23 (21.3%)	0.157
Education level	Diploma Bachelor's degree Master's degree and higher	46 (79.3%) 84 (74.3%) 10 (62.5%)	12 (20.7%) 29 (25.7%) 6 (37.5%)	0.382
Work experience	<5 years 5–9 years 10–14 years >15 years	120 (76.4%) 1 (33.3%) 1 (100%) 18 (69.2%)	37 (23.6%) 2 (66.7%) 0 (0%) 8 (30.8%)	0.292
Workplace	General hospital Private Clinic/Hospital University clinics/hospitals Others including rehabilitation centers	88 (79.3%) 14 (63.6%) 3 (50%) 35 (72.9%)	23 (20.7%) 8 (36.4%) 3 (50%) 13 (27.1%)	0.196
Nature of work	Full time Part time	112 (78.9%) 28 (62.2%)	30 (21.1%) 17 (37.8%)	0.025 *
Hours with patients/week	<10 10–19 20–29 30–39 >40	7 (87.5%) 18 (78.3%) 11 (78.6%) 50 (74.6%) 54 (72%)	1 (12.5%) 5 (21.7%) 3 (21.43%) 17 (25.4%) 21 (28%)	0.870

* $p < 0.05$.

Among the 187 participants, 140 complained of LBP, whereas 47 did not. Accordingly, more non-Saudi nurses had LBP (67.8%) compared to their Saudi counterparts irrespective of sex, though the difference was not significant ($p < 0.05$). Moreover, the majority of the nurses (76.2%) who developed some type of LBP were between 26 to 40 years old, with only 7.5% and 1.8% of those aged 41–50 and >50 years developing LBP, respectively. However, no significant association was found between age and LBP (Table 2). Furthermore, LBP was significantly more prevalent among female (60.8%) than male (39.2%) nurses (* $p < 0.05$) (Table 2).

Among nursing professionals with LBP, nearly all (92.8%) had a diploma and a bachelor's degree, whereas only 7.2% had a master's degree and higher. However, no significant difference in educational level was noted.

Our data showed that place of work, nature of work, and direct contact hours with patient per week, but not work experience, were statistically associated with LBP (Table 2). Overall, among nursing professionals, 80% of those who developed LBP were employed full time, whereas only 20% were employed part time, with the difference being significant (* $p < 0.05$). Interestingly, our results showed that increased contact hours with patients per week was significantly associated with an increased number of nurses with LBP (* $p < 0.05$).

The final part of the study aimed at exploring the characteristics of LBP reported by nurses from Najran region.

A majority of the nurses (89.3%) reported no past medical conditions, whereas 3.6%, 2.9%, and 4.3% reported having cardiac conditions, hypertension, and other associated medical conditions, respectively (Table 3). Moreover, 59.3% and 40.7% of the participants reported having acute and chronic LBP, with 58.4%, 25%, and 18.6% reporting an average pain duration of 1 week, 2–4 weeks, and >4 weeks, respectively.

Table 3. Characteristics of low back pain among the included participants.

Characteristics	Characteristics	Number of Participants with LBP (n = 140)	Frequency (%)
Past medical condition:	None	125	89.3%
	Cardiac conditions	5	3.6%
	Hypertension	4	2.9%
	Others	6	4.3%
Nature of lower back pain (LBP):	Acute	83	59.3%
	Chronic	57	40.7%
Average duration of LBP:	1 week	79	58.4%
	2–4 weeks	35	25%
	>4 weeks	26	18.6%
Severity of LBP:	Mild	63	45%
	Moderate	52	37.2%
	Severe	25	17.8%
Functional limitation resulting from LBP:	None	93	66.4%
	Mild	33	23.6%
	Moderate	10	7.1%
	Severe	4	2.9%
Effect of LBP on normal activities:	Yes	103	73.6%
	No	37	26.4 %
Anatomical location of pain on a body chart:	Lower back	72	51.4%
	Lower back and buttocks	54	38.6%
	Lower back and thighs	5	3.5%
	Lower back and leg	4	3%
	Lower back and both legs	5	3.5%
Regular activities affected by LBP: n = 103	Lifting, carrying	28	27.2%
	Patient handling	21	20.3%
	Prolonged sitting	10	9.7%
	Prolonged standing	25	24.2%
	Pulling, pushing	19	18.6%

A majority of the participants (88.2%) reported having mild to moderate LBP, whereas the rest (17.8%) reported severe LBP. Moreover, a majority (66.4%) reported having no functional limitations, while 23.6%, 7.1%, and 2.9% reported having mild, moderate, and severe functional limitation, respectively. Furthermore, a majority (73.6%, n = 103) of the participants reported that LBP had an effect on the execution of normal daily activities (Table 3). Our results showed that the majority of the participants (51.4%) suffered pain localized in the lower back, whereas 38.6% reported having pain in both the lower back and buttocks. However, 10% of the nurses reported having radiating LBP, which suggested peripheralization (Table 3). Our data revealed that 27.2% of the nurses experienced difficulty in lifting and carrying weight, 24.2% reported having problems in prolonged standing, and 20.3% reported having problems in handling patients (Table 3).

4. Discussion

The present study focused on work-related factors affecting LBP among nursing staff. Among the various health care professionals, nurses experience tremendous physical stress by virtue of their work responsibilities. Najran, an important city located in the Southwestern part of the Kingdom of Saudi Arabia sharing a border with Yemen, has a number of important hospitals and other medical institutions. Nurses, who have been considered the backbone of the health care system, are prone to LBP given the work-related stressors they experience. Quite a large number of studies have shown that work-related injuries are quite common among members of the allied health care team. Moreover, studies revealed that low backache has been ranked third among the conditions nursing professionals experience [7,11,14,16]. Our results have been consistent with those presented in another study recently conducted in Zimbabwe that evaluated and reported the effects of various work-related factors on work-related musculoskeletal disorders among registered nurses in Hospitals across Harare [15]. The current study found that 74.8% of nursing professionals suffered from LBP, which was similar to that reported by other studies in other parts of the world. In a Nigerian study, Tinubu et al. reported a LBP prevalence of 78% among Nigerian nurses [16]. Yet another study conducted among Chinese nurses revealed a LBP prevalence of 77.4% among Chinese nurses [20]. Moreover, a series of studies in a large university hospital in Switzerland reported a high prevalence of LBP (73–76%) among nurses [21].

Among the various work-related factors investigated herein, such as education level, years of experience, place of work, nature of work, and direct contact hours per week with patients, only the last three were found to be significantly associated with LBP ($p < 0.05$). Though many of the symptoms and etiology of LBP remain unclear, investigations have linked work-related factors to LBP onset [12,18]. The manual tasks that most nurses perform daily have been shown to contribute toward LBP [19,22,23]. Stressful trunk postures that frequently occur due to direct patient contact during prolonged working conditions can provoke low back symptoms. The results presented herein clearly showed that the nature of work (i.e., 80% of the nurses who participated in this study in Najran with LBP reported working full time, while 74.2% reported having more than 30–40 h of direct patient contact) was a major work-related factor associated with LBP among nurses.

Nurses have increased susceptibility for developing back pain due to various stressors associated with long working hours. A series of studies found that LBP was positively related to the number of working hours [13,14,24,25].

The current study reported that LBP was more prevalent among female (60.8%) than male (39.2%) nurses. Another study conducted in Nigeria observed that among the 148 and 260 male and female nurses analyzed, 96 and 204 reported to have LBP, respectively. Our results also showed that that majority of nurses (76.2%) who developed some type of LBP were between the ages of 26 to 40 years, with only 7.5% and 1.8% of those aging 41–50 and >50 years developing LBP, respectively. However, no significant association has been observed between age and LBP (Table 2). This finding is similar to that presented in another set of studies conducted in Nigeria wherein age was not correlated with work-related musculoskeletal disorders among nursing professionals [16]. However, some studies have reported that the prevalence of LBP increases with age. Accordingly, Kassebaum et al. previously reported that susceptibility to the development of chronic diseases typically increases with age. This phenomenon is a reflection of genetic risk factor exposure and physiological changes along with the cumulative effect of environmental stress (occupation) [7]. An interesting finding observed herein was that a majority (76.2%) of nurses who reported having LBP were in the 26 to 40 year age group, which can be considered quite young by any standards. Thus, the reported prevalence of LBP among the relatively young population may be assumed to be caused by work-related stresses rather than actual chronic diseases or age-related changes, which could enhance the severity and prevalence.

Apart from nature of work, the current study found that place of work, working hours, poor working habits, and incorrect lifting postures can be associated with LBP. Another point emphasized herein is that more female nurses (60.8%) reported having LBP compared to male nurses (39.2%). This could perhaps be explained by the higher amount of work pressure in obstetrics and gynecology units, including labor wards, which are major parts of general hospitals, compared to that in other areas, such as university teaching hospitals or rehabilitation centers.

Our results found that 89.3% of nurses reported no past medical conditions. Considering that the majority of the nurses were relatively young (26–40 years), no significant association has been observed (Table 3). Our findings also determined that 59.3% of the nurses reported having acute LBP, while almost 84% reported having experienced LBP for only one to four weeks. This could have been caused by working without changing positions for a prolonged period, as well as lifting/transferring patients and increased patient load, which have been previously linked to acute LBP which can be reversed by taking rests.

Another important finding reported herein is that 88.2% of nursing professionals had developed mild to moderate LBP, with 66.4% reporting no functional limitations. This may have been due to the fact that 90% of the nurses had localized LBP without radiation. Our findings were similar to those presented in a study conducted on physical therapists in Kuwait, which reported that the phenomenon of peripheralization could adversely affect functional movements [26]. Lastly, the present study found that 27.2% of nurses experienced difficulty in lifting and carrying weight, 24.2% experienced difficulty with prolonged standing, 20.3% experienced difficulty in handling patients, and 18.6% reported having problems pulling and pushing weights (Table 3). This might be associated with decreasing nurses' work capacity, which might lead to sick leave, and might encourage managers to do something about the situation. The aforementioned difficulties are inherent in the various work stressors associated with the nursing profession. Accordingly, a number of previous studies have reported that LBP was strongly associated with working in the same position for prolonged periods, lifting/transferring of patients, and increased patient load. Our findings are consistent with those of the Zimbabwean study, which found that repeated performance of various work-related tasks, caring for a large number of patients daily, awkward bending or twisting of the back, lifting or transferring dependent patients, and heavy equipment and materials were significantly associated with the incidence of LBP [15].

There are several limitations in our study, one of them regarding selection bias. We know little about which individuals wanted to answer the questionnaires: maybe those with LBP were more interested in answering the study than those without back pain. Another limitation is the relatively small sample size of the participants in this study.

5. Conclusions

The present study concluded that nursing professionals working across various institutions in the Najran region of Saudi Arabia had a high prevalence of LBP. Moreover, our findings showed that various work-related characteristics, including place and nature of work, might be associated with the onset of LBP. The result presented herein will be of considerable help to institutional heads in their establishment of related policies and appropriate measures in managing associated work-related LBP among not only nursing professionals but also other related health care professionals.

Acknowledgments: The author expresser his thanks to the Ministry of Education and the Deanship of Scientific Research, Najran University, Najran, Saudi Arabia for sponsoring this study (project number NU/MID/17/114), as well as to all participants for their collaboration.

References

1. Dionne, C.E.; Dunn, K.M.; Croft, P.R. Does back pain prevalence really decrease with increasing age? A systematic review. *Age Ageing* **2006**, *35*, 229–234. [CrossRef] [PubMed]
2. Ganasegeran, K.; Perianayagam, W.; Nagaraj, P.; Al-Dubai, S. Psycho-behavioural risks of low back pain in railway workers. *Occup. Med.* **2014**, *64*, 372–375. [CrossRef] [PubMed]
3. Foster, N.E. Barriers and progress in the treatment of low back pain. *BMC Med.* **2011**, *9*, 108. [CrossRef] [PubMed]

4. Leboeuf-Yde, C.; Klougart, N.; Lauritzen, T. How Common Is Low Back Pain in the Nordic Population? Data From a Recent Study on a Middle-Aged General Danish Population and Four Surveys Previously Conducted in the Nordic Countries. *Spine* **1996**, *21*, 1518–1525. [CrossRef] [PubMed]
5. Manzini, F.; Cesana, G.; Manzini, C.; Riva, M.A. A pioneering patient lift: Prevention of low Back pain in health care workers in the 18th century. *Spine* **2015**, *40*, 126–127. [CrossRef] [PubMed]
6. Reigo, T.; Timpka, T.; Tropp, H. The epidemiology of back pain in vocational age groups. *Scand. J. Prim. Health Care* **1999**, *17*, 17–21. [CrossRef] [PubMed]
7. Kassebaum, N.J.; Arora, M.; Barber, R.M.; Bhutta, Z.A.; Brown, J.; Carter, A.; Casey, D.C.; Charlson, F.J.; Coates, M.M.; Coggeshall, M.; et al. Global, regional, and national disability-adjusted life-years (DALYs) for 315 diseases and injuries and healthy life expectancy (HALE), 1990–2015: A systematic analysis for the Global Burden of Disease Study 2015. *Lancet* **2016**, *388*, 1603–1658. [CrossRef]
8. Walker, B.; Muller, R.; Grant, W. Low back pain in Australian adults: The economic burden. *Asia Pac. J. Public Health* **2003**, *15*, 79–87. [CrossRef]
9. Kim, L.H.; Vail, D.; Azad, T.D.; Bentley, J.P.; Zhang, Y.; Ho, A.L.; Fatemi, P.; Feng, A.; Varshneya, K.; Desai, M.; et al. Expenditures and health care utilization among adults with newly diagnosed low back and lower extremity pain. *JAMA Netw. Open* **2019**, *2*, e193676. [CrossRef]
10. Jackson, T.; Thomas, S.; Stabile, V.; Shotwell, M.; Han, X.; McQueen, K. A systematic review and meta-analysis of the global burden of chronic pain without clear etiology in low- and middle-income countries: Trends in heterogeneous data and a proposal for new assessment methods. *Anesth. Analg.* **2016**, *123*, 739–748. [CrossRef]
11. Homaid, M.B.; Abdelmoety, D.; Alshareef, W.; Alghamdi, A.; Alhozali, F.; Alfahmi, N.; Hafiz, W.; Alzahrani, A.; Elmorsy, S. Prevalence and risk factors of low back pain among operation room staff at a tertiary care center, Makkah, Saudi Arabia: A cross-sectional study. *Ann. Occup. Environ. Med.* **2016**, *28*, 1. [CrossRef]
12. Chaffin, D.B.; Park, K.S. A longitudinal study of low-back pain as associated with occupational weight lifting factors. *Am. Ind. Hyg. Assoc. J.* **1973**, *34*, 513–525. [CrossRef]
13. Mukhtad, A.A.; Mohamed, H.A. Lower Back Pain among Health Care Workers in Operating Room at Al-Fateh Children's Hospital: Prevalence and Risk Factors. *Asian J. Res. Nurs. Health* **2018**, *1*, 1–11.
14. Karahan, A.; Kav, S.; Abbasoglu, A.; Dogan, N. Low back pain: Prevalence and associated risk factors among hospital staff. *J. Adv. Nurs.* **2009**, *65*, 516–524. [CrossRef]
15. Chiwaridzo, M.; Makotore, V.; Dambi, J.M.; Munambah, N.; Mhlanga, M. Work-related musculoskeletal disorders among registered general nurses: A case of a large central hospital in Harare, Zimbabwe. *BMC Res. Notes* **2018**, *11*, 315. [CrossRef] [PubMed]
16. Tinubu, B.M.; Mbada, C.E.; Oyeyemi, A.L.; Fabunmi, A.A. Work-related musculoskeletal disorders among nurses in Ibadan, South-west Nigeria: A cross-sectional survey. *BMC Musculoskelet. Disord.* **2010**, *11*, 12. [CrossRef] [PubMed]
17. Gaowgzeh, R.A.M. Low back pain among nursing professionals in Jeddah, Saudi Arabia: Prevalence and risk factors. *J. Back Musculoskelet. Rehabil.* **2019**, *32*, 555–560. [CrossRef] [PubMed]
18. Alzidani, T.H.; Alturkistani, A.M.; Alzahrani, B.S.; Aljuhani, A.M.; Alzahrani, K.M. Prevalence and risk factors of low back pain among Taif surgeons. *Saudi J. Health Sci.* **2018**, *7*, 172–177.
19. Dionne, C.E.; Dunn, K.M.; Croft, P.R.; Nachemson, A.L.; Buchbinder, R.; Walker, B.F.; Wyatt, M.; Cassidy, J.D.; Rossignol, M.; Leboeuf-Yde, C.; et al. A consensus approach toward the standardization of back pain definitions for use in prevalence studies. *Spine* **2008**, *33*, 95–103. [CrossRef] [PubMed]
20. Chiou, W.-K.; Wong, M.-K.; Lee, Y.-H. Epidemiology of low back pain in Chinese nurses. *Int. J. Nurs. Stud.* **1994**, *31*, 361–368. [CrossRef]
21. Genevay, S.; Cedraschi, C.; Courvoisier, D.S.; Perneger, T.V.; Grandjean, R.; Griesser, A.C.; Monnin, D. Work-related characteristics of back and neck pain among employees of a Swiss University Hospital. *Joint Bone Spine* **2011**, *78*, 392–397. [CrossRef] [PubMed]
22. Cargnin, Z.A.; Schneider, D.G.; Vargas, M.A.O.; Machado, R.R. Non-specific low back pain and its relation to the nursing work process. *Rev. Lat. Am. Enferm.* **2019**, *27*, e3172. [CrossRef]
23. Yip, Y.B. A study of work stress, patient handling activities and the risk of low back pain among nurses in Hong Kong. *J. Adv. Nurs.* **2001**, *36*, 794–804. [CrossRef]
24. June, K.J.; Cho, S.H. Low back pain and work—Related factors among nurses in intensive care units. *J. Clin. Nurs.* **2011**, *20*, 479–487. [CrossRef]

25. Sikiru, L.; Hanifa, S. Prevalence and risk factors of low back pain among nurses in a typical Nigerian hospital. *Afr. Health Sci.* **2010**, *10*, 26. [PubMed]
26. Shehab, D.; Al-Jarallah, K.; Moussa, M.A.; Adham, N. Prevalence of low back pain among physical therapists in Kuwait. *Med. Princ. Pract.* **2003**, *12*, 224–230. [CrossRef] [PubMed]

3

Eye Gaze Markers Indicate Visual Attention to Threatening Images in Individuals with Chronic Back Pain

Zoë C. Franklin [1,*], Paul S. Holmes [1] and Neil E. Fowler [2]

1 Musculoskeletal Science and Sports Medicine Research Centre, Manchester Metropolitan University, Manchester M15 6BH, UK; p.s.holmes@mmu.ac.uk
2 Vice Chancellor's Office, University of Salford, Salford M5 4WT, UK; n.fowler1@salford.ac.uk
* Correspondence: z.franklin@mmu.ac.uk

Abstract: Research into attentional biases and threatening, pain-related information has primarily been investigated using reaction time as the dependent variable. This study aimed to extend previous research to provide a more in depth investigation of chronic back pain and individuals' attention to emotional stimuli by recording eye movement behavior. Individuals with chronic back pain (n = 18) were recruited from a back rehabilitation program and age and sex matched against 17 non-symptomatic controls. Participants' eye movements were recorded whilst they completed a dot probe task, which included back pain specific threatening images and neutral images. There were no significant differences between chronic pain and control participants in attentional biases recorded using reaction time from the dot probe task. Chronic pain participants, however, demonstrated a significantly higher percentage of fixations, larger pupil diameter, a longer average fixation duration and faster first fixation to threatening compared to neutral images. They also had a significantly longer average fixation duration and larger pupil diameter to threatening images compared to control participants. The findings of this study suggest eye gaze metrics may provide a more sensitive measure of attentional biases in chronic pain populations. These findings may have important therapeutic implications for the patient and therapist.

Keywords: chronic pain; attentional biases; eye gaze

1. Introduction

Attentional biases are a selective attention towards or away from a stimulus, which is both specific and salient to an individual's current environment and situation [1] and can result in a variety of cognitive, behavioral and physiological responses. Excessive attentional biases towards pain have been hypothesized to contribute towards the promotion of pain-related anxiety, fear of pain-related activity, physical disability and exacerbations in the pain experience [2]. Attentional biases towards pain-related stimuli have been proposed in theories of attention and pain [3,4]. The pain-specific models explain an individual's attentional response to the presence of pain-related stimuli. Todd et al. [5] proposed the threat interpretation model of attentional biases, suggesting that there is a relationship between an individual's interpretation of threat, which then influences their attentional bias towards it. As threat interpretation increases, initial vigilance towards pain-related stimuli increases; the level of the threat then influences whether the individual is able to disengage from the threat or avoid the threat.

Meta-analyses [6–8] have reported that pain participants have an attentional bias towards threat related information compared to controls, although with low effect sizes of 0.1–0.3 which may be due, in part, to the lack of consistency with the type of pain-related stimuli (e.g., words or pictures; sensory or affective pain). Within the most recent review [8], the majority of studies used word-based stimuli or pain-related faces, rather than pictures associated with movement. Kourtzi and Kanwasher [9] have identified that pictures which have implied physical movement lead to greater activation of the extended motor system, compared to images without implied movement. Therefore, it could be suggested that the increased motor activity associated with movement-related images might represent a marker of a more valid cognitive response to movement-related emotional stimuli.

Attentional biases have been assessed, traditionally, using the dot probe paradigm [10]. This technique captures a momentary cross-section of attention at the stimulus offset. Therefore, the method does not indicate duration of attention or attentional exertion to stimuli [11]. The use of eye-tracking equipment, however, can address some of these limitations and allows researchers to record location and duration of gaze fixations. In addition, eye-tracking also provides the opportunity to measure pupil diameter as an index of attentional effort [12]. Eye gaze markers can, therefore, provide researchers with a range of additional metrics to improve the understanding of attentional biases in chronic pain patients.

Several studies have utilised the dot probe method in conjunction with eye tracking and identified a bias towards pain-related information. Unfortunately, however, these studies were all conducted with pain-free undergraduate students, using pain-related words [13,14] or faces [15–17]. While these studies do provide some insight into the mechanisms associated with attention to pain-related information, further research is needed to be conducted in patients suffering from chronic pain. To our knowledge, only three studies have used eye movements to examine attentional biases to pictorial stimuli, and these were with chronic headache populations [18,19] and mixed chronic pain groups [20]. Both Liossi et al. [18] and Schoth et al. [19] used a visual search task to assess the attentional biases of chronic headache patients. Participants were shown four facial expressions (pain, angry, happy and neutral). Both studies [18,19] identified that the pain group demonstrated a significantly higher proportion of initial fixations on the pain face, compared to the other facial expressions. Furthermore, Liossi et al. [18] found that patients had an initial shift in their attention towards pain stimuli, but then maintained their gaze on happy" images. There was no evidence that pain patients maintained their gaze on pain related images. These findings support the theoretical models of pain and attentional biases [3–5] and propose that attentional biases may play an important role in the maintenance of chronic headache. Fashler and Katz [20] investigated the attentional biases of undergraduate students who were experiencing a variety of chronic pain conditions (e.g., neck/back, migraine, ankle/knee, stomach, hip, arm, eye and jaw pain). Participants completed a dot probe task using injury related (e.g., needle being inserted into the skin, black eye, open wound, burned skin) and neutral images while their eye movements were recorded. Reaction time results revealed that chronic pain individuals responded faster to neutral stimuli in contrast to the injury related images. In contrast, the eye tracking data demonstrated that chronic pain individuals maintained attention towards injury related pictures. Supporting Todd et al.'s [5] theory that as the interpretation of threat increases, vigilance towards the threat also increases. To date, however, no study has investigated the attentional biases of a chronic back pain patient population using both the dot probe paradigm and eye tracking approaches.

The aim of this study, therefore, was to provide a more in depth investigation of chronic back pain patients' attention to pain-related images in comparison to non-symptomatic controls by recording eye movement behavior whilst participants also completed a dot probe task. We hypothesized that chronic back pain participants would have: (i) a significantly higher percentage of fixations to threatening stimuli compared to controls; (ii) a longer average fixation duration to threatening images; and (iii) exhibit a faster reaction time to threatening images in the dot probe task.

2. Method

2.1. Participants

Participants were recruited from a back rehabilitation program at a UK NHS trust (n = 18) and an age and sex matched non-symptomatic control group was recruited from the university and local area ($n = 17$). Chronic pain participants had been suffering from back pain for a minimum of three months. Non-symptomatic controls were recruited through advertisements through unsolicited noticeboards and electronic advertising. Ethical approval was granted by NRES Committee North West Greater Manchester Central and by Manchester Metropolitan University Ethics Committee. All participants provided written informed consent to take part in this study. Inclusion criteria for the back pain group were: (i) over 18 years of age; (ii) a referral to a hospital-based back pain management program for non-specific musculoskeletal pain; (iii) pain duration of >3 months; and (iv) normal or corrected to normal vision. Inclusion criteria for the control group were: (i) over 18 years of age; and (ii) normal or corrected to normal vision. Exclusion criteria for the control group were: (i) any form of current or recent chronic or recurrent pain; and (ii) regular (daily or near daily) use of any form of analgesic medication.

2.2. Materials

2.2.1. Dot Probe Paradigm

All participants completed a dot probe task comprising 20 practice trials and 150 experimental trials (100 threat-neutral, 50 neutral-neutral). The threat images were taken from the Photograph Series of Daily Activities (PHODA) image bank [21] (back pain specific and showing movements known to be associated as threatening and evoking pain or pain-related fear, for example lifting or bending tasks). The neutral images were taken from the International Affective Picture System (IAPS) [22] and included images of neutral activities, faces and inanimate objects. The presentation of images were randomized for each participant. Dot probe stimuli were presented on a 23-inch screen (HP EliteDisplay E231, Hewlett-Packard Company, Palo Alto, CA, USA) with a 1920 × 1080-pixel resolution and a 100 Hz refresh rate. Participants were told to engage actively with the pictures that were presented to them on the screen. Each trial began with a central fixation cross presented for 500 ms, followed by an image pair on the left and right side of the screen, either threat-neutral or neutral-neutral pairs presented for 500 ms. Following presentation of the image pair, a probe stimulus (a pair of dots either vertical or horizontal) was presented in the location of either the emotional or the neutral image and remained displayed until the patient/participant responded (see Figure 1). Participants were instructed to press, as quickly and accurately as possible, one of two keys to identify the probe presented. The inter-trial interval varied randomly between 500 and 1250 ms. Response times shorter than 200 ms or longer than 1200 ms were removed from the data. Incorrect responses were also excluded from the analysis. Errors and outliers accounted for 2.5% of the data.

Congruent (e.g., the target followed the emotional picture) and incongruent (e.g., the target followed the neutral picture) attentional bias scores for threatening images relative to neutral were calculated for each participant from the response time data using the formula:

$$\text{Congruent} = ((\text{Trpr} + \text{Tlpl})/2) - ((\text{Nrpr} + \text{Nlpr} + \text{Nrpl} + \text{Nlpl})/4) \quad (1)$$

$$\text{Incongruent} = ((\text{Tlpr} + \text{Trpl})/2) - ((\text{Nrpr} + \text{Nlpr} + \text{Nrpl} + \text{Nlpl})/4) \quad (2)$$

T = threat, N = neutral, p = probe, r = right position, l = left position.

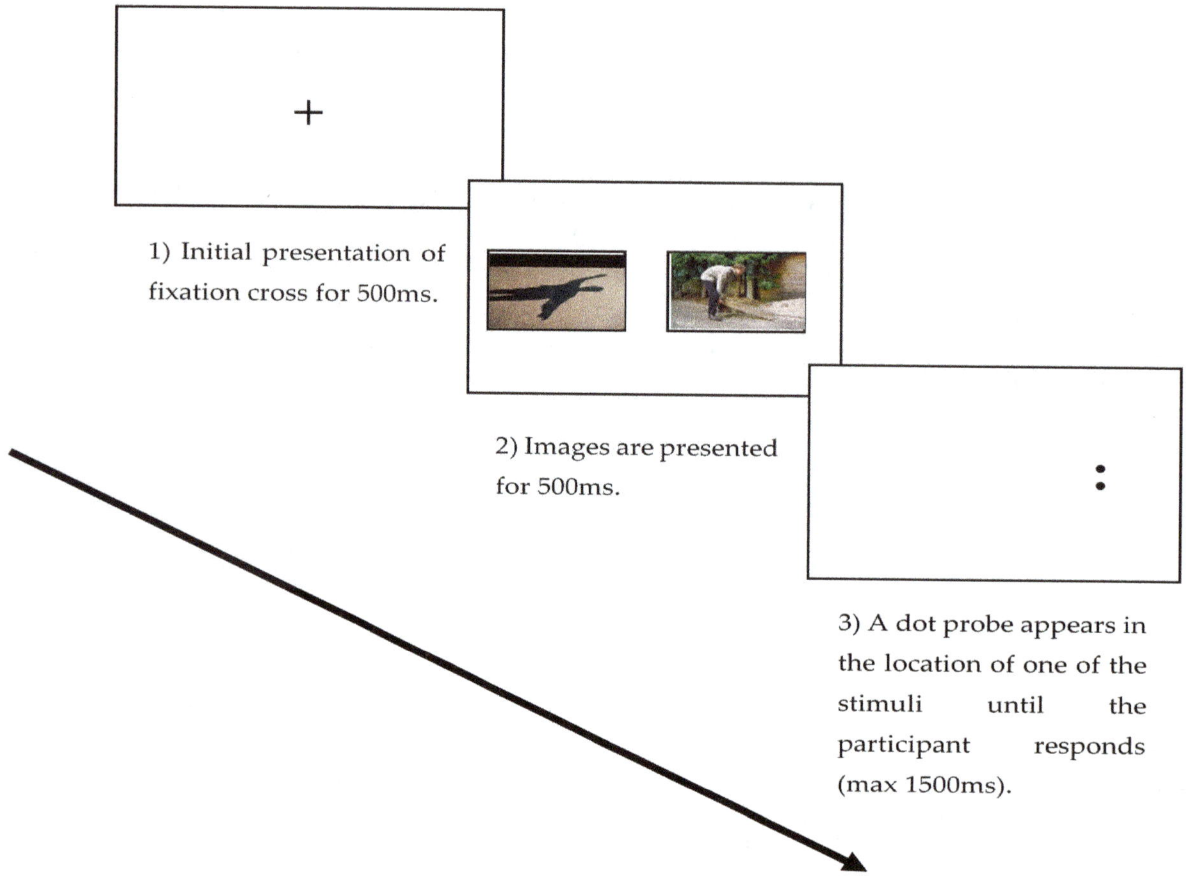

Figure 1. An example of the three stages of the dot probe task in the neutral threat condition.

2.2.2. Eye-Gaze

While participants completed the dot probe paradigm, their eye movements were also recorded. Eye movement data were recorded with an Applied Science Laboratories Mobile Eye System (ASL; Bedford, MA, USA) using a dark pupil tracking technique throughout the dot probe paradigm. This method uses the relationship between the pupil and a reflection from the cornea to calculate the point of gaze in relation to an external scene camera. The ASL software computes the relationship between the pupil and cornea to locate gaze within a scene at a sampling rate of 30 Hz. The system has an accuracy of 0.5° of visual angle, a resolution of 0.10° of visual angle, and a visual range of 50° horizontal and 40° vertical.

Previous eye gaze research has assessed: (i) percentage of fixations on the threat or neutral stimuli; (ii) average pupil diameter when fixating on the threat and neutral stimuli; (iii) average time spent fixating on the threat or neutral stimuli; and (iv) first fixation time on either the threat or the neutral stimuli. In this study, visual fixations were defined as maintaining gaze on a specific location on the screen for at least 100ms and a maximum fixation radius of 1°, as employed in previous studies [13,16].

2.3. Procedures

Participants were asked to sit at a desk in a black booth and facing the screen approximately 60 cm in front of them and at eye level. A desk mounted chin rest was used to reduce participants' head movements ensuring that participants' eyes were level with the middle of the monitor on which the stimuli were presented. This ensured that each participant's eyes were in the same location relative to the camera and monitor. A 9-point calibration check was used prior to the start of testing. A drift check was conducted before each trial and recalibration performed when necessary. Participants were instructed to look at the fixation cross before each trial to standardize the starting location of their eye gaze and were told to engage actively with the pictures that were presented to them on the screen. Participants provided demographic information after testing was completed to allow for age and sex matching.

2.4. Preparation of Eye Gaze Data

Eye gaze data were analyzed using ASL Results Plus (Applied Science Laboratories, Bedford, MA, USA). Each trial was parsed into 150 (100 threat-neutral, 50 neutral-neutral) separate trials. Individual trials were then analyzed by drawing two separate areas of interest (AOIs) around the threatening and neutral images. From this, the number of fixations, average fixation duration, and pupil diameter when fixating in each AOI were calculated. A fixation was defined as any gaze that remained stable (within 1 degree of visual angle) for a duration of over 100 ms. In accordance with previous studies [23], participants with missing data of more than 15% over the 150 trials were excluded from the study. Based on this criterion, no participants were excluded from the study. Due to technical difficulties with the eye tracking equipment, no eye movement data were recorded for one of the non-symptomatic control participants and this participant was excluded from further analysis.

2.5. Data Analysis

A series of 2 × 2 analysis of variances (ANOVA) were conducted on the eye gaze data (percentage fixation, average pupil diameter, average fixation duration, first fixation time), with group (patient, control) as a between participants independent variable, and image type (threat or neutral image) as a within participants variable. A 2 × 2 ANOVA of the probe response time data with group (patient, controls) as the between variable, and probe position (probe in same versus different location to threatening image) as the within participants variable. Bonferroni *post hoc* analyses were used where needed to clarify significant main effects and interactions. Alpha was set at $p < 0.05$ and effect sizes were calculated using Cohen's d.

3. Results

3.1. Group Characteristics

The chronic pain and control groups did not differ significantly in sex ratio (chronic pain: 12 (66%) female, control group 11 (64%) female, $\chi^2 = 0.15$, $p = 0.90$) or age (chronic pain group: M = 46.72, SD ± 9.97 years; control group: M = 40.47, SD ± 9.23 years, $t(33) = -1.92$, $p = 0.07$).

3.2. Power Analysis

Post-hoc power analyses [24] were conducted for the dot probe and eye movement data. The power analysis results for the dot probe data were: power = 0.64 ($\alpha = 0.05$; $\beta = 0.36$) $d = 0.6$, for number of fixations to threat; power = 0.82 ($\alpha = 0.05$; $\beta = 0.18$) $d = 0.8$, and neutral images; power = 0.83 ($\alpha = 0.05$; $\beta = 0.17$) $d = 0.9$. The power analysis results for the average pupil diameter; power = 0.76 ($\alpha = 0.05$; $\beta = 0.24$) $d = 0.8$; average fixation duration; power = 0.86 ($\alpha = 0.05$; $\beta = 0.14$) $d = 0.9$; and for total fixation duration; power = 0.99 ($\alpha = 0.05$; $\beta = 0.01$) $d = 1.6$. Therefore, despite the relatively modest sample size there was sufficient power to have confidence in the findings from the study.

3.3. Eye Gaze Reliability Analysis

Internal consistency, reflecting the interrelatedness of items on a test was calculated using Cronbach's alpha for both the control group and the patient group for each outcome variable. For both patient and control groups there was high reliability for percentage fixation count, pupil diameter and first fixation time (Cronbach's $\alpha = 0.73$–0.93). Average fixation duration subscale, however, had a relatively low reliability, Cronbach's $\alpha = 0.62$–0.64 (see Table 1).

Table 1. Internal consistency measured with Cronbach's alpha for each outcome variable in the patient and control group.

Group	Outcome Measure	Cronbach's α
Patient	Percentage fixation count	0.750
	Pupil diameter	0.802
	Average fixation duration	0.644
	First fixation time	0.722
Control	Percentage fixation count	0.927
	Pupil diameter	0.743
	Average fixation duration	0.616
	First fixation time	0.725

3.4. Percentage Fixation Count

The results of the two way mixed ANOVA showed a significant interaction between participant group and image type, (F (1, 33) = 32.01, $p < 0.001$) and a significant main effect of stimuli type, (F (1, 33) = 11.05, $p = 0.002$). Pairwise comparisons indicated that chronic pain individuals attended to threat images (M = 34.07, SD $\pm$ 10.58) significantly more than neutral stimuli (M = 18.27, SD $\pm$ 9.32); $t(17) = 6.25$, $p < 0.001$, $d = 1.57$, 95% CI [0.80, 2.29] (see Figure 2). For the control group, there was no significant difference between the percentage fixation count to threat (M = 21.61, SD = 5.97) or neutral (M = 25.72, SD $\pm$ 8.39) stimuli; $t(16) = -1.69$, $p = 0.11$, d= 0.5, 95% CI [−1.24, 0.13].

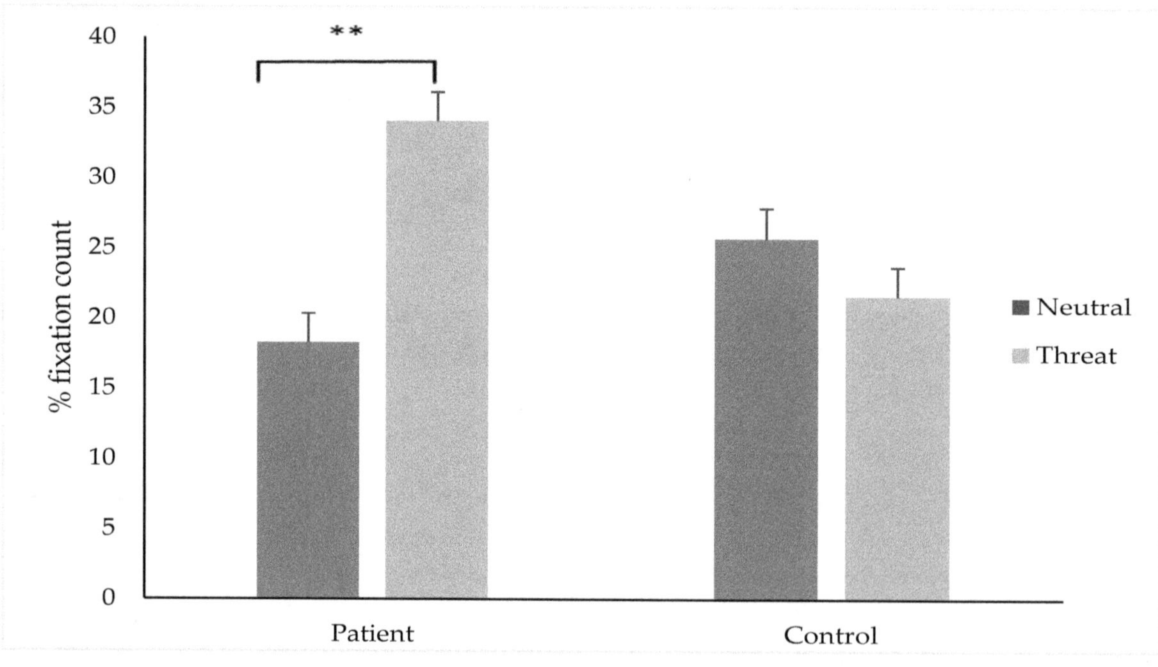

Figure 2. The percentage of fixations ($\pm$SE) on threatening or neutral stimuli in the patient and control group. ** indicates $p < 0.01$.

3.5. Average Pupil Diameter

A significant main effect of group was found (F (1,33) = 23.71, $p = 0.0001$); t-tests revealed that individuals in the pain group (M = 5.69, SD $\pm$ 0.18 mm) had a significantly larger pupil diameter compared to controls (M = 4.62, SD $\pm$ 0.18 mm), $d = 0.5$, 95% CI [4.29, 7.32]. A significant main effect for stimuli type was found (F (1, 33) = 11.65, $p = 0.002$); t-tests showed that participants had a significantly larger pupil diameter when attending to threatening (M = 5.30, SD $\pm$ 1.33 mm) compared to neutral (M = 4.64, SD $\pm$ 1.23mm) stimuli, $t(34) = 2.71$, $p = 0.01$, d= 0.9, 95% CI [−0.16, 1.17] (Figure 3). There was no significant interaction effect found (F (1,33) = 0.10, $p = 0.749$).

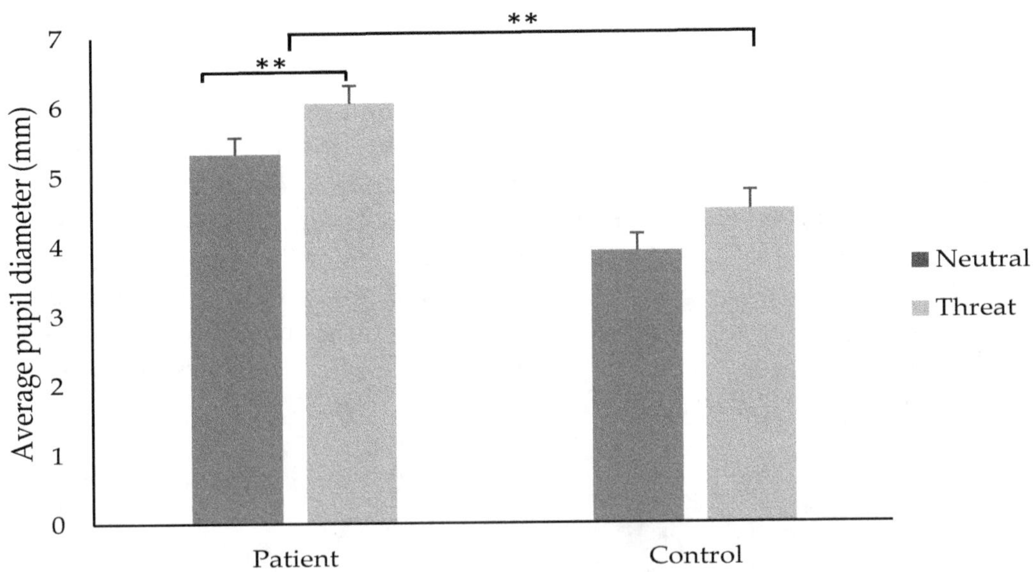

Figure 3. The average pupil diameter (mm) (±SE) for the patient and control groups when attending to threatening and neutral stimuli. ** indicates $p < 0.01$.

3.6. *Average Fixation Duration*

A significant group x image type interaction F (1, 33) = 10.90, p = 0.02, and a significant main effect of group F (1, 33) = 4.72, p = 0.03 was found. T-tests revealed that pain participants demonstrated a significantly higher average fixation duration on threatening (M = 219.18, SD ± 53.06 ms) compared to neutral stimuli (M = 185.04, SD ± 38.68 ms); $t(34) = -2.16$, $p = 0.03$, $d = 0.8$, 95% CI [−0.06, −0.001] (Figure 4). There was no significant difference between the control group's average fixation duration towards threatening or neutral stimuli. T-tests revealed that the pain group (M = 219.18, SD ± 53.06 ms) had a significantly longer average fixation duration to threatening stimuli compared to controls (M = 174.88, SD ± 17.36 ms); $t(68) = -3.35$, $p = 0.03$, $d = 0.9$, 95% CI [−0.04, −0.004].

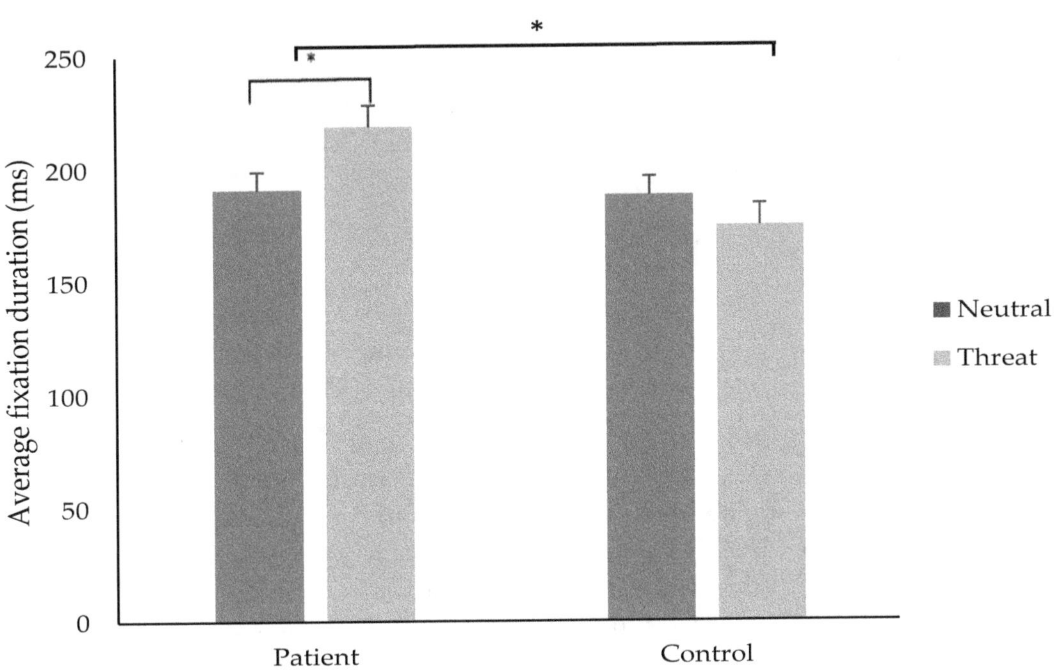

Figure 4. The average fixation (ms) duration (±SE) to threatening and neutral stimuli for the patient and control group. * indicates $p < 0.05$.

3.7. First Fixation Time

There was a significant interaction of group x first fixation time (F (1,33) = 35.21, p = 0.0001), and a significant main effect of group (F (1,33) = 27.00, p = 0.0001. Pairwise comparisons indicated that patients made significantly faster first fixations to threatening images, (t(33) = 8.90, p = 0.0001, d = 0.7, 95% CI [−3.59, −1.76] compared to controls (patient M = 124.98 ms, SD = 65.67; control M = 210.24, SD = 28.21) (Figure 5). The control group made significantly faster first fixations to the neutral stimuli compared to the threatening, (t(16) = 3.97, p = 0.001, d = 1.02, 95% CI [0.28, 1.71]). In contrast, the pain patients made significantly faster first fixations to the threatening image type compared to the neutral image type (t(17) = 4.44, p = 0.0001, d = 0.9, 95% CI [−1.47, −0.27]). There was no significant main effect of image type (F (1,33) = 5.36, p = 0.469).

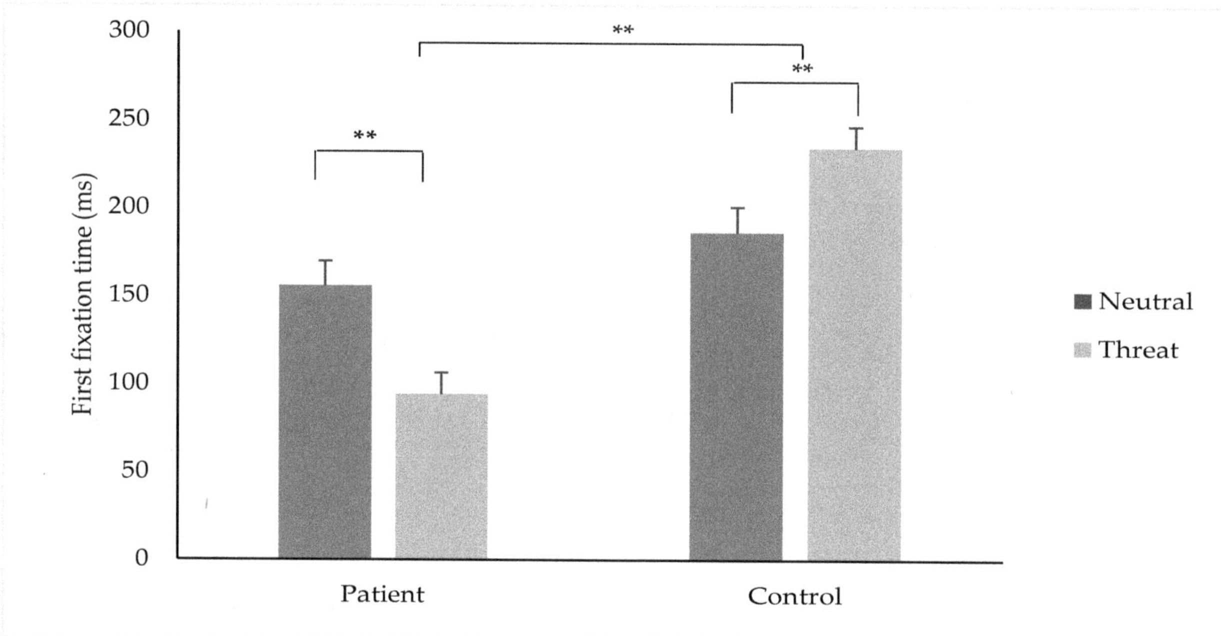

Figure 5. First fixation time (ms) (±SE) to threatening and neutral stimuli for the patient and control group. ** indicates $p < 0.01$.

3.8. Dot Probe Response Time Measures

There was no significant interaction of group x attentional bias (F (1,33) = 3.17, p = 0.08), and no significant main effect of group (F (1, 33) = 1.69, p = 0.20) or probe position (F (1, 33) = 4.60, p = 0.12). There was no significant difference between attentional bias to threatening images for either congruent (t(33) = 1.79, p = 0.08, d = 0.6, 95% CI [−3.35, 51.14]) or incongruent (t(33) = 0.47, p = 0.64, d = 0.6, 95% CI [−17.61, 28.29]) trials for the pain group (congruent, M= −14.23, SD ± 48.50 ms; incongruent, M = 6.22, SD ± 39.46 ms) and controls (congruent, M = 9.66, SD ± 27.09 ms; incongruent, M = 11.56, SD ± 25.32 ms). Table 2 shows the mean response times for the congruent, incongruent and neutral trials for the chronic pain and control groups.

Table 2. Mean reaction times of congruent and incongruent trials (in ms; standard deviations in brackets) for the threat and neutral images in the dot probe task for participants with chronic low back pain and the non-symptomatic control group.

	Stimuli	Chronic Pain Group	Non-Symptomatic Control Group
Congruent	Threat (ms)	595.79 (59.40)	548.74 (49.08)
	Neutral (ms)	591.32 (65.10)	540.44 (49.65)
Incongruent	Threat (ms)	597.31 (59.64)	552.69 (48.36)
	Neutral (ms)	591.32 (65.10)	540.44 (49.65)

4. Discussion

This study used an eye gaze protocol to consider the attentional biases of individuals with chronic back pain to threatening and neutral images using a modified dot probe paradigm. The eye gaze data highlight important new findings about the differences in attentional bias to threatening and neutral images between individuals with chronic pain and non-symptomatic controls that cannot be identified by using the standard dot probe paradigm.

Within-group analysis demonstrated that the chronic pain individuals had a significantly higher percentage of fixations, larger pupil diameter and longer average fixation duration on threatening compared to neutral images. There were no significant differences in eye gaze metrics to threatening or neutral images in non-symptomatic controls; the absence of attentional bias suggesting that the back pain specific images were not perceived as threatening for the non-symptomatic controls. Between-group analysis revealed that chronic pain participants also had a longer average fixation duration and larger pupil diameter to threatening images compared to the non-symptomatic controls. Chronic pain patients also had a faster initial fixation to the pain related image compared to the neutral image; the opposite pattern was found for the non-symptomatic controls. In contrast, and of concern to the validity of the standard dot probe procedure, there were no significant differences in attentional biases for the dot probe task between the chronic pain group and non-symptomatic controls. Taken together, the findings of this study suggest that eye gaze metrics may provide a more sensitive measure of attentional bias compared to the dot probe response time.

The majority of previous research investigating pain-related attentional biases using eye gaze has been within a non-symptomatic population and used word-based stimuli or pain-related faces [13–16]. To our knowledge, only three studies have previously used back pain-specific images in a dot probe task [25–27], but none have used eye-tracking markers concurrent with the dot probe test with pain-related physical activity movements. Consistent with the findings of Roelofs et al. [25] the dot probe data indicated that there was no difference between chronic pain participants and non-symptomatic controls for attention to threatening images in congruent trials. Whereas, the eye gaze behavior in this study demonstrated that chronic pain participants attended to the pain-related images significantly faster, more often and for a significantly longer average duration than neutral images compared to non-symptomatic controls. The attentional bias to threatening stimuli in the pain group may have been due to the implied motion cues within the image. Kourtzi et al. [9] found greater activation of the medial temporal/medial superior temporal cortex (MT/MST) when viewing photographs with implied movement and imaging studies have supported the role of these brain areas in the analysis of movement, but not object, recognition [28]. Action understanding depends, in part, on prior knowledge about the movement's goal and intention with predictions about an object's (or body's) future position being made from the motion implied in the static image [29]. Participant's memorial biases modulate the increase in attentional bias to threatening information and, therefore, they perceive implied painful motion in the image (e.g., rotation of the back, which causes them pain); the dynamic images accessing a more meaningful motor representation that is presented for analysis through the variety of eye gaze metrics employed in this study.

Eye tracking studies within healthy populations have identified vigilance towards pain-related words and faces [14,15]. In line with previous research [18,19], we identified that chronic pain patients attended to pain related images significantly faster than neutral images and in contrast to the profiles of non-symptomatic controls. Todd et al. [5] have proposed the Threat Interpretation Model of pain that can be used to consider some of the study's findings. Specifically, there is an initial vigilance towards the threat-related stimuli; as the threat continues, there is an avoidance of the threatening cues. Further, Fashler and Katz [20] identified that both pain and control participants responded faster to neutral images in the dot probe task, whereas the eye movement data demonstrated that in the early phase of the trial, participants attended to the neutral images, then in the later phases, gaze duration was maintained on the injury-related images. These findings are in contrast to those presented here; there were no differences found for reaction time data and chronic pain patients only made faster first fixations to pain related images. Due to the short presentation time used in this study, we were unable to assess whether participants would maintain their gaze on the pain stimuli or, in line with Todd et al., [5] the patients showed an active avoidance of the threatening cues. One possible explanation for the differences could be due to the specificity of the images. Fashler and Katz [20] used images for which both individuals with, and without pain could perceive as threatening (e.g., an open wound, needle inserted into the skin etc.). In contrast, our study used images that were specific to back pain and were not deemed threatening for the control group. Todd et al. [5] propose that initial vigilance occurs when participants interpret the stimuli as threatening. The specificity of the image, and using a homogenous pain group, may, therefore, have influenced the attentional bias to pain related stimuli. Furthermore, the differences between the studies could be due to the image presentation time and type of probe stimulus. In the current study, the images were presented for 500 ms and the dot probe was either.. or : and each probe could appear on either side. In contrast, Fashler and Katz [20] presented the images for 2000 ms and participants were shown a single dot, the response required participants to press one of two buttons to indicate the side of the screen the dot was on. The significant differences in the methods between the studies may explain the differences in the reaction time data. In contrast to Fashler and Katz [20], Yang et al. [30] found that chronic pain participants had an early attentional bias towards catastrophe-based words, followed by avoidance of pain words. Due to the short stimuli presentation time within our study, we were only able to assess initial vigilance, consistent with previous research in pain populations [18]. This bottom up process is considered to be automatic in anxious individuals. In contrast to other studies identifying a vigilance-avoidance pattern [18,30], this study used images of physical activity (rather than words) associated with pain. Images with implied movement provide elements of action understanding. They may give more personal meaning, agency, ownership and motor response [31] for the viewed activity for chronic back pain participants compared to words, pain faces or images of an individual experiencing pain (e.g., someone grimacing while they are completing an activity). Future studies should present pain-related images for a longer duration to identify whether chronic back pain participants maintain vigilance or attend then avoid threatening images. Using images that are specific to the pain condition may also provide researchers with the ability to alter biases to allow for top down processing of attending to goal directed information. This enhanced attention to goal related information may reduce avoidance of activity and disability levels. Although a greater understanding of attention in this context is needed, preliminary evidence has supported the therapeutic benefits of attentional bias modification in pain populations [32,33].

In this study, chronic pain participants showed a significantly larger pupil diameter to threatening images compared to controls. As well as for light intensity, the pupil dilates under conditions of high attentional allocation and also in response to emotionally-congruent information [34,35]. In this regard, it has been suggested that pupil dilation is a physiological response that can indicate brain mechanisms associated with the processing of emotional information [36]. When viewing threatening, emotional images pupil dilation has also been found to be mediated by increased sympathetic activity (e.g., increased heart rate and skin conductance) [34]. According to the biopsychosocial model of pain [37], there is both a psychological and physiological response to pain. If individuals attend to their physiological reaction to emotional information, it increases their worry-based anxiety, based on schemas, causing them to associate the increased arousal with the pain and lead to active avoidance behaviors. The results from this study suggest that not only are individuals with chronic pain attending to pain-related images more than controls, but they are also allocating greater visual attention to them indicating that the stimuli having greater emotional congruence and meaning. This study suggests that investigating pupil diameter could be a useful addition to the study of chronic pain.

The eye gaze data from this study provides support for current models of attention and extends the current chronic pain literature. Models of attentional bias within chronic pain attribute slightly different roles to the process of attention. In general, they propose that individuals in pain are fearful of, and threatened by, pain [2,3,38], which causes them to over attend to pain-related information. Pain is prioritized over other demands for attention [39], which interferes with movement, leads to higher levels of anxiety, catastrophizing and ultimately exacerbation of levels of disability [40]. Understanding the mechanisms of attention to information which is perceived as threatening, is essential to better understand approaches to effective intervention.

The longer duration of attention to pain-related images in this study may be a function of the schemas associated with the movements. During experimental debriefs, some of the chronic pain participants commented that the images they viewed reminded them of activities in which they would expect to experience pain. Beck [41] proposed that maladaptive schemas cause individuals to have a preoccupation with threatening information and subsequently catastrophize due to a negative interpretive and attentional bias. Pincus and Morley [4] proposed the schema enmeshment model of pain (SEMP) in an attempt to explain recall bias in chronic pain patients through the operation of schemas. Pain schemas contain sensory, intensity, spatial and temporal features of pain, while illness schemas contain information about the consequences of illness, and self-schemas contain information about the self. The chronic pain experience may have illness related schemas about the implications of self-future activity, which causes enmeshment with the pain sensory, self and illness schemas. The anxiety experienced by the pain participants with particular activities they perceive as pain threatening leads to different behavioral and cognitive reactions [1]. The misinterpretation of pain stimuli leads to excessive fear of physical activity and avoidance of physical activity. This may be due to their negative cognitions and increased somatic anxiety about completing the activity, which leads to physical avoidance behavior [42]. Current interventions in the UK tend to focus on reducing a patient's disability through improved education about their pain and the opportunity to discuss problems with particular activities [43]. Understanding the cognitive and emotional mechanisms behind a patient's initial activity avoidance behavior may allow for more specific interventions that modify the way chronic pain patients not only attend to activity-related information, but also the way they interpret the planned movement. The interaction of these two cognitive biases will affect the processing of information, lead to behavior change and, potentially, reduce the patient's disability.

There were some limitations in the study. First, the PHODA images used were not assessed for their affective content (valence and arousal) or whether the images were personally meaningful to the individual. The images have, however, been used successfully in previous dot probe studies and to assess perceived harmfulness of daily activities [44,45] suggesting they have good ecological validity. Although we did not ask chronic pain participants to rate the images directly, in follow up manipulation checks, pain participants reported that they could attribute the images to behaviors in their daily life and that the activities would be difficult and painful for them to complete at home. Similarly, verbal follow up checks with the control group demonstrated that the PHODA images represented a "neutral" image set and they showed no bias to either image type. Therefore, the biases predicted in the chronic pain group can be attributed to the pain-specific content of the image set. Future studies should assess the valence and arousal of the images in larger and more varied pain populations. Future research should also consider asking patients to rate their personal relevance to them; there may be different attentional biases towards images that are more personally-relevant, compared to those that are not (e.g., see Lang's meaning propositions within Bioinformational Theory [46]).

Due to the recruitment strategy, there may be some selection bias. It has been suggested that pain patients who take part in research are often highly motivated, have more severe pain and respond better to treatment [47]. This is a continuing issue for pain research. We were, however, interested in the patients' cognitive response to threatening stimuli and did not implement an intervention. Future research may wish to consider comparing the health status of patients who volunteer, compared to those who decline to take part in a study.

Although the power analysis indicated there was sufficient power for this study, the sample size was low in comparison to other studies investigating attentional biases. Therefore, future research should aim to include a larger sample size. It should be noted that although the use of eye gaze is regarded as a more direct assessment of attention, it does not reflect overt attentional engagement. For example, visual attention can occur in the absence of eye movements [48] and eye tracking technology does not measure peripheral vision, which can be used to complete the dot-probe task accurately [17].

Despite these limitations, the present study provides further support for attentional biases towards pain-related images in chronic back pain participants. This finding is supported by additional data from eye gaze measurement techniques that provide a richer and more detailed analysis of the attentional biases in this population. Future studies should be conducted which investigate whether images that involve movement are more reliable at identifying attentional biases in chronic pain patients compared to pain-related words within a dot probe paradigm. Future research should also investigate the relationship between attention and interpretation of pain to provide an updated model to explain the mechanisms associated with patient responses to chronic pain. If the cognitive mechanisms of attention cause individuals with chronic pain to attend and dwell on painful stimuli, interventions that focus on modifying a patient's attention to goal-related outcomes (e.g., attentional bias modification) may have important beneficial effects on future quality of life.

Author Contributions: Conceptualization, Z.C.F., P.S.H. and N.E.F.; Formal analysis, Z.C.F.; Investigation, Z.C.F.; Methodology, Z.C.F., P.S.H. and N.E.F.; Project administration, Z.C.F.; Supervision, P.S.H. and N.E.F.; Writing—original draft, Z.C.F., P.S.H. and N.E.F.; Writing—review & editing, Z.C.F. and P.S.H.

Acknowledgments: The authors would like to thank the physiotherapy and administration staff at Kingsgate House in Stockport for their support throughout this project and allowing us to conduct this study in the clinic.

References

1. Eysenck, M.W. *Anxiety and Cognition: A Unified Theory*; Psychology Press: Hove, UK, 1997.
2. Vlaeyen, J.W.; Linton, S.J. Fear-avoidance and its consequences in chronic musculoskeletal pain: A state of the art. *Pain* **2000**, *85*, 317–332. [CrossRef]
3. Van Damme, S.; Legrain, V.; Vogt, J.; Crombez, G. Keeping pain in mind: A motivational account of attention to pain. *Neurosci. Biobehav. Rev.* **2010**, *34*, 204–213. [CrossRef] [PubMed]
4. Pincus, T.; Morley, S. Cognitive-processing bias in chronic pain: A review and integration. *Psychol. Bull.* **2001**, *127*, 599–617. [CrossRef] [PubMed]
5. Todd, J.; Sharpe, L.; Johnson, A.; Perry, K.N.; Colagiuri, B.; Dear, B.F. Towards a new model of attentional biases in the development, maintenance, and management of pain. *Pain* **2015**, *156*, 1589–1600. [CrossRef] [PubMed]
6. Crombez, G.; Van Ryckeghem, D.M.L.; Eccleston, C.; Van Damme, S. Attentional bias to pain-related information: A meta-analysis. *Pain* **2013**, *154*, 497–510. [CrossRef]
7. Schoth, D.E.; Nunes, V.D.; Liossi, C. Attentional bias towards pain-related information in chronic pain; a meta-analysis of visual-probe investigations. *Clin. Psychol. Rev.* **2012**, *32*, 13–25. [CrossRef]
8. Todd, J.; van Ryckeghem, D.M.; Sharpe, L.; Crombez, G. Attentional bias to pain-related information: A meta-analysis of dot-probe studies. *Health Psychol. Rev.* **2018**, *12*, 419–436. [CrossRef]
9. Kourtzi, Z.; Kanwisher, N. Activation in human mt/mst by static images with implied motion. *J. Cogn. Neurosci.* **2000**, *12*, 48–55. [CrossRef]

10. MacLeod, C.; Mathews, A.; Tata, P. Attentional bias in emotional disorders. *J. Abnorm. Psychol.* **1986**, *95*, 15–20. [CrossRef]
11. Mogg, K.; Bradley, B.P. Attentional bias in generalized anxiety disorder versus depressive disorder. *Cogn. Ther. Res.* **2005**, *29*, 29–45. [CrossRef]
12. Derakshan, N.; Salt, M.; Koster, E.H.W. Attentional control in dysphoria: An investigation using the antisaccade task. *Biol. Psychol.* **2009**, *80*, 251–255. [CrossRef] [PubMed]
13. Sharpe, L.; Brookes, M.; Jones, E.; Gittins, C.; Wufong, E.; Nicholas, M. Threat and fear of pain induces attentional bias to pain words: An eye-tracking study. *Eur. J. Pain* **2017**, *21*, 385–396. [CrossRef] [PubMed]
14. Yang, Z.; Jackson, T.; Gao, X.; Chen, H. Identifying selective visual attention biases related to fear of pain by tracking eye movements within a dot-probe paradigm. *Pain* **2012**, *153*, 1742–1748. [CrossRef] [PubMed]
15. Priebe, J.; Messingschlager, M.; Lautenbacher, S. Gaze behaviour when monitoring pain faces: An eye-tracking study. *Eur. J. Pain* **2015**, *19*, 817–825. [CrossRef] [PubMed]
16. Todd, J.; Sharpe, L.; Colagiuri, B.; Khatibi, A. The effect of threat on cognitive biases and pain outcomes: An eye-tracking study. *Eur. J. Pain* **2016**, *20*, 1357–1368. [CrossRef] [PubMed]
17. Vervoort, T.; Trost, Z.; Prkachin, K.M.; Mueller, S.C. Attentional processing of other's facial display of pain: An eye tracking study. *Pain* **2013**, *154*, 836–844. [CrossRef]
18. Liossi, C.; Schoth, D.E.; Godwin, H.J.; Liversedge, S.P. Using eye movements to investigate selective attention in chronic daily headache. *Pain* **2014**, *155*, 503–510. [CrossRef]
19. Schoth, D.E.; Godwin, H.; Liversedge, S.P.; Liossi, C. Eye movements during visual search for emotional faces in individuals with chronic headache. *Eur. J. Pain* **2015**, *19*, 722–732. [CrossRef]
20. Fashler, S.R.; Katz, J. Keeping an eye on pain: Investigating visual attention biases in individuals with chronic pain using eye-tracking methodology. *J. Pain Res.* **2016**, *9*, 551–561. [CrossRef]
21. Kugler, K.; Wijn, J.; Geilen, M.; de Jong, J.; Vlaeyen, J. *The Photograph Series of Daily Activities (Phoda). Cd-Rom Version 1.0*; Institute for Rehabilitation Research and School for Physiotherapy: Heerlen, The Netherlands, 1999.
22. Lang, P.J.; Bradley, M.M.; Cuthbert, B.N. *International Affective Picture System (IAPS): Affective Ratings of Pictures and Instruction Manual*; Technical Report A-8l; University of Florida: Gainesville, FL, USA, 2008.
23. Mogg, K.; Bradley, B.P.; Field, M.; De Houwer, J. Eye movements to smoking-related pictures in smokers: Relationship between attentional biases and implicit and explicit measures of stimulus valence. *Addiction* **2003**, *98*, 825–836. [CrossRef]
24. Cohen, J. *Statistical Power Analysis for the Behavioral Sciences*, 2nd ed.; Lawrence Earlbaum Associates: Hillsdale, NJ, USA, 1988.
25. Roelofs, J.; Peters, M.L.; Fassaert, T.; Vlaeyen, J.W. The role of fear of movement and injury in selective attentional processing in patients with chronic low back pain: A dot-probe evaluation. *J. Pain* **2005**, *6*, 294–300. [CrossRef] [PubMed]
26. Dear, B.F.; Sharpe, L.; Nicholas, M.K.; Refshauge, K. Pain-related attentional biases: The importance of the personal relevance and ecological validity of stimuli. *J. Pain* **2011**, *12*, 625–632. [CrossRef] [PubMed]
27. Franklin, Z.C.; Holmes, P.S.; Smith, N.C.; Fowler, N.E. Personality type influences attentional bias in individuals with chronic back pain. *PLoS ONE* **2016**, *11*, e0147035. [CrossRef] [PubMed]
28. Peelen, M.V.; Wiggett, A.J.; Downing, P.E. Patterns of fmri activity dissociate overlapping functional brain areas that respond to biological motion. *Neuron* **2006**, *49*, 815–822. [CrossRef] [PubMed]
29. Açık, A.; Bartel, A.; Koenig, P. Real and implied motion at the center of gaze. *J. Vis.* **2014**, *14*, 2. [CrossRef] [PubMed]
30. Yang, Z.; Jackson, T.; Chen, H. Effects of chronic pain and pain-related fear on orienting and maintenance of attention: An eye movement study. *J. Pain* **2013**, *14*, 1148–1157. [CrossRef] [PubMed]
31. Riach, M.; Wright, D.J.; Franklin, Z.C.; Holmes, P.S. Screen Position Preference Offers a New Direction for Action Observation Research: Preliminary Findings Using TMS. *Front. Hum. Neurosci.* **2018**, *12*, 26. [CrossRef]
32. Schoth, D.E.; Georgallis, T.; Liossi, C. Attentional bias modification in people with chronic pain: A proof of concept study. *Cogn. Behav. Ther.* **2013**, *42*, 233–243. [CrossRef]
33. Sharpe, L.; Ianiello, M.; Dear, B.F.; Perry, K.N.; Refshauge, K.; Nicholas, M.K. Is there a potential role for attention bias modification in pain patients? Results of 2 randomised, controlled trials. *Pain* **2012**, *153*, 722–731. [CrossRef]

34. Bradley, M.M.; Miccoli, L.; Escrig, M.A.; Lang, P.J. The pupil as a measure of emotional arousal and autonomic activation. *Psychophysiology* **2008**, *45*, 602–607. [CrossRef]
35. Duque, A.; Sanchez, A.; Vazquez, C. Gaze-fixation and pupil dilation in the processing of emotional faces: The role of rumination. *Cogn. Emot.* **2014**, *28*, 1347–1366. [CrossRef] [PubMed]
36. Siegle, G.J.; Steinhauer, S.R.; Thase, M.E.; Stenger, V.A.; Carter, C.S. Can't shake that feeling: Event-related fmri assessment of sustained amygdala activity in response to emotional information in depressed individuals. *Biol. Psychiatry* **2002**, *51*, 693–707. [CrossRef]
37. Waddell, G. 1987 Volvo award in clinical sciences. A new clinical model for the treatment of low-back pain. *Spine* **1987**, *12*, 632–644. [CrossRef]
38. Vlaeyen, J.W.; Linton, S.J. Fear-avoidance model of chronic musculoskeletal pain: 12 years on. *Pain* **2012**, *153*, 1144–1147. [CrossRef] [PubMed]
39. Eccleston, C.; Crombez, G. Pain demands attention: A cognitive–affective model of the interruptive function of pain. *Psychol. Bull.* **1999**, *125*, 356. [CrossRef] [PubMed]
40. Franklin, Z.C.; Smith, N.C.; Fowler, N.E. Influence of defensiveness on disability in a chronic musculoskeletal pain population. *Pain Pract.* **2016**, *16*, 882–889. [CrossRef]
41. Beck, A.T. *Cognitive Therapy and the Emotional Disorders*; International Universities Press: New York, NY, USA, 1976.
42. Crombez, G.; Eccleston, C.; Van Damme, S.; Vlaeyen, J.W.S.; Karoly, P. Fear-avoidance model of chronic pain: The next generation. *Clin. J. Pain* **2012**, *28*, 475–483. [CrossRef]
43. British Pain Society. Guidance for Pain Management Programmes for Adults. Available online: http://www.britishpainsociety.org/book_pmp2013_main.pdf (accessed on 8 July 2015).
44. Leeuw, M.; Goossens, M.E.J.B.; van Breukelen, G.J.P.; Boersma, K.; Vlaeyen, J.W.S. Measuring perceived harmfulness of physical activities in patients with chronic low back pain: The photograph series of daily activities—Short electronic version. *J. Pain* **2007**, *8*, 840–849. [CrossRef]
45. Barke, A.; Baudewig, J.; Schmidt-Samoa, C.; Dechent, P.; Kröner-Herwig, B. Neural correlates of fear of movement in high and low fear-avoidant chronic low back pain patients: An event-related fmri study. *Pain* **2012**, *153*, 540–552. [CrossRef]
46. Lang, P.J. A bio-informational theory of emotional imagery. *Psychophysiology* **1979**, *16*, 495–512. [CrossRef]
47. Nijs, J.; Inghelbrecht, E.; Daenen, L.; Hachimi-Idrissi, S.; Hens, L.; Willems, B.; Roussel, N.; Cras, P.; Wouters, K.; Bernheim, J. Recruitment bias in chronic pain research: Whiplash as a model. *Clin. Rheumatol.* **2011**, *30*, 1481. [CrossRef] [PubMed]
48. Zhao, M.; Gersch, T.M.; Schnitzer, B.S.; Dosher, B.A.; Kowler, E. Eye movements and attention: The role of pre-saccadic shifts of attention in perception, memory and the control of saccades. *Vis. Res.* **2012**, *74*, 40–60. [CrossRef] [PubMed]

4

The Evolving Case Supporting Individualised Physiotherapy for Low Back Pain

Jon Ford [1,2,*], Andrew Hahne [1], Luke Surkitt [2], Alexander Chan [2] and Matthew Richards [2]

1 School of Allied Health, La Trobe University, Kingsbury Drive, Bundoora 3086, Australia
2 Advance Healthcare, 157 Scoresby Road, Boronia 3155, Australia
* Correspondence: J.Ford@latrobe.edu.au

Abstract: Low-back pain (LBP) is one of the most burdensome health problems in the world. Guidelines recommend simple treatments such as advice that may result in suboptimal outcomes, particularly when applied to people with complex biopsychosocial barriers to recovery. Individualised physiotherapy has the potential of being more effective for people with LBP; however, there is limited evidence supporting this approach. A series of studies supporting the mechanisms underpinning and effectiveness of the Specific Treatment of Problems of the Spine (STOPS) approach to individualised physiotherapy have been published. The clinical and research implications of these findings are presented and discussed. Treatment based on the STOPS approach should also be considered as an approach to individualised physiotherapy in people with LBP.

Keywords: low-back pain; physiotherapy; individualisation

---

1. Introduction

Low-back pain (LBP) is recognised as a common and costly problem in the Western world, with a global prevalence of 0.5 billion, the highest ranking cause of years lived with disability contributing 57·6 million years [1], and an increase in prevalence and disease burden of nearly 20% over the last 10 years [2]. People with LBP have historically been described as having a favourable natural history [3]; however, systematic reviews of primary care studies show that 28%–79% of people with acute LBP experience persistent or recurrent symptoms at 12 months [4,5]. Higher rates are supported by one large general population study which is likely to be a more accurate measure of persistency/recurrence than samples recruited from primary care settings [6].

Syntheses of clinical guidelines suggest international consensus in recommending initial exclusion of red flags and radiculopathy, and subsequent management of LBP as a "non-specific" condition on the basis that a nociceptive cause of symptoms cannot be identified [7–9]. Guideline-based treatment (Table 1) aims to minimise potential harm of treatments such as surgery or medication and maximise cost-effectiveness by utilising simple treatments such as advice [10,11]. However, the randomised controlled trials (RCTs) upon which guideline recommendations are based typically show small effect sizes of questionable clinical importance [8,9,12].

A potential reason for the limited effects demonstrated in RCTs on LBP is a false assumption that non-specific LBP is a homogeneous group. It has been postulated that multiple subgroups exist within the non-specific LBP population that are likely to respond differently to generic treatment [13]. In such circumstances, a false assumption of sample homogeneity in RCTs may lead to a treatment being inappropriately applied, resulting in either failure to respond or exacerbation of the condition. Based on this understanding, identifying valid subgroups for the purposes of an RCT has been described as a high research priority [14,15]. Meaningful subgroups enable treatment to be individualised to the patient presentation, potentially increasing the size of the effect [16]. An example of the value of individualised treatment is the management of inflammation in people with LBP. Guidelines suggest that non-steroidal anti-inflammatory drugs (NSAIDs) have small and short-term positive effects for LBP [8], yet these recommendations are based on RCTs selecting people with non-specific LBP. It is unlikely that every patient in this population has LBP with inflammatory processes as a contributing factor. It is, therefore, plausible that RCTs sampling populations with a greater likelihood of an inflammatory component to their LBP would show larger effects.

Table 1. Overview of interventions endorsed for non-specific low-back pain in evidence-based clinical practice guidelines (adapted from Foster et al. 2018) [9].

	Acute LBP (<6 weeks)	**Persistent LBP (>12 weeks)**
First line care	Advice Education	Advice Education Exercise CBT
Second line or adjunctive care	NSAIDs Superficial heat Manual therapy Massage Acupuncture	NSAIDs Selective norepinephrine reuptake inhibitors Manual therapy Acupuncture Yoga Mindfulness Interdisciplinary rehabilitation Discectomy or laminectomy for disc herniation with associated radiculopathy
Limited use in selected patients	Opioids Skeletal muscle relaxants Exercise CBT	Opioids Epidural injection
Not recommended	Paracetamol Systemic glucocorticoids Epidural injection	Paracetamol Systemic glucocorticoids
Insufficient evidence	Mindfulness Interdisciplinary rehabilitation Selective norepinephrine reuptake inhibitors Antiseizure medication Any surgery	Superficial heat Skeletal muscle relaxants

CBT = cognitive behavioural therapy, NSAIDs = non-steroidal anti-inflammatory drugs.

The argument for the importance of individualised treatment is further strengthened by considering the multi-dimensional nature of LBP. Clinical guidelines for LBP [9], the World Health Organisation's International Classification of Functioning, Disability and Health [17] and internationally accepted standards on clinical reasoning [18] all emphasise multiple factors that are relevant for the management of LBP including the pathoanatomical (e.g., nociceptive source of symptoms), psychosocial (e.g., fear avoidance), neurophysiological (e.g., central sensitisation and neuropathic pain) and genetic dimensions. The complexity of LBP is also reflected in the wide range of subgrouping approaches reported in systematic and narrative reviews [13,19–21]. Given the multidimensional and complex nature of LBP, it is almost axiomatic that a "one size fits all" approach to treatment provision in RCTs is likely to yield suboptimal results [13].

Based on the scale of the LBP problem, the limited data on treatment effectiveness, and the potential value of individualised treatment, the aim of this paper was to overview the evidence on individualised physiotherapy, including a contextualised presentation and discussion of a series of studies on the Specific Treatment of Problems of the Spine (STOPS) approach.

2. The Evidence on Individualised Physiotherapy for Low-Back Pain

A search on the evidence supporting individualised physiotherapy for LBP was conducted on PubMed using the Boolean term OR for individ*, subgroup*, classif* AND back pain AND "review" in the title. Reference lists of the retrieved papers, as well as recent clinical guidelines [7–9], were also checked for relevant evidence. A total of 546 citations were identified from PubMed, with 12 being deemed relevant for this overview.

Individualising treatment for LBP has been identified as a high research priority by a series of international expert panels [14,15] and a methodological framework for future research suggested [19,22]. However, research investigating the large number of heterogenous approaches for individualising treatment are of variable methodological quality [20,23–27]. Individualising physiotherapy based on movement is recommended in a professional guideline [28] but is not supported by recent clinical trials [29]. The STarT Back approach to individualising physiotherapy has been extensively researched in different contexts [30–42], and is recommended in clinical guidelines based on cost effectiveness [8,9]. However, the STarT Back approach only confers small clinical effects on activity limitation, and no long-term effects on pain compared to usual care [33].

Given the limited evidence supporting attempts to develop effective individualised physiotherapy approaches for LBP, exploration of alternative methods has merit.

3. A Series of Studies Supporting Individualised Physiotherapy for Low-Back Pain

The STOPS trial was a randomised controlled trial (n = 300) published in 2016 that concluded individualised physiotherapy was more effective than guideline-based advice for early persistent LBP [43]. This trial was part of a series of studies that will be overviewed to inform a discussion on the STOPS approach to individualised physiotherapy for LBP.

3.1. *Prognosis in Identifying Potential Targets for Individualised Physiotherapy*

Identification of prognostic factors can improve clinical decision making, understanding of disease processes, definitions of risk groups, and prediction of clinical outcomes [44]. Prognostic factors can also assist in identifying treatment targets to improve the effectiveness of individualised treatment [45,46]. Exploring and identifying gaps in the prognostic literature for LBP has been recommended as a research priority [47].

Prognostic studies and systematic reviews on LBP commonly evaluate specific prognostic factors [47,48] such as psychosocial distress [49–52], clinical features [53–56] and physical activity [57]. We are unaware of any high-quality studies evaluating a comprehensive range of biomedical (including pathoanatomical), psychological and social prognostic factors using multivariate methods in a large sample of people with LBP [46,58,59].

We, therefore, conducted a study that aimed to develop a multivariate prognostic model for back pain, leg pain and activity limitation in patients with LBP based on a comprehensive range of commonly used prognostic factors reflective of the biopsychosocial model of health [60]. Following univariate analyses of a range of variables from 300 participants in the STOPS trial, 58 variables progressed to multivariate analysis (Table A1). Five indicators of positive outcome (belonging to either the reducible discogenic pain or disc herniation with associated radiculopathy subgroups, below waist paraesthesia, walking as an easing factor and low transversus abdominis tone) and 10 indicators of negative outcome (both parents born overseas, deep leg symptoms, higher sick leave duration on the Örebro Musculoskeletal Pain Questionnaire [61], high multifidus tone, clinically determined inflammation [62,63], higher back and leg pain severity, lower Oswestry Disability Index [64] lifting capacity, lower capacity for light work (Örebro item) and higher Pain Drawing [65] scores based on percentage body chart coverage) were identified (Table 2).

Table 2. Back related healthcare utilization and costs per patient.

Resource	Resource Use: Units/Patient (SD), % of Patients Utilizing		Cost/Patient (SD) in US$		
	IP	Advice	IP	Advice	Between-Group Cost Difference (95% CI) *
Study physiotherapy	8.9 (2.1), 100%	1.8 (2.4), 99%	379.35 (87.10)	81.93 (18.46)	**297.72 (282.85 to 312.01)**
Medical consultations	1.7 (5.3), 32%	2.0 (4.2), 40%	86.95 (280.78)	110.55 (238.03)	−23.61 (−85.61 to 38.40)
Medical intervention					
Surgery (discectomy)	0.01 (0.08), 0.7%	0.02 (0.12), 1.5%	35.81 (434.18)	80.99 (650.40)	−45.18 (−174.68 to 84.32)
Injections	0.1 (0.3), 3.4%	0.1 (0.5), 7.7	5.87 (36.32)	13.82 (56.10)	−7.95 (−19.01 to 3.10)
Allied health consultations	3.3 (6.3), 38.8%	7.9 (12.3), 60.8%	152.38 (292.15)	324.47 (480.14)	**−172.09 (−264.94 to −79.25)**
Medication	57.0%	54.6%	59.87 (140.54)	85.60 (207.93)	−25.73 (−69.16 to 17.69)
Total Healthcare cost (95%CI)			782.82 (623.82 to 941.82)	755.79 (592.84 to 918.75)	27.03 (−200.29 to 254.35)
Work absence: Mean (95%CI), %	10.8 (4.6 to 17.1) days, 36%	20.5 (13.3 to 27.6) days, 44%	$1889.16 (680.86 to 3097.46)	$3884.67 (2497.22 to 5272.12)	**$ −1995.51 (−3847.03 to −143.98)**

IP = individualised physiotherapy; SD = standard deviation; *, Between-group comparisons analysed via linear mixed models, with positive values representing a higher cost in the individualised physiotherapy group relative to the advice group, significant between-group differences in bold.

Researchers and clinical practice guidelines [66] have suggested that biomedical factors are less relevant in the management of non-specific LBP and few studies have identified biomedical or physical factors of prognostic value [67]. However biomedical factors are commonly used by clinicians in decision making [68]. In our study, nine of the 15 prognostic factors related primarily to pathoanatomical mechanisms. In addition, previously reported psychosocial predictors such as depression, fear avoidance and recovery expectations were not prognostic when analysed in a multi-variate model of a comprehensive range of prognostic factors. These results provide support for the validity of the STOPS approach of individualised treatment based on a range of biomedical, psychological and social factors.

3.2. Development of an Individualised Physiotherapy Treatment Program

Identifying subgroups of different types of LBP is one way of individualising physiotherapy, and treatment targeting specific features or causal mechanisms underpinning the nature of the subgroup has the potential of being more effective in RCTs [13,16]. However, developing a LBP subgrouping system is challenging and the review literature shows that a wide array of approaches exist [13,19–21,25–27,29,69–72]. Historically, subgrouping systems have been developed by experts combining the best available evidence with their own clinical experience [73–77]. More recently, a standardised approach to subgroup development used in the medical domain [78] has been extrapolated to LBP [19,79] involving: initial evaluation of assessment methods of potential utility for subgrouping, hypothesis setting studies using a range of methodologies, a priori hypothesis testing studies and a series of further validation stages including analysis of impact of the subgrouping system on routine care (Figure 1). A key component of the hypothesis generation, hypothesis testing and subgroup validation studies is evaluation of treatment effect modifiers within a RCT. Treatment effect modifier studies aim to assess whether the effect of a treatment (relative to a comparison treatment) is different in people with certain characteristics (which are of potential use in defining a subgroup), compared to those without [80]. However, to be adequately powered treatment effect modifiers studies need to be around four times larger than studies investigating overall treatment effect [81,82]. Given the complexity of LBP, a relatively large number of variables require exploration for relevance to subgrouping, which further increases the necessary sample size in treatment effect modifier studies [83]. These issues mean that treatment effect modifier RCTs, with the associated high costs, are of questionable feasibility, particularly in certain research funding contexts such as Australia [71,84,85].

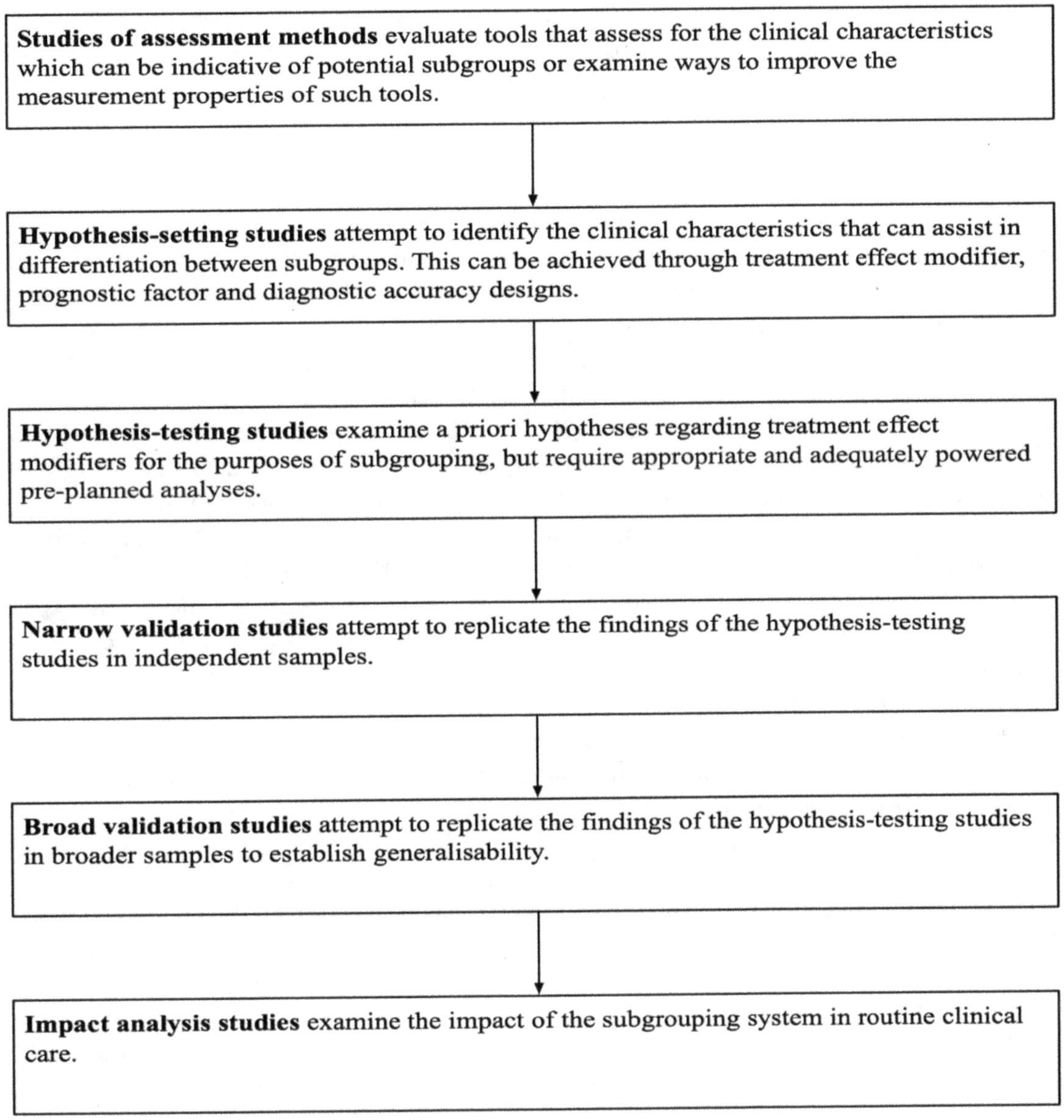

Figure 1. Conceptual phases of subgrouping research (adapted from Kent et al [19]).

A range of methodologies other than treatment effect modifiers can be used in the hypothesis setting stage of subgroup development, although each approach has significant limitations. Studies evaluating the diagnostic accuracy of different subgroup features/clinical measures are limited by the absence of suitable reference standards [7]. Commonly used reference standards such as imaging, discography and diagnostic blocks have all demonstrated significant false positives due, at least in part, to the complexity of LBP including psychosocial and neurophysiological influences [86]. Despite growing popularity [87] and defined methodological rigour, 'data driven' analyses for identifying and developing subgroups also have significant limitations. Statistical processes can result in artificial subgroups [88] of limited clinical use and/or meaningfulness [20,21,83] and a degree of judgement is required in undertaking the analyses with the potential for bias [20,88–90].

Contemporary methodologies for the development and validation of subgrouping systems work well in certain medical contexts to allow greater individualisation of treatment [78]. Yet, as described above, extrapolation of these principles to the complex domain of LBP has limited feasibility and methodological shortcomings. An alternative approach is the principle of "convergence of validity" described as when " ... evidence supporting or refuting the (subgrouping) system (is) gathered from different sources and from the use of different methods. In the best case scenario, these sources converge and indicate similar meanings of the underlying constructs being studied." [91] (p. 312). Implicit in this approach is an acceptance of the limitations of all research designs in relation to subgroup development.

As an alternative subgrouping strategy, convergence of validity is consistent with the original definitions of evidence-based practice that emphasise the constructive interaction between the research literature and clinical perspectives [92]. It also aligns with expert recommendations from the field of epidemiology [93] and mirrors the approach taken in other complex medical domains such as the classification of headache [94] and non-Hodgkin's lymphoma [95].

In essence, a convergence of validity approach is the equivalent to the hypothesis setting phase where a range of research methodologies are considered in developing a subgrouping system. In applying a convergence of validity approach, it is accepted that the complete validation of such a system, particularly through repeated treatment effect modifier studies, is not likely to be feasible. Yet this limitation in achieving full validation should not prohibit the use of the subgrouping system in other research designs, such as RCTs, provided the limitations of system validity are acknowledged.

Four papers [83,96–98] have been published in relation to the STOPS trial justifying and outlining detailed individualised treatment protocols on the basis of convergence of validity supporting five subgroups. This process has been further supported by two expert panels [99,100] and five systematic reviews [20,101–104]. Four of the subgroups were primarily based on clinical features indicative of a pathoanatomical diagnosis of the LBP and comprised: reducible discogenic pain, zygapophyseal joint pain, non-reducible discogenic pain, and disc herniation with associated radiculopathy. A fifth subgroup (multi-factorial persistent pain) captured people without a clear pathoanatomical classification along with likely psychosocial contributors to their delayed recovery as measured on the Örebro Musculoskeletal Pain Questionnaire [61].

Participants with reducible discogenic pain were prescribed a home program based on mechanical loading strategies that led to improvement or centralisation of symptoms. This included repeated/sustained movement exercises, a walking program, taping and postural advice [83]. Participants with zygapophysial joint dysfunction received targeted manual therapy comprising unilateral mobilisation ± manipulation applied with a rigorous clinical reasoning approach [96]. All participants apart from those in the MFP group received motor-control training targeting local muscles such as transversus abdominus leading into a pain contingent graded functional exercise program [96]. This was the primary treatment for participants with disc herniation with associated radiculopathy or non-reducible discogenic pain. Those with multifactorial persistent pain received physiotherapy focusing on psychosocial and neurophysiological rather than pathoanatomical mechanisms [98]. Progression of functional exercise in this subgroup was time-contingent, and cognitive restructuring/behavioural strategies were used targeting key barriers identified on the Örebro Musculoskeletal Pain Questionnaire.

Although subgroup membership determined the primary treatment approach, a range of other treatment components were also provided depending on identification of other pathoanatomical, psychosocial or neurophysiological barriers to recovery. All participants receiving individualised physiotherapy engaged in an explanation/discussion regarding: the nature/source of their symptoms, treatment options available outside of the RCT and timeframes for recovery. Participants also worked with the trial physiotherapists on goal setting, cognitive restructuring of counterproductive beliefs, behavioural strategies to support and reinforce the education program, as well as modifying unproductive behaviours and discharge planning. A range of optional treatment components were provided including: pain management strategies (pharmacological and non-pharmacological), management of inflammation in participants with a clinically determined inflammatory component to their pain, management of work issues, sleep strategies, relaxation and dealing with increases in pain (flare-ups). In participants failing to improve with a pathoanatomical approach initially, the trial physiotherapist determined whether transfer to the MFP treatment protocol was required. These treatment strategies were all applied in a manner individualised to the participant's presentation as determined by the trial physiotherapist.

3.3. *Effectiveness of Individualised Physiotherapy*

Based on the above-described research, the STOPS trial aimed to evaluate the effectiveness of individualised physiotherapy compared to guideline-based advice. Advice regarding prognosis and resuming normal activities is recommended in all clinical guidelines for people with LBP of over 6-weeks duration [8]. Prior to our clinical trials, there had been few published RCTs evaluating the effectiveness of individualised physiotherapy compared to guideline-based advice.

Other recent subgrouping approaches based on risk stratification such as STarT Back [33] and physical examination findings (i.e., movement patterns) do not address pathoanatomical factors despite this approach being common in clinical practice and the convergence of evidence that it may be important in clinical decision making for LBP [16,83,96–98].

Using the STOPS individualised physiotherapy protocol including manual therapy, directional preference management, postural re-education, motor control training, and graded functional exercise [83,96–98] we evaluated the effectiveness of individualised physiotherapy compared to guideline-based advice for 300 participants with early persistent LBP (6-weeks to 6-months duration) [43].

Results (Figure 2) showed that individualised physiotherapy was more effective than advice in improving activity limitation (at 10, 26 and 52-weeks) as well as back pain and leg pain (at 5, 10 and 26-weeks). Between-group mean differences were statistically significant in 71% of the primary and secondary outcomes measured in the trial. Participants receiving individualised physiotherapy took 5-8 weeks to achieve the same pain rating as those receiving advice at 12 months indicating a more rapid rate of recovery. Satisfaction with individualised treatment was high, and 92.3% of individualised physiotherapy participants completed the intervention. Based on contemporary definitions, these results are clinically important [105,106].

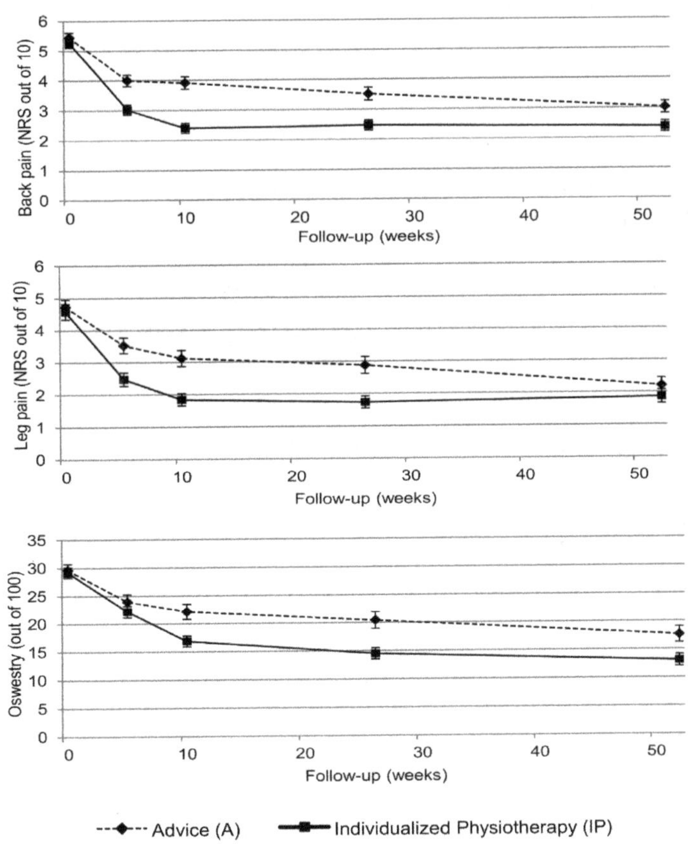

Figure 2. Group mean scores (error bars indicate standard errors) for primary outcomes at baseline and 5-, 10-, 26- and 52-week follow-up in the STOPS Trial (adapted from Ford et al. [43], permission admitted).

3.4. Cost-Effectiveness of Individualised Physiotherapy

Direct healthcare costs attributable to people with LBP in Western countries seeking healthcare is estimated at billions of dollars annually [107,108] and is predicted to rise [109,110]. Treatments that improve clinical outcomes such as pain and activity at a sustainable cost are urgently needed [111].

Guideline-based advice is a low-cost treatment that is commonly prescribed by medical practitioners [112] and physiotherapists [113]. However, low cost does not necessarily correspond to cost-effectiveness when treatment effects and all relevant costs (healthcare and other) are considered. There is insufficient evidence regarding the cost-effectiveness of advice for LBP according to one systematic review [111].

The STOPS trial showed that individualised physiotherapy was clinically more effective than guideline-based advice [43]. Given the treatment cost of delivering individualised physiotherapy (10 sessions) was higher than advice (2 sessions), consideration is required as to whether the larger effects were worth the additional cost. We therefore investigated the cost-effectiveness of individualised physiotherapy versus advice in people with LBP enrolled in the STOPS trial [114].

The results showed that total health care costs were similar for both groups despite individualised physiotherapy being more expensive than guideline-based advice (Table 2). This was due to 61% of participants receiving advice seeking further non-medical treatment outside the trial compared to 39% of participants receiving individualised physiotherapy (Table 2). Health benefits favoured individualised physiotherapy over advice (incremental Quality Adjusted Life Years = 0.06 (95%CI: 0.02 to 0.10)). Cost-effectiveness was established by the achievement of an Incremental Cost Effectiveness ratio of $US 422 per quality adjusted life year gained [114]. In addition, lower work absence across the 12-month follow-up resulted in income savings of $US 1995 (95%CI: 144 to 3847) per working participant in the individualised physiotherapy group compared to the advice group (Table 2).

3.5. Who Benefits Most from Individualised Physiotherapy Versus Advice?

Treatment effect modifier studies are helpful for determining characteristics of patients who respond best to a particular treatment relative to another in an RCT [19]. The STOPS treatment effect modifier study investigated several patient characteristics identified a priori and listed on the trial register [115] based on the hypothesis that participants with more severe, persistent or complex LBP would derive the largest benefits from individualised physiotherapy relative to advice. This hypothesis was supported by the results showing that participants with higher back pain intensity, higher Örebro scores (indicative of higher risk of persistent pain) or longer duration of symptoms derived the largest benefits from individualised physiotherapy relative to advice. These findings are of particular importance because the presence of these characteristics has been associated with a worse prognosis as well as higher treatment and societal costs [107,116,117]. Targeting individualised physiotherapy towards these higher risk groups may, therefore, result in even stronger treatment effectiveness and cost-effectiveness than those reported for the whole sample involved in the STOPS trial.

4. Discussion

Research into individualised physiotherapy is a high research priority that has, to date, yielded disappointing results in RCTs. The series of studies described in this paper support the development and validity of the STOPS subgrouping approach. In addition, three studies on the effectiveness, cost-effectiveness and treatment effect modifiers provide further support for the individualised eatment of LBP using the STOPS approach. We are unaware of any similar body of research on the ity of individualised physiotherapy based on a comprehensive biopsychosocial-based treatment el. There are a range of possible factors that may have contributed to the above-described results.

4.1. The Definition of Clinical Importance

Most RCTs on LBP demonstrating statistically significant results show small effects of questionable clinical importance [8,9]. However, the traditional definition of clinical importance based on the minimal clinically important difference (MCID) has been questioned given it was developed for use on individuals rather than group data and may not be appropriate for people with lower severity symptoms [105,118]. Authoritative contemporary guidelines recommend determining clinical importance using multiple methods of analysis including consistency of results across multiple primary and secondary outcome measures, risks/benefits of the treatments, consideration of the population being sampled, and the proportion of individual patients who demonstrate change in outcome measures in excess of the MCID *in addition* to between-group differences in mean scores [106,119,120].

The STOPS trial did not demonstrate clinically important between-group mean differences based on the MCID. However, in accordance with our a priori statistical plan [121], a primary outcome responder analysis was conducted. This analysis showed that participants receiving individualised physiotherapy had 1.8 and 1.6 times the chance of improving by at least 50% from baseline on back and leg pain, respectively, at the 10-week follow-up compared with those receiving advice alone. By 52 weeks, those having individualised physiotherapy also had 1.5 times the chance of improving by 50% from baseline on the Oswestry Disability Questionnaire compared with those receiving advice. All secondary outcomes favoured individualised physiotherapy, with the exception of work interference, but the cost-effectiveness study showed significantly lower work absence (and associated lost income) in the individualised physiotherapy group. In the secondary-outcomes responder analysis, participants receiving individualised physiotherapy had 1.3–4.1 times the chance of achieving a clinically important change compared with those receiving advice. Participant satisfaction was significantly greater and non-medical co-interventions significantly lower in the individualised physiotherapy group. All between-group comparisons should be interpreted in the context of large *within-group* improvements on all primary outcomes for both treatment groups [33]. Given the population sampled were ≥6-weeks post-injury where spontaneous recovery is limited [4,5], it is likely that both treatments were helpful, with individualised physiotherapy conferring additional benefits over and above advice. There were no serious adverse events in either group and with detailed published clinical protocols available, the STOPS approach to LBP is potentially accessible worldwide without extensive training common to other individualised physiotherapy approaches [33,122].

The clinical importance of the between-group differences as a measure of significance in the STOPS trial is further strengthened by the cost-effectiveness analysis. Results showed an incremental cost-effectiveness ratio (ICER) of US$422 per quality-adjusted life year (QALY), which compares favourably to other relevant RCTs in the field. Cognitive behavioural therapy is recommended in all clinical guidelines for LBP [8,9], but has an ICER of US$2773 per QALY gained for group cognitive behavioural therapy along with advice versus advice alone [123]. In another relevant RCT [124] five sessions of physiotherapy were not cost-effective compared with one session of advice as there were no significant differences in health outcomes. These data further support the clinical importance of the STOPS trial results by way of cost-effectiveness compared to guideline-based advice.

Another potential indicator of clinical importance from RCTs is the proportion of participants who complete the intervention. High drop-out rates in clinical trials may indicate that the intervention is not acceptable to participants on the basis of ineffectiveness, patient preferences, the required commitment to comply with treatment, or side-effects. Drop-out rates exceeding 15% have been reported for multiple LBP trials of graded activity [125], anticonvulsants [126], and in one trial of individualised physiotherapy [122]. The individualised physiotherapy group in the STOPS trial had a 7.7% drop-out rate, suggesting that the treatment was acceptable for most participants and giving further support to the clinical importance of the STOPS trial results.

4.2. Comparison Group Selection and Advice

When designing and interpreting RCTs, it is important for the researcher and consumer to carefully consider the comparison group. Common trial designs in LBP use no treatment, placebo treatment, advice, usual medical care or various types of physiotherapy interventions. There is no right or wrong approach to designing a comparison group in an RCT; it simply informs the hypothesis being tested. For example, a RCT comparing manual therapy to placebo manual therapy is designed to test the specific effect of manual therapy independent of any non-specific effects such as patient expectations, learning/conditioning effects and neurophysiological effects [127].

It is worth reflecting on the use of guideline-based advice in designing a RCT. Advice to stay active and reassurance regarding prognosis is recommended as first-line treatment in all clinical guidelines for acute and persistent LBP as described in Table 1 [9]. The evidence directly supporting the effectiveness and cost-effectiveness of guideline-based advice is sparse [111,128–130]. Nevertheless, it has been asserted that this treatment is just as effective as more costly and complex treatments [10,11]. Although not commonly used as the sole treatment approach by practitioners in the field [131], guideline-based advice is being advocated strongly as first line treatment ahead of other physiotherapeutic treatments such as manual therapy as well as medical treatments such as NSAIDs [8,9,131,132]. Given the low-quality evidence supporting guideline-based advice, it is possible that this approach is counterproductive, particularly if second-line treatments are more effective without being prohibitively more expensive. On this basis, guideline-based advice is an important comparison group in a RCT evaluating the effectiveness of commonly used second-line treatments (Table 1).

4.3. Use of a Pathoanatomical Approach

A major difference between the STOPS trial and the majority of the LBP research was the incorporation of pathoanatomical factors into the subgrouping approach and pathoanatomical-based decision making in the clinical protocol. Definitive criteria for pathoanatomical-based diagnosis and/or clinical decision making in LBP are not available [8]. It has been suggested that further research into and clinicians hypothesising about pathoanatomical barriers to recovery is likely to be at best, futile and, at worst, counterproductive to patient outcomes [66,133,134]. However, there is sparse evidence supporting this contention [16] and a pathoanatomical approach is common in clinical practice [68]. In addition, although there are likely to be benefits from addressing exercise/activity, lifestyle and psychosocial factors, the prognostic and treatment effects are small [134]. On this basis, it does not seem sensible to abandon clinical and research-based hypothesising on the role of pathoanatomy unless compelling evidence to do so is provided. Guideline-based advice is not informed by pathoanatomy and the mechanisms of effect are likely to be non-specific. As such, it is possible that a reason for the significant between-group differences in the STOPS trial was that assessment and treatment incorporated hypothesised pathoanatomical diagnoses and related clinical decision making. This premise was supported by the prevalence of pathoanatomical factors in the STOPS prognostic study and the convergence of results from a range of other research designs [83,96–98]

One example of this approach is the STOPS protocol, where treatment was individualised based on the hypothesised presence or absence of an inflammatory component to the LBP. The lumbar intervertebral disc is a biologically plausible contributor to LBP [135]. The mechanisms underpinning the symptoms of disc related pain and activity limitation are unclear, however substantial evidence exists supporting the role of inflammation in disc degeneration and disc herniation with associated radiculopathy (DHR) [136,137]. Studies investigating the composition and structure of lumbar discs have shown fibrosis, vascular invasion, inflammatory granulation tissue formation and extensive innervation along fissures in the posterior annulus fibrosis in painful degenerative discs and around symptomatic nerve roots. Such changes are not observed in non-painful degenerative or herniated discs [138,139].

Further evidence on the presence of and potential importance of inflammatory processes in degenerative discs and DHR [140] can be seen in disc tissue histologically [141–145], in the disc tissue using other inflammatory markers [146–151] and as measured by serum biomarkers in people with LBP [152]. A recent study showed that high serum tumour necrosis factor in acute LBP predicted poor recovery of pain and activity limitation at 6-months, providing further evidence of the relevance of inflammation [153].

Significant evidence suggests that inflammatory processes are a potential treatment target in clinical trials [136,137,154–156], particularly in people who may have discogenic pain [141–145]. Clinical features of inflammatory back pain such as spondyloarthropathy have been validated using practitioner surveys, expert panels and diagnostic accuracy studies [63,157–160]. These features include age <40 years, insidious onset, improvement with exercise, no improvement with rest and pain at night with improvement upon getting up from bed [161]. These results are similar to studies on the clinical features of disc related LBP and associated inflammation [144,145,147].

Although systematic reviews and guidelines suggest that NSAIDs are only a second-line treatment option for the management of LBP (Table 1), the literature above suggests that management of inflammatory processes might be more effective if targeted to individuals with clinical symptoms indicative of inflammation, particularly with a combination of pharmacological and other relevant management strategies. The clinical features suggestive of the presence of inflammation informed clinical decision making in the STOPS trial regarding when to implement anti-inflammatory treatment such as medication, taping, postural management and gentle walking. The identification of an inflammatory component was also important where inflammation may have hindered the effectiveness of mechanically based treatment approaches such as exercise, manual therapy or directional preference management [162,163]. The STOPS trial was unique in identifying clinically determined inflammation as a reason for exercising caution with mechanical treatment and simultaneously, treating inflammatory problems using anti-inflammatory treatment. The guideline-based advice comparison treatment gave no consideration to the role of inflammation. Therefore, clinical decision making based on the possible presence/absence of inflammation may have been a factor contributing to the significant between-group differences. This premise is further supported by the significance of clinically determined inflammation identified in the STOPS prognosis study.

4.4. *Treatment Fidelity in Randomised Controlled Trials*

Methods to maximise treatment fidelity in RCTs for physiotherapy interventions are highly variable and often poorly reported [164–169]. The STOPS trial employed a range of evidence-based methods [170] to enhance treatment fidelity including: specification regarding the treatment program design (140 page clinical manual with full detail on all aspects of individualised treatment); 16 hours of standardised practitioner training; review of practitioner treatment and practitioner feedback during the RCT (by way of study researchers reviewing the clinical notes followed by verbal feedback and group-based monthly case reviews); and evaluation of the participant's perspective/understanding of the treatment provided (qualitative exit interviews). Participants also completed exercise diaries that were checked by the physiotherapist at each visit. Similar methods were put in place with the advice treatment program. Given the relative complexity of the individualised physiotherapy, it is plausible that the treatment fidelity program would have had greater impact on patient outcomes in the individualised physiotherapy group. This could, therefore, have been an additional factor for the significant between-group differences observed in the STOPS trial.

4.5. *The Importance of Motor Control*

Motor control retraining focusing on posture, movement and muscle activation was a significant component of individualised physiotherapy for all participants apart from those in the multifactorial persistent pain (MFP) subgroup. The relevance and effectiveness of this approach is contentious [171] and there are significant inconsistencies in systematic review results [172–174]. Nevertheless, as the advice group did not receive motor control training this treatment component could have been responsible in part for the significant between-group effects. This premise is supported by the significance of suboptimal motor control identified in the STOPS prognosis study as well as the biological plausibility and potential pathoanatomical relevance of optimising motor control in people with LBP [175–178].

5. Clinical Implications

The clinical implications of the research presented in this paper are potentially substantial but need to be contextualised within an evidence-based framework. In order to make strong recommendations to practitioners, the findings need to be replicated in independent samples and/or systematic reviews updated to incorporate the relevant data into meta-analyses. However, the significance and consistency of the results are sufficient to challenge some of the common perceptions around evidence-based practice for LBP.

Guidelines routinely state that the vast majority of LBP patients should be considered as a non-specific condition where consideration of pathoanatomy is not possible or necessary [8,9]. Some guidelines go so far as to state that clinical decision making based on pathoanatomy may be harmful [66] despite sparse data to support this assertion. The results presented in this paper support the notion that hypothesising on and clinical decision making with regard to pathoanatomical considerations cannot be discounted and may lead to superior outcomes compared to a less targeted approach.

There is sparse data supporting the effectiveness of simple guideline-based advice. It is of interest that the RCT with the largest effect sizes in favour of advice incorporated a pathoanatomical explanation [179]. Despite this, advice in the absence of a pathoanatomical explanation is being recommended as first-line treatment for LBP of any duration [8,9]. The series of studies described in this paper suggest that further consideration and evaluation of guideline-based advice as a first-line treatment is required.

The generalisability of the STOPS trial results should be superior to most recent RCTs on individualised physiotherapy, where only a few experienced practitioners were used [122] and/or detailed clinical protocols were not published [33,122]. The treatment used in the STOPS trial was provided by physiotherapists with a range of experience, none of whom had a post-graduate qualification. It encompassed the most commonly used methods by physiotherapists [113,180,181] however the published treatment protocols have the potential to improve the quality of existing standards in clinical practice due to the detailed explanations and clinical decision making processes provided.

On the basis of the STOPS trial, practitioners can provide their patients with an average timeframe for expected treatment outcomes when receiving individualised physiotherapy. Patients are likely to experience rapid reductions in back/leg pain in the first 10 weeks of treatment, but optimal improvements in activity limitation are likely to take longer. Patients will also be reassured regarding the cost-effectiveness of the treatment, particularly with regards to minimising time off work.

6. Future Research

The results of this series of studies should be highly impactful on future research. Much of the research in LBP develop study designs, eligibility criteria, prognostic factors or treatment protocols that are relatively simplistic in nature. Whilst this approach renders research projects more feasible and potentially more methodologically rigorous, it does not reflect the real-world complexity of LBP and the associated treatment options that are likely to be most effective.

A pathoanatomical approach should be considered when planning future clinical research within the context of a truly biopsychosocial model for LBP.

More research is required on the relative importance of different components of individualised physiotherapy. Individualised physiotherapy also needs to be compared to other comparison groups and on different populations, particularly persistent LBP where more entrenched psychosocial and neurophysiological barriers to recovery are likely to be relevant.

Researchers should be encouraged by the clinical importance of the results in the STOPS trial and be emboldened to develop ambitious research hypotheses based on an in-depth understanding of both clinical and research perspectives.

Greater rigour should be applied to the development of clinical guidelines to ensure that low-quality evidence such as the sparse data and questionable cost-effectiveness supporting simple advice is acknowledged.

Researchers should follow the lead of the STOPS trial in providing detailed clinical protocols that are feely available in full-text. Such an approach would greatly accelerate the dissemination of evidence-based information to practitioners in the field and substantially improve external validity.

7. Conclusions

LBP is the most burdensome health problem in the world. Prior to the publication of the studies in this body of research, there was limited evidence for the effectiveness of individualised physiotherapy and a focus in clinical guidelines on advice as first-line treatment for LBP. Our series of studies challenge the role of advice alone in early persistent pain and suggests that the concept of non-specific LBP needs to be reconsidered. Furthermore, there are now detailed clinical protocols and quality evidence to support the STOPS approach to individualised physiotherapy in clinical practice and future research studies.

Author Contributions: Conceptualization, J.F. and A.H.; methodology, J.F., A.H., L.S., A.C. and M.R.; formal analysis, A.H. and J.F.; data curation, J.F., A.H., L.S., A.C. and M.R.; writing—original draft preparation, J.F. and A.H.; writing—review and editing, J.F., A.H., L.S., A.C. and M.R.; supervision, J.F.; project administration, J.F., A.H., L.S., A.C. and M.R.; funding acquisition, J.F.

Acknowledgments: We wish to acknowledge the physiotherapists who treated participants in the STOPS Trial free of charge.

Appendix A

Table A1. Prognostic factors for Oswestry, back pain and leg pain obtained from the multivariate model.

	Oswestry (0–100)			Back Pain (0–10)			Leg Pain (0–10)		
Prognostic factor	*N*	B Coefficient (95% CI)	*p*-value	*N*	B Coefficient (95% CI)	*p*-value	*N*	B Coefficient (95% CI)	*p*-value
Intercept		−0.2 (−14.4 to 13.9)	0.975		0.0 (−1.962 to 2.019)	0.977		−2.0 (−4.3 to 0.4)	0.095
Subgroup									
Disc herniation/radiculopathy *	54	−1.3 (−5.0 to 2.3)	0.473 +	54	**−0.6 (−1.2 to −0.1)**	**0.029 +**	54	−0.3 (−0.9 to 0.3)	0.312 +
Reducible discogenic pain *	78	−3.2 (−5.9 to −0.6)	0.017 +	78	**−0.9 (−1.3 to −0.4)**	**<0.001 +**	70	**−0.7 (−1.2 to −0.2)**	**0.005 +**
Manual therapy group *	64	−2.6 (−5.5 to 0.3)	0.082 +	64	−0.5 (−1.0 to 0.0)	0.050 +	49	−0.2 (−0.7 to 0.4)	0.560 +
Multifactorial persistent pain *	8	−1.3 (−7.8 to 5.1)	0.683 +	8	0.2 (−0.5 to 0.8)	0.647	7	−0.2 (−1.4 to 0.9)	0.725 +
Parents born overseas									
Both born overseas #	165	**3.4 (1.1 to 5.7)**	**0.004**	165	**0.6 (0.2 to 0.9)**	**0.003**	141	**0.5 (0.1 to 0.9)**	**0.026**
One born overseas #	21	0.7 (−3.7 to 5.1)	0.761	21	0.2 (−0.4 to 0.8)	0.570	18	0.1 (−0.5 to 0.8)	0.723
Paresthesia below waist	134	**−3.3 (−6.0 to −0.6)**	**0.016 +**	134	−0.1 (−0.5 to 0.3)	0.607 +	125	−0.2 (−0.6 to 0.3)	0.498 +
Deep leg symptoms	145	2.5 (0.0 to 4.9)	0.053	145	0.2 (−0.2 to 0.6)	0.286	145	**0.6 (0.2 to 1.0)**	**0.002**
Walking eases symptoms	160	−2.0 (−4.2 to 0.2)	0.073 +	160	**−0.5 (−0.9 to −0.2)**	**0.005 +**	138	−0.2 (−0.6 to 0.2)	0.273 +
Lateral flexion limited by pain	116	1.0 (−1.3 to 3.4)	0.382	116	0.1 (−0.3 to 0.5)	0.536	106	0.4 (0.0 to 0.8)	0.055
Transversus abdominis low tone	109	**−3.0 (−5.3 to −0.7)**	**0.012 +**	109	**−0.8 (−1.1 to −0.4)**	**<0.001 +**	91	−0.4 (−0.9 to 0.0)	0.051
Multifidus high tone	60	2.0 (−1.2 to 5.1)	0.215	60	0.0 (−0.4 to 0.5)	0.918	47	**0.7 (0.1 to 1.4)**	**0.019**
Clinical inflammation	182	1.1 (−1.1 to 3.3)	0.342	182	**0.4 (0.1 to 0.8)**	**0.020**	165	−0.2 (−0.6 to −0.2)	0.311 +
Back pain severity	300	0.2 (−0.5 to 0.8)	0.556	300	**0.3 (0.2 to 0.4)**	**<0.001**	261	0.1 (0.0 to 0.2)	0.245
Leg pain severity	300	0.1 (−0.5 to 0.6)	0.764	300	0.0 (−0.1 to 0.1)	0.896	261	**0.3 (0.2 to 0.4)**	**<0.001**
Örebro sick leave duration (0–10)	300	**1.1 (0.4 to 1.7)**	**0.002**	300	0.1 (0.0 to 0.2)	0.112	261	0.1 (0.0 to 0.2)	0.219

*, relative to "non-reducible discogenic pain"' #, relative to "both parents born in Australia"; +, Positive prognostic indicator. Results are independent of time point, significant p-values in bold. Negative B-coefficients represent lower outcome scores and therefore a better outcome at follow-up in participants with the listed prognostic factor. Predicted outcome for a given patient can be calculated by applying the patient's score on each baseline factor to the B-coefficients, and adding the scores from each item together (including the intercept).

References

1. Global Burden of Disease 2016 Disease and Injury Incidence and Prevalence Collaborators. Global, regional, and national incidence, prevalence, and years lived with disability for 328 diseases and injuries for 195 countries, 1990–2016: A systematic analysis for the Global Burden of Disease Study 2016. *Lancet* **2017**, *390*, 1211–1259. [CrossRef]
2. Hurwitz, E.L.; Randhawa, K.; Yu, H.; Cote, P.; Haldeman, S. The Global Spine Care Initiative: a summary of the global burden of low back and neck pain studies. *Eur. Spine J.* **2018**, *27*, 796–801. [CrossRef] [PubMed]
3. Waddell, G. A new clinical model for the treatment of low back pain. *Spine* **1987**, *12*, 632–654. [CrossRef] [PubMed]
4. Itz, C.J.; Geurts, J.W.; van Kleef, M.; Nelemans, P. Clinical course of non-specific low back pain: a systematic review of prospective cohort studies set in primary care. *Eur. J. Pain* **2013**, *17*, 5–15. [CrossRef] [PubMed]
5. Costa, L.M.; Maher, C.G.; Hancock, M.J.; McAuley, J.H.; Herbert, R.D.; Costa, L.O. The prognosis of acute and persistent low-back pain: a meta-analysis. *CMAJ* **2012**, *184*, E613–E624. [CrossRef]
6. Vasseljen, O.; Woodhouse, A.; Bjorngaard, J.H.; Leivseth, L. Natural course of acute neck and low back pain in the general population: The HUNT study. *Pain* **2013**, *154*, 1237–1244. [CrossRef] [PubMed]
7. Hartvigsen, J.; Hancock, M.J.; Kongsted, A.; Louw, Q.; Ferreira, M.L.; Genevay, S.; Hoy, D.; Karppinen, J.; Pransky, G.; Sieper, J.; et al. What low back pain is and why we need to pay attention. *Lancet* **2018**, *391*, 2356–2367. [CrossRef]
8. Oliveira, C.B.; Maher, C.G.; Pinto, R.Z.; Traeger, A.C.; Lin, C.C.; Chenot, J.F.; van Tulder, M.; Koes, B.W. Clinical practice guidelines for the management of non-specific low back pain in primary care: An updated overview. *Eur. Spine J.* **2018**, *27*, 2791–2803. [CrossRef]
9. Foster, N.E.; Anema, J.R.; Cherkin, D.; Chou, R.; Cohen, S.P.; Gross, D.P.; Ferreira, P.H.; Fritz, J.M.; Koes, B.W.; Peul, W.; et al. Prevention and treatment of low back pain: Evidence, challenges, and promising directions. *Lancet* **2018**, *391*, 2368–2383. [CrossRef]
10. Michaleff, Z.A.; Maher, C.G.; Lin, C.W.; Rebbeck, T.; Jull, G.; Latimer, J.; Connelly, L.; Sterling, M. Comprehensive physiotherapy exercise programme or advice for chronic whiplash (PROMISE): A pragmatic randomised controlled trial. *Lancet* **2014**, *384*, 133–141. [CrossRef]
11. Machado, L.A.; Maher, C.G.; Herbert, R.D.; Clare, H.; McAuley, J.H. The effectiveness of the McKenzie method in addition to first-line care for acute low back pain: A randomized controlled trial. *BMC Med.* **2010**, *8*, 10. [CrossRef] [PubMed]
12. O'Keeffe, M.; Purtill, H.; Kennedy, N.; Conneely, M.; Hurley, J.; O'Sullivan, P.; Dankaerts, W.; O'Sullivan, K. Comparative Effectiveness of Conservative Interventions for Nonspecific Chronic Spinal Pain: Physical, Behavioral/Psychologically Informed, or Combined? A Systematic Review and Meta-Analysis. *J. Pain* **2016**, *17*, 755–774. [CrossRef] [PubMed]
13. Ford, J.J.; Hahne, A.J. Complexity in the physiotherapy management of low back disorders: Clinical and research implications. *Man. Ther.* **2013**, *18*, 438–442. [CrossRef] [PubMed]
14. Foster, N.E.; Dziedzic, K.S.; Windt, D.; Fritz, J.M.; Hay, E.M. Research priorities for non-pharmacological therapies for common musculoskeletal problems: Nationally and internationally agreed recommendations. *BMC Muscul. Disord.* **2009**, *10*, 3. [CrossRef] [PubMed]
15. Costa, L.; Koes, B.; Pransky, G.; Borkan, J.; Maher, C.; Smeets, R. Primary care research priorities in low back pain: An update. *Spine* **2013**, *38*, 148–156. [CrossRef] [PubMed]
16. Ford, J.J.; Hahne, A.J. Pathoanatomy and classification of low back disorders. *Man. Ther.* **2013**, *18*, 165–168. [CrossRef] [PubMed]
17. World Health Organization. *International Classification of Functioning, Disability and Health: ICF*; World Health Organization: Geneva, Switzerland, 2001.
18. Jones, M. Clinical reasoning: From the Maitland Concept and beyond. In *Maitland's Vertebral Manipulation. Management of Neuromusculoskeletal Disorders*, 8th ed.; Elsevier: Edinburgh, UK, 2014; pp. 14–54.
19. Kent, P.; Keating, J.L.; Leboeuf-Yde, C. Research methods for subgrouping low back pain. *BMC Med. Res. Methodol.* **2010**, *10*, 62. [CrossRef]
20. Ford, J.; Story, I.; O'Sullivan, P.; McMeeken, J. Classification systems for low back pain: A review of the methodology for development and validation. *Physical Therapy Rev.* **2007**, *12*, 33–42. [CrossRef]

21. Karayannis, N.; Jull, G.; Hodges, P. Physiotherapy movement based classification approaches to low back pain: comparison of subgroups through review and developer/expert survey. *BMC Muscull Disord.* **2012**, *13*, 24. [CrossRef]
22. Kent, P.; Hancock, M.; Petersen, D.H.; Mjosund, H.L. Clinimetrics corner: choosing appropriate study designs for particular questions about treatment subgroups. *J. Manipulative Physiol. Ther.* **2010**, *18*, 147–152. [CrossRef]
23. Fairbank, J.; Gwilym, S.E.; France, J.C.; Daffner, S.D.; Dettori, J.; Hermsmeyer, J.; Andersson, G. The role of classification of chronic low back pain. *Spine* **2011**, *36*, 19–42. [CrossRef] [PubMed]
24. Stynes, S.; Konstantinou, K.; Dunn, K.M. Classification of patients with low back-related leg pain: A systematic review. *BMC Muscul. Disord.* **2016**, *17*, 226. [CrossRef] [PubMed]
25. Saragiotto, B.T.; Maher, C.G.; Moseley, A.M.; Yamato, T.P.; Koes, B.W.; Sun, X.; Hancock, M.J. A systematic review reveals that the credibility of subgroup claims in low back pain trials was low. *J. Clin. Epidemiology* **2016**, *79*, 3–9. [CrossRef] [PubMed]
26. Kent, P.; Mjosund, H.L.; Petersen, D.H. Does targeting manual therapy and/or exercise improve patient outcomes in nonspecific low back pain? A systematic review. *BMC Med.* **2010**, *8*, 22. [CrossRef] [PubMed]
27. Kent, P.; Kjaer, P. The efficacy of targeted interventions for modifiable psychosocial risk factors of persistent nonspecific low back pain—A systematic review. *Man. Ther.* **2012**, *17*, 385–401. [CrossRef] [PubMed]
28. American Physical Therapy Association. Guide to physical therapy practice 3.0. In *Guide to Physical Therapist Practice 3.0*; APTA: Alexandria, Egypt, 2014.
29. Riley, S.P.; Swanson, B.T.; Dyer, E. Are movement-based classification systems more effective than therapeutic exercise or guideline based care in improving outcomes for patients with chronic low back pain? A systematic review. *J. Manual Manipulative Therapy* **2019**, *27*, 5–14. [CrossRef] [PubMed]
30. Hill, J.C.; Dunn, K.M.; Main, C.J.; Hay, E.M. Subgrouping low back pain: A comparison of the STarT Back Tool with the Orebro Musculoskeletal Pain Screening Questionnaire. *Eur. J. Pain* **2010**, *14*, 83–89. [CrossRef]
31. Hill, J.C.; Vohora, K.; Dunn, K.M.; Main, C.J.; Hay, E.M. Comparing the STarT back screening tool's subgroup allocation of individual patients with that of independent clinical experts. *Clin. J. Pain* **2010**, *26*, 783–787. [CrossRef]
32. Fritz, J.M.; Beneciuk, J.M.; George, S.Z. Relationship between categorization with the STarT Back Screening Tool and prognosis for people receiving physical therapy for low back pain. *Phys. Ther.* **2011**, *91*, 722–732. [CrossRef]
33. Hill, J.C.; Whitehurst, D.G.; Lewis, M.; Bryan, S.; Dunn, K.M.; Foster, N.E.; Konstantinou, K.; Main, C.J.; Mason, E.; Somerville, S.; et al. Comparison of stratified primary care management for low back pain with current best practice (STarT Back): A randomised controlled trial. *Lancet* **2011**, *378*, 1560–1571. [CrossRef]
34. Main, C.J.; Sowden, G.; Hill, J.C.; Watson, P.J.; Hay, E.M. Integrating physical and psychological approaches to treatment in low back pain: The development and content of the STarT Back trial's 'high-risk' intervention (StarT Back; ISRCTN 37113406). *Physiotherapy* **2012**, *98*, 110–116. [CrossRef] [PubMed]
35. Morso, L.; Kent, P.; Manniche, C.; Albert, H.B. The predictive ability of the STarT Back Screening Tool in a Danish secondary care setting. *Eur. Spine J.* **2013**, *23*, 120–128. [CrossRef] [PubMed]
36. Hill, J.C.; Afolabi, E.K.; Lewis, M.; Dunn, K.M.; Roddy, E.; van der Windt, D.A.; Foster, N.E. Does a modified STarT Back Tool predict outcome with a broader group of musculoskeletal patients than back pain? A secondary analysis of cohort data. *BMJ Open* **2016**, *6*, e012445. [CrossRef] [PubMed]
37. Mansell, G.; Hill, J.C.; Main, C.; Vowles, K.E.; van der Windt, D. Exploring what factors mediate treatment effect: Example of the STarT Back study high-risk intervention. *J. Pain* **2016**, *17*, 1237–1245. [CrossRef] [PubMed]
38. Morso, L.; Kongsted, A.; Hestbaek, L.; Kent, P. The prognostic ability of the STarT Back Tool was affected by episode duration. *Eur. Spine J.* **2016**, *25*, 936–944. [CrossRef] [PubMed]
39. Bier, J.D.; Sandee-Geurts, J.J.W.; Ostelo, R.; Koes, B.W.; Verhagen, A.P. Can primary care for back and/or neck pain in the Netherlands benefit from stratification for risk groups according to the STarT Back Tool-classification? *Arch. Phys. Med. Rehabil.* **2017**, *99*, 65–71. [CrossRef] [PubMed]
40. Magel, J.; Fritz, J.M.; Greene, T.; Kjaer, P.; Marcus, R.L.; Brennan, G.P. Outcomes of Patients With Acute Low Back Pain Stratified by the STarT Back Screening Tool: Secondary Analysis of a Randomized Trial. *Phys. Ther.* **2017**, *97*, 330–337. [CrossRef] [PubMed]

41. Suri, P.; Delaney, K.; Rundell, S.D.; Cherkin, D.C. Predictive Validity of the STarT Back Tool for Risk of Persistent Disabling Back Pain in a U.S. Primary Care Setting. *Arch. Phys. Med. Rehabil.* **2018**, *99*, 1533–1539. [CrossRef]
42. Rabey, M.; Kendell, M.; Godden, C.; Liburd, J.; Netley, H.; O'Shaughnessy, C.; O'Sullivan, P.; Smith, A.; Beales, D. STarT Back Tool risk stratification is associated with changes in movement profile and sensory discrimination in low back pain: A study of 290 patients. *Eur. J. Pain* **2019**, *23*, 823–834. [CrossRef]
43. Ford, J.J.; Hahne, A.J.; Surkitt, L.D.; Chan, A.Y.; Richards, M.C.; Slater, S.L.; Hinman, R.S.; Pizzari, T.; Davidson, M.; Taylor, N.F. Individualised physiotherapy as an adjunct to guideline-based advice for low back disorders in primary care: A randomised controlled trial. *Br. J. Sports Med.* **2016**, *50*, 237–245. [CrossRef]
44. Verkerk, K.; Luijsterburg, P.A.; Miedema, H.S.; Pool-Goudzwaard, A.; Koes, B.W. Prognostic factors for recovery in chronic nonspecific low back pain: A systematic review. *Phys. Ther.* **2012**, *92*, 1093–1108. [CrossRef] [PubMed]
45. Pincus, T.; Burton, A.K.; Vogel, S.; Field, A.P. A systematic review of psychological factors as predictors of chronicity/disability in prospective cohorts of low back pain. *Spine* **2002**, *5*, E109–E120. [CrossRef] [PubMed]
46. Ashworth, J.; Konstantinou, K.; Dunn, K.M. Prognostic factors in non-surgically treated sciatica: A systematic review. *BMC Muscul. Disord.* **2011**, *12*, 208. [CrossRef] [PubMed]
47. Hayden, J.A.; Chou, R.; Hogg-Johnson, S.; Bombardier, C. Systematic reviews of low back pain prognosis had variable methods and results: Guidance for future prognosis reviews. *J. Clin. Epidemiol.* **2009**, *62*, 781–796. [CrossRef] [PubMed]
48. Kent, P.; Keating, J. Can we predict poor recovery from recent-onset nonspecific low back pain? A systematic review. *Man. Ther.* **2008**, *13*, 12–28. [CrossRef] [PubMed]
49. Ramond, A.; Bouton, C.; Richard, I.; Roquelaure, Y.; Baufreton, C.; Legrand, E.; Huez, J.F. Psychosocial risk factors for chronic low back pain in primary care: A systematic review. *Fam. Pract.* **2011**, *28*, 12–21. [CrossRef] [PubMed]
50. Gray, H.; Adefolarin, A.T.; Howe, T.E. A systematic review of instruments for the assessment of work-related psychosocial factors (Blue Flags) in individuals with non-specific low back pain. *Man. Ther.* **2011**, *16*, 531–543. [CrossRef]
51. Iles, R.A.; Davidson, M.; Taylor, N.F. Psychosocial predictors of failure to return to work in non-chronic non-specific low back pain: A systematic review. *Occup. Environ. Med.* **2008**, *65*, 507–517. [CrossRef]
52. Hartvigsen, J.; Lings, S.; Leboeuf-Yde, C.; Bakketeig, L. Psychosocial factors at work in relation to low back pain and consequences of low back pain; a systematic, critical review of prospective cohort studies. *Occup. Environ. Med.* **2004**, *61*, e2.
53. Wong, A.Y.; Parent, E.C.; Funabashi, M.; Stanton, T.R.; Kawchuk, G.N. Do various baseline characteristics of transversus abdominis and lumbar multifidus predict clinical outcomes in non-specific low back pain? A systematic review. *Pain* **2013**, *154*, 2589–2602. [CrossRef]
54. Konstantinou, K.; Hider, S.L.; Jordan, J.L.; Lewis, M.; Dunn, K.M.; Hay, E.M. The Impact of Low Back-related Leg Pain on Outcomes as Compared With Low Back Pain Alone: A Systematic Review of the Literature. *Clin. J. Pain* **2013**, *29*, 644–654. [CrossRef] [PubMed]
55. Chorti, A.; Chortis, A.G.; Strimpakos, N.; McCarthy, C.J.; Lamb, S.E. The prognostic value of symptom responses in the conservative management of spinal pain: A systematic review. *Spine* **2009**, *34*, 2686–2699. [CrossRef] [PubMed]
56. Borge, J.; Leboeuf-Yde, C.; Lothe, J. Prognostic values of physical examination findings in patients with chronic low back pain treated conservatively: A systematic literature review. *J. Manipulative Physiol. Ther.* **2001**, *24*, 292–295. [CrossRef] [PubMed]
57. Hendrick, P.; Milosavljevic, S.; Hale, L.; Hurley, D.A.; McDonough, S.; Ryan, B.; Baxter, G.D. The relationship between physical activity and low back pain outcomes: A systematic review of observational studies. *Eur. Spine J.* **2011**, *20*, 464–474. [CrossRef] [PubMed]
58. Van Oort, L.; van den Berg, T.; Koes, B.W.; de Vet, R.H.; Anema, H.J.; Heymans, M.W.; Verhagen, A.P. Preliminary state of development of prediction models for primary care physical therapy: A systematic review. *J. Clin. Epidemiol.* **2012**, *65*, 1257–1266. [CrossRef]
59. Hilfiker, R.; Bachmann, L.M.; Heitz, C.A.; Lorenz, T.; Joronen, H.; Klipstein, A. Value of predictive instruments to determine persisting restriction of function in patients with subacute non-specific low back pain. Systematic review. *Eur. Spine J.* **2007**, *16*, 1755–1775. [CrossRef] [PubMed]

60. Ford, J.J.; Richards, M.C.; Surkitt, L.D.; Chan, A.Y.P.; Slater, S.L.; Taylor, N.F.; Hahne, A.J. Development of a Multivariate Prognostic Model for Pain and Activity Limitation in People With Low Back Disorders Receiving Physiotherapy. *Arch. Phys. Med. Rehabil.* **2018**, *99*, 2504–2512. [CrossRef]
61. Linton, S.; Boersma, K. Early identification of patients at risk of developing a persistent back problem: The predictive validity of the Örebro musculoskeletal pain questionnaire. *Clin. J. Pain* **2003**, *19*, 80–86. [CrossRef]
62. Walker, B.F.; Williamson, O.D. Mechanical or inflammatory low back pain. What are the potential signs and symptoms? *Man. Ther.* **2009**, *14*, 314–320. [CrossRef]
63. Keeling, S.O.; Majumdar, S.R.; Conner-Spady, B.; Battie, M.C.; Carroll, L.J.; Maksymowych, W.P. Preliminary validation of a self-reported screening questionnaire for inflammatory back pain. *J. Rheumatol.* **2012**, *39*, 822–829. [CrossRef]
64. Fairbank, J.C.; Pynsent, P.B. The Oswestry Disability Index. *Spine* **2000**, *25*, 2940–2952. [CrossRef] [PubMed]
65. Ransford, A.; Cairns, D.; Mooney, V. The pain drawing as an aid to the psychologic evaluation of patients with low-back pain. *Spine* **1976**, *1*, 127–134. [CrossRef]
66. Dagenais, S.; Tricco, A.C.; Haldeman, S. Synthesis of recommendations for the assessment and management of low back pain from recent clinical practice guidelines. *Spine J.* **2010**, *10*, 514–529. [CrossRef] [PubMed]
67. Hayden, J.A.; Dunn, K.M.; van der Windt, D.A.; Shaw, W.S. What is the prognosis of back pain? *Best Practice Res. Clin.l Rheumatol.* **2010**, *24*, 167–179. [CrossRef] [PubMed]
68. Kent, P.; Keating, J.L. Classification in non-specific low back pain: What methods do primary care clinicians currently use? *Spine* **2005**, *30*, 1433–1440. [CrossRef] [PubMed]
69. Haskins, R.; Rivett, D.A.; Osmotherly, P.G. Clinical prediction rules in the physiotherapy management of low back pain: A systematic review. *Man. Ther.* **2012**, *17*, 9–21. [CrossRef] [PubMed]
70. Patel, S.; Friede, T.; Froud, R.; Evans, D.W.; Underwood, M. Systematic review of randomized controlled trials of clinical prediction rules for physical therapy in low back pain. *Spine* **2013**, *38*, 762–769. [CrossRef]
71. Mistry, D.; Patel, S.; Hee, S.W.; Stallard, N.; Underwood, M. Evaluating the quality of subgroup analyses in randomized controlled trials of therapist-delivered interventions for nonspecific low back pain: A systematic review. *Spine* **2014**, *39*, 618–629. [CrossRef]
72. Haskins, R.; Osmotherly, P.G.; Rivett, D.A. Diagnostic clinical prediction rules for specific subtypes of low back pain: A systematic review. *J. Ortho. Sports Phys. Thera.* **2015**, *45*, 61–76. [CrossRef]
73. McKenzie, R.; May, S. *The Lumbar Spine: Mechanical Diagnosis and Therapy*, 2nd ed.; Orthopedic Physical Therapy Products: Waikanae, New Zealand, 2003.
74. Sahrmann, S. *Diagnosis and Treatment of Movement Impairment Syndromes*, 1st ed.; Mosby Inc: St Louis, MI, USA, 2002.
75. Petersen, T.; Laslett, M.; Thorsen, H.; Manniche, C.; Ekdahl, C.; Jacobsen, S. Diagnostic classification of non-specific low back pain. A new system integrating patho-anatomic and clinical categories. *Physiother. Theory Pract.* **2003**, *19*, 213–237. [CrossRef]
76. O'Sullivan, P. Lumbar segmental 'instability': Clinical presentation and specific stabilizing exercise management. *Man. Ther.* **2000**, *5*, 2–12. [CrossRef] [PubMed]
77. O'Sullivan, P. Diagnosis and classification of chronic low back pain disorders: Maladaptive movement and motor control impairments as underlying mechanism. *Man. Ther.* **2005**, *10*, 242–255. [CrossRef] [PubMed]
78. McGinn, T.; Guyatt, G.; Wyer, P.; Naylor, C.; Stiell, I.; Richardson, W. Users' guides to the medical literature XXII: How to use articles about clinical decision rules. *J. Am. Med. Assoc.* **2000**, *284*, 79–84. [CrossRef] [PubMed]
79. Kamper, S.J.; Maher, C.G.; Hancock, M.J.; Koes, B.W.; Croft, P.R.; Hay, E. Treatment-based subgroups of low back pain. A guide to appraisal of research studies and a summary of current evidence. *Best Practice Res. Clin. Rheumatology* **2010**, *24*, 181–191. [CrossRef] [PubMed]
80. Hancock, M.J.; Kjaer, P.; Korsholm, L.; Kent, P. Interpretation of subgroup effects in published trials. *Phys. Ther.* **2013**, *93*, 852–859. [CrossRef] [PubMed]
81. Hancock, M.; Herbert, R.D.; Maher, C.G. A guide to interpretation of studies investigating subgroups of responders to physical therapy interventions. *Phys. Ther.* **2009**, *89*, 698–704. [CrossRef] [PubMed]
82. Brookes, S.T.; Whitely, E.; Egger, M.; Smith, G.D.; Mulheran, P.A.; Peters, T.J. Subgroup analyses in randomized trials: Risks of subgroup-specific analyses; power and sample size for the interaction test. *J. Clin. Epidemiology* **2004**, *57*, 229–236. [CrossRef] [PubMed]

83. Ford, J.J.; Surkitt, L.D.; Hahne, A.J. A classification and treatment protocol for low back disorders. Part 2: directional preference management for reducible discogenic pain. *Physical Therapy Rev.* **2011**, *16*, 423–437. [CrossRef]
84. Gurung, T.; Ellard, D.R.; Mistry, D.; Patel, S.; Underwood, M. Identifying potential moderators for response to treatment in low back pain: A systematic review. *Physiotherapy* **2015**, *101*, 243–251. [CrossRef]
85. Maher, C.G. Natural course of acute neck and low back pain in the general population: The HUNT study. *Pain* **2013**, *154*, 1480–1481. [CrossRef]
86. Carragee, E.; Hannibal, M. Diagnostic evaluation of low back pain. *Orthop. Clin. North Am.* **2004**, *35*, 7–16. [CrossRef]
87. Stanton, T.; Hancock, M.; Maher, C.; Koes, B. Critical appraisal of clinical prediction rules that aim to optimize treatment selection for musculoskeletal conditions. *Phys. Ther.* **2010**, *90*, 843–854. [CrossRef] [PubMed]
88. Feinstein, A. Clinical biostatistics XIII: On homogeneity, taxonomy, and nosography. *Clin. Pharmacol. Ther.* **1972**, *13*, 114–129. [CrossRef] [PubMed]
89. Heinrich, I.; O'Hare, H.; Sweetman, B.; Anderson, J. Validation aspects of an empirically derived classification for "non-specific" low back pain. *Statistician* **1985**, *34*, 215–230. [CrossRef]
90. Klapow, J.; Slater, M.; Patterson, T.; Doctor, J.; Atkinson, J.; Garfin, S. An empirical evaluation of multidimensional clinical outcome in chronic low back pain patients. *Pain* **1993**, *55*, 107–118. [CrossRef]
91. George, S.; Delitto, A. Clinical examination variables discriminate among treatment-based classification groups: A study of construct validity in patients with acute low back pain. *Phys. Ther.* **2005**, *85*, 306–314.
92. Sackett, D.; Straus, S.; Richardson, W.; Rosenberg, W.; Haynes, R. *Evidence-Based Medicine*; Churchill Livingstone: London, UK, 2000.
93. Reitsma, J.B.; Rutjes, A.W.S.; Khan, K.S.; Coomarasamy, A.; Bossuyt, P.M. A review of solutions for diagnostic accuracy studies with an imperfect or missing reference standard. *J. Clin. Epidemiol.* **2009**, *62*, 797–806. [CrossRef] [PubMed]
94. International Headache Society. Headache Classification Committee of the International Headache Society (IHS) The International Classification of Headache Disorders, 3rd edition. *Cephalalgia* **2018**, *38*, 1–211. [CrossRef]
95. Swerdlow, S.H.; Campo, E.; Pileri, S.A.; Harris, N.L.; Stein, H.; Siebert, R.; Advani, R.; Ghielmini, M.; Salles, G.A.; Zelenetz, A.D.; et al. The 2016 revision of the World Health Organization classification of lymphoid neoplasms. *Blood* **2016**, *127*, 2375–2390. [CrossRef]
96. Ford, J.J.; Thompson, S.L.; Hahne, A.J. A classification and treatment protocol for low back disorders. Part 1: Specific manual therapy. *Physical Therapy Rev.* **2011**, *16*, 168–177. [CrossRef]
97. Ford, J.J.; Hahne, A.J.; Chan, A.Y.P.; Surkitt, L.D. A classification and treatment protocol for low back disorders. Part 3: functional restoration for intervertebral disc related disorders. *Physical Therapy Rev.* **2012**, *17*, 55–75. [CrossRef]
98. Ford, J.J.; Richards, M.J.; Hahne, A.J. A classification and treatment protocol for low back disorders. Part 4: Functional restoration for low back disorders associated with multifactorial persistent pain. *Physical Therapy Rev.* **2012**, *17*, 322–334. [CrossRef]
99. Wilde, V.; Ford, J.; McMeeken, J. Indicators of lumbar zygapophyseal joint pain: Survey of an expert panel with the Delphi Technique. *Phys. Ther.* **2007**, *87*, 1348–1361. [CrossRef] [PubMed]
100. Chan, A.Y.; Ford, J.J.; McMeeken, J.M.; Wilde, V.E. Preliminary evidence for the features of non-reducible discogenic low back pain: Survey of an international physiotherapy expert panel with the Delphi technique. *Physiotherapy* **2013**, *99*, 212–220. [CrossRef] [PubMed]
101. Hahne, A.J.; Ford, J.J.; McMeeken, J.M. Conservative management of lumbar disc herniation with associated radiculopathy: A systematic review. *Spine* **2010**, *35*, E488–E504. [CrossRef] [PubMed]
102. Richards, M.C.; Ford, J.J.; Slater, S.L.; Hahne, A.J.; Surkitt, L.D.; Davidson, M.; McMeeken, J.M. The effectiveness of physiotherapy functional restoration for post-acute low back pain: A systematic review. *Man. Ther.* **2012**, *18*, 4–25. [CrossRef] [PubMed]
103. Slater, S.L.; Ford, J.J.; Richards, M.C.; Taylor, N.F.; Surkitt, L.D.; Hahne, A.J. The effectiveness of sub-group specific manual therapy for low back pain: A systematic review. *Man. Ther.* **2012**, *17*, 201–212. [CrossRef] [PubMed]
104. Surkitt, L.D.; Ford, J.J.; Hahne, A.J.; Pizzari, T.; McMeeken, J.M. Efficacy of directional preference management for low back pain: a systematic review. *Phys. Ther.* **2012**, *92*, 652–665. [CrossRef] [PubMed]

105. Dworkin, R.H.; Turk, D.C.; McDermott, M.P.; Peirce-Sandner, S.; Burke, L.B.; Cowan, P.; Farrar, J.T.; Hertz, S.; Raja, S.N.; Rappaport, B.A.; et al. Interpreting the clinical importance of group differences in chronic pain clinical trials: IMMPACT recommendations. *Pain* **2009**, *146*, 238–244. [CrossRef] [PubMed]
106. Deyo, R.A.; Dworkin, S.F.; Amtmann, D.; Andersson, G.; Borenstein, D.; Carragee, E.; Carrino, J.; Chou, R.; Cook, K.; DeLitto, A.; et al. Report of the NIH Task Force on research standards for chronic low back pain. *J. Pain* **2014**, *15*, 569–585. [CrossRef] [PubMed]
107. Dagenais, S.; Caro, J.; Haldeman, S. A systematic review of low back pain cost of illness studies in the United States and internationally. *Spine J.* **2008**, *8*, 8–20. [CrossRef] [PubMed]
108. Maniadakis, N.; Gray, A. The economic burden of back pain in the UK. *Pain* **2000**, *84*, 95–103. [CrossRef]
109. Murray, C.J.; Vos, T.; Lozano, R.; Naghavi, M.; Flaxman, A.D.; Michaud, C.; Ezzati, M.; Shibuya, K.; Salomon, J.A.; Abdalla, S.; et al. Disability-adjusted life years (DALYs) for 291 diseases and injuries in 21 regions, 1990–2010: A systematic analysis for the Global Burden of Disease Study 2010. *Lancet* **2012**, *380*, 2197–2223. [CrossRef]
110. Hoy, D.; March, L.; Brooks, P.; Blyth, F.; Woolf, A.; Bain, C.; Williams, G.; Smith, E.; Vos, T.; Barendregt, J.; et al. The global burden of low back pain: estimates from the Global Burden of Disease 2010 study. *Ann. Rheum. Dis.* **2014**, *73*, 968–974. [CrossRef] [PubMed]
111. Lin, C.W.; Haas, M.; Maher, C.G.; Machado, L.A.; van Tulder, M.W. Cost-effectiveness of guideline-endorsed treatments for low back pain: A systematic review. *Eur. Spine J.* **2011**, *20*, 1024–1038. [CrossRef] [PubMed]
112. Britt, H.; Miller, G.C.; Henderson, J.; Bayram, C.; Valenti, L.; Harrison, C.; Charles, J.; Pan, Y.; Zhang, C.; Pollack, A.J.; et al. *General Practice Activity in Australia 2012–2013. General Practice Series No.33.*; Sydney University Press: Sydney, Austrilia, 2013.
113. Liddle, D.; Baxter, D.; Gracey, J. Physiotherapists' use of advice and exercise for the management of chronic low back pain: A national survey. *Man. Ther.* **2009**, *14*, 189–196. [CrossRef] [PubMed]
114. Hahne, A.J.; Ford, J.J.; Surkitt, L.D.; Richards, M.C.; Chan, A.Y.; Slater, S.L.; Taylor, N.F. Individualized Physical Therapy is Cost Effective Compared to Guideline-Based Advice for People with Low Back Disorders. *Spine* **2017**, *42*, E169–E176. [CrossRef] [PubMed]
115. Hahne, A.J.; Ford, J.J.; Richards, M.C.; Surkitt, L.D.; Chan, A.Y.P.; Slater, S.L.; Taylor, N.F. Who Benefits Most From Individualized Physiotherapy or Advice for Low Back Disorders? A Preplanned Effect Modifier Analysis of a Randomized Controlled Trial. *Spine* **2017**, *42*, E1215–E1224. [CrossRef]
116. Celestin, J.; Edwards, R.; Jamison, R. Pretreatment psychosocial variables as predictors of outcomes following lumbar surgery and spinal cord stimulation: A systematic review and literature synthesis. *Pain Med.* **2009**, *10*, 639–653. [CrossRef]
117. Hockings, R.L.; McAuley, J.H.; Maher, C.G. A systematic review of the predictive ability of the Orebro Musculoskeletal Pain Questionnaire. *Spine* **2008**, *33*, E494–E500. [CrossRef]
118. Ferreira, M.L.; Herbert, R.D. What does 'clinically important' really mean? *Aust. J. Physiother.* **2008**, *54*, 229–230. [CrossRef]
119. Guyatt, G.H.; Thorlund, K.; Oxman, A.D.; Walter, S.D.; Patrick, D.; Furukawa, T.A.; Johnston, B.C.; Karanicolas, P.; Akl, E.A.; Vist, G.; et al. GRADE guidelines: 13. Preparing summary of findings tables and evidence profiles-continuous outcomes. *J. Clin. Epidemiol.* **2013**, *66*, 173–183. [CrossRef] [PubMed]
120. Dworkin, R.H.; Turk, D.C.; Farrar, J.T.; Haythornthwaite, J.A.; Jensen, M.P.; Katz, N.P.; Kerns, R.D.; Stucki, G.; Allen, R.R.; Bellamy, N.; et al. Core outcome measures for chronic pain clinical trials: IMMPACT recommendations. *Pain* **2005**, *113*, 9–19. [CrossRef] [PubMed]
121. Hahne, A.J.; Ford, J.J.; Surkitt, L.D.; Richards, M.C.; Chan, A.Y.; Thompson, S.L.; Hinman, R.S.; Taylor, N.F. Specific treatment of problems of the spine (STOPS): Design of a randomised controlled trial comparing specific physiotherapy versus advice for people with subacute low back disorders. *BMC Muscul. Disord.* **2011**, *12*, 104. [CrossRef] [PubMed]
122. Vibe Fersum, K.; O'Sullivan, P.; Skouen, J.S.; Smith, A.; Kvale, A. Efficacy of classification-based cognitive functional therapy in patients with non-specific chronic low back pain: A randomized controlled trial. *Eur. J. Pain* **2013**, *17*, 916–928. [CrossRef] [PubMed]
123. Lamb, S.E.; Hansen, Z.; Lall, R.; Castelnuovo, E.; Withers, E.J.; Nichols, V.; Potter, R.; Underwood, M.R. Group cognitive behavioural treatment for low-back pain in primary care: A randomised controlled trial and cost-effectiveness analysis. *Lancet* **2010**, *375*, 916–923. [CrossRef]

124. Rivero-Arias, O.; Gray, A.; Frost, H. Cost-utility analysis of physiotherapy treatment compared with physiotherapy advice in low back pain. *Spine* **2006**, *31*, 1381–1387. [CrossRef]
125. Macedo, L.G.; Smeets, R.J.; Maher, C.G.; Latimer, J.; McAuley, J.H. Graded activity and graded exposure for persistent nonspecific low back pain: A systematic review. *Phys. Ther.* **2010**, *90*, 860–879. [CrossRef]
126. Enke, O.; New, H.A.; New, C.H.; Mathieson, S.; McLachlan, A.J.; Latimer, J.; Maher, C.G.; Lin, C.C. Anticonvulsants in the treatment of low back pain and lumbar radicular pain: A systematic review and meta-analysis. *Can. Med. Association J.* **2018**, *190*, E786–E793. [CrossRef]
127. Bialosky, J.E.; Bishop, M.D.; George, S.Z.; Robinson, M.E. Placebo response to manual therapy: Something out of nothing? *J. Manipulative Physiol. Ther.* **2011**, *19*, 11–19. [CrossRef]
128. Dahm, K.; Brurberg, K.G.; Jamtvedt, G.; Hagen, K.B. Advice to rest in bed versus advice to stay active for acute low-back pain and sciatica. *Cochrane. Database Syst. Rev.* **2010**, *6*, CD007612. [CrossRef] [PubMed]
129. Liddle, S.; Gracey, J.; Baxter, G. Advice for the management of low back pain: A systematic review of randomised controlled trials. *Man. Ther.* **2007**, *12*, 310–327. [CrossRef] [PubMed]
130. Abdel Shaheed, C.; Maher, C.G.; Williams, K.A.; McLachlan, A.J. Interventions available over the counter and advice for acute low back pain: Systematic review and meta-analysis. *J. Pain* **2014**, *15*, 2–15. [CrossRef] [PubMed]
131. Buchbinder, R.; van Tulder, M.; Öberg, B.; Costa, L.M.; Woolf, A.; Schoene, M.; Croft, P.; Buchbinder, R.; Hartvigsen, J.; Cherkin, D.; et al. Low back pain: A call for action. *Lancet* **2018**, *391*, 2384–2388. [CrossRef]
132. National Guideline Centre. National Guideline Centre. National Institute for Health and Care Excellence: Clinical Guidelines. In *Low Back Pain and Sciatica in Over 16s: Assessment and Management*; National Institute for Health and Care Excellence: London, UK, 2016.
133. O'Sullivan, P. It's time for change with the management of non-specific chronic low back pain. *Br. J. Sports Med.* **2012**, *46*, 224–227. [CrossRef] [PubMed]
134. O'Sullivan, K.; O'Sullivan, P.B.; O'Keeffe, M. The Lancet series on low back pain: reflections and clinical implications. *Br. J. Sports Med.* **2019**, *53*, 392–393. [CrossRef]
135. Bogduk, N. *Clinical and Radiological Anatomy of the Lumbar Spine*, 5th ed.; Churchill Livingstone: New York, NY, USA, 2012.
136. Peng, B.G. Pathophysiology, diagnosis, and treatment of discogenic low back pain. *World J. Orthpedics* **2013**, *4*, 42–52. [CrossRef] [PubMed]
137. Adams, M.A.; Stefanakis, M.; Dolan, P. Healing of a painful intervertebral disc should not be confused with reversing disc degeneration: Implications for physical therapies for discogenic back pain. *Clin. Biomech.* **2010**, *25*, 961–971. [CrossRef]
138. Peng, B.; Wu, W.; Hou, S.; Li, P.; Zhang, C.; Yang, Y. The pathogenesis of discogenic low back pain. *J. Bone Joint Surg. Br.* **2005**, *87*, 62–67. [CrossRef]
139. Peng, B.; Hao, J.; Hou, S.; Wu, W.; Jiang, D.; Fu, X.; Yang, Y. Possible pathogenesis of painful intervertebral disc degeneration. *Spine* **2006**, *31*, 560–566. [CrossRef]
140. Van den Berg, R.; Jongbloed, E.M.; de Schepper, E.I.T.; Bierma-Zeinstra, S.M.A.; Koes, B.W.; Luijsterburg, P.A.J. The association between pro-inflammatory biomarkers and nonspecific low back pain: A systematic review. *Spine J.* **2018**, *18*, 2140–2151. [CrossRef] [PubMed]
141. Gronblad, M.; Virri, J.; Tolonen, J.; Seitsalo, S.; Kaapa, E.; Kankare, J. A controlled immunohistochemical study of inflammatory cells in disc herniation tissue. *Spine* **1994**, *19*, 2744–2751. [CrossRef] [PubMed]
142. Habtemariam, A.; Gronglad, M.; Virri, J.; Seitsala, S.; Ruuskanen, M.; Karaharju, E. Immunocytochemical localization of immunoglobulins in disc herniations. *Spine* **1996**, *21*, 1864–1869. [CrossRef] [PubMed]
143. Habtemariam, A.; Gronglad, M.; Virri, J.; Seitsala, S.; Karaharju, E. A comparative immunohistochemical study of inflammatory cells in acute-stage and chronic-stage disc herniations. *Spine* **1998**, *23*, 2159–2166. [CrossRef] [PubMed]
144. Rothoerl, R.D.; Woertgen, C.; Holzschuh, M.; Rueschoff, J.; Brawanski, A. Is there a clinical correlate to the histologic evidence of inflammation in herniated lumbar disc tissue? *Spine* **1998**, *23*, 1197–1200. [CrossRef] [PubMed]
145. Virri, J.; Grönblad, M.; Seitsalo, S.; Habtemariam, A.; Kääpä, E.; Karaharju, E. Comparison of the prevalence of inflammatory cells in subtypes of disc herniations and associations with straight leg raising. *Spine* **2001**, *26*, 2311–2315. [CrossRef] [PubMed]

146. Miyamoto, H.; Saura, R.; Harada, T.; Doita, M.; Mizuno, K. The role of cyclooxygenase-2 and inflammatory cytokines in pain induction of herniated lumbar intervertebral disc. *Kobe J. Med. Sci.* **2000**, *46*, 13–28. [PubMed]
147. Piperno, M.; le Graverand, M.; Reboul, P.; Mathieu, P.; Tron, A. Phospholipase A2 activity in herniated lumbar discs: Clinical correlations and inhibition by piroxicam. *Spine* **1997**, *22*, 2061–2063. [CrossRef]
148. Jimbo, K.; Park, J.S.; Yokosuka, K.; Sato, K.; Nagata, K. Positive feedback loop of interleukin-1beta upregulating production of inflammatory mediators in human intervertebral disc cells in vitro. *J. Neurosurg. Spine* **2005**, *2*, 589–595. [CrossRef]
149. Brisby, H.; Byrod, G.; Olmarke, R.; Miller, V.; Aoki, Y.; Rydevik, B. Nitric oxide as a mediator of nucleus pulposus-induced effects on spinal nerve roots. *J. Orthop. Res.* **2000**, *18*, 815–820. [CrossRef]
150. Burke, J.; Watson, R.; McCormack, D.; Dowling, F.; Walsh, M.; Fitzpatrick, J. Intervertebral discs which cause low back pain secrete high levels of proinflammatory mediators. *J.f Bone Joint Surgery* **2002**, *84B*, 196–201.
151. Kang, J.; Georgescu, H.; McIntyre-Larkin, L.; Stefanovic-Racic, M.; Donaldson, W.r.; CH, E. Herniated lumbar intervertebral discs spontaneously produce matrix metalloproteinases, nitric oxide, interleukin-6, and prostaglandin E2. *Spine* **1996**, *21*, 271–277. [CrossRef] [PubMed]
152. Khan, A.N.; Jacobsen, H.E.; Khan, J.; Filippi, C.G.; Levine, M.; Lehman, R.A., Jr.; Riew, K.D.; Lenke, L.G.; Chahine, N.O. Inflammatory biomarkers of low back pain and disc degeneration: A review. *Ann. N. Y. Acad. Sci.* **2017**, *1410*, 68–84. [CrossRef] [PubMed]
153. Klyne, D.M.; Barbe, M.F.; van den Hoorn, W.; Hodges, P.W. ISSLS PRIZE IN CLINICAL SCIENCE 2018: longitudinal analysis of inflammatory, psychological, and sleep-related factors following an acute low back pain episode-the good, the bad, and the ugly. *Eur. Spine J.* **2018**, *27*, 763–777. [CrossRef] [PubMed]
154. Podichetty, V.K. The aging spine: The role of inflammatory mediators in intervertebral disc degeneration. *Cell. Mol. Biol.* **2007**, *53*, 4–18. [CrossRef] [PubMed]
155. Zhou, Y.; Abdi, S. Diagnosis and minimally invasive treatment of lumbar discogenic pain: A review of the literature. *Clin. J. Pain* **2006**, *22*, 468–481. [CrossRef]
156. Ross, J.S. Non-mechanical inflammatory causes of back pain: current concepts. *Skeletal Radiol.* **2006**, *35*, 485–487. [CrossRef]
157. Adizie, T.; Elamanchi, S.; Prabu, A.; Pace, A.V.; Laxminarayan, R.; Barkham, N. Knowledge of features of inflammatory back pain in primary care in the West Midlands: A cross-sectional survey in the United Kingdom. *Rheumatol. Int.* **2018**, *38*, 1859–1863. [CrossRef]
158. Sieper, J.; van der Heijde, D.; Landewe, R.; Brandt, J.; Burgos-Vagas, R.; Collantes-Estevez, E.; Dijkmans, B.; Dougados, M.; Khan, M.A.; Leirisalo-Repo, M.; et al. New criteria for inflammatory back pain in patients with chronic back pain: A real patient exercise by experts from the Assessment of SpondyloArthritis international Society (ASAS). *Ann. Rheum. Dis.* **2009**, *68*, 784–788. [CrossRef]
159. Calin, A.; Porta, J.; Fries, J.F.; Schurman, D.J. CLinical history as a screening test for ankylosing spondylitis. *JAMA* **1977**, *237*, 2613–2614. [CrossRef]
160. Underwood, M.R.; Dawes, P. Inflammatory back pain in primary care. *Br. J. Rheumatol.* **1995**, *34*, 1074–1077. [CrossRef] [PubMed]
161. Weisman, M.H. Inflammatory back pain: the United States perspective. *Rheum. Dis. Clin. North Am.* **2012**, *38*, 501–512. [CrossRef] [PubMed]
162. McKenzie, R. *The Lumbar Spine: Mechanical Diagnosis and Therapy*; Spinal Publication: Waikanae, New Zealand, 1981.
163. Maitland, G.D. *Vertebral Manipulation*, 5th ed.; Butterworth-Heinemann: Oxford, UK, 1986.
164. Van der Windt, D.; Hay, E.; Jellema, P.; Main, C. Psychosocial interventions for low back pain in primary care: lessons learned from recent trials. *Spine* **2008**, *33*, 81–89. [CrossRef] [PubMed]
165. Borrelli, B.; Sepinwall, D.; Ernst, D.; Bellg, A.J.; Czajkowski, S.; Breger, R.; DeFrancesco, C.; Levesque, C.; Sharp, D.L.; Ogedegbe, G.; et al. A new tool to assess treatment fidelity and evaluation of treatment fidelity across 10 years of health behavior research. *J. Consult. Clin. Psychol.* **2005**, *73*, 852–860. [CrossRef] [PubMed]
166. Perepletchikova, F.; Treat, T.A.; Kazdin, A.E. Treatment integrity in psychotherapy research: Analysis of the studies and examination of the associated factors. *J. Consulting Clin. Psychol.* **2007**, *75*, 829–841. [CrossRef] [PubMed]

167. Helmhout, P.; Staal, J.; Maher, C.; Petersen, T.; Rainville, J.; Shaw, W. Exercise therapy and low back pain: Insights and proposals to improve the design, conduct, and reporting of clinical trials. *Spine* **2008**, *33*, 1782–1788. [CrossRef] [PubMed]
168. Herbert, R.D.; Bo, K. Analysis of quality of interventions in systematic reviews. *Br. Med. J.* **2005**, *331*, 507–509. [CrossRef]
169. Karas, S.; Plankis, L. Consideration of treatment fidelity to improve manual therapy research. *J. Man. Manip. Ther.* **2016**, *24*, 233–237. [CrossRef]
170. Borrelli, B. The Assessment, Monitoring, and Enhancement of Treatment Fidelity In Public Health Clinical Trials. *J. Public Health Dent.* **2011**, *71*, S52–S63. [CrossRef]
171. Hodges, P.W.; van Dieen, J.H.; Cholewicki, J. Time to Reflect on the Role of Motor Control in Low Back Pain. *J. Orthop. Sports Phys. Ther.* **2019**, *49*, 367–369. [CrossRef]
172. Macedo, L.G.; Saragiotto, B.T.; Yamato, T.P.; Costa, L.O.; Menezes Costa, L.C.; Ostelo, R.W.; Maher, C.G. Motor control exercise for acute non-specific low back pain. *Cochrane Database Syst. Rev.* **2016**, *2*, cd012085. [CrossRef] [PubMed]
173. Saragiotto, B.T.; Maher, C.G.; Yamato, T.P.; Costa, L.O.; Menezes Costa, L.C.; Ostelo, R.W.; Macedo, L.G. Motor control exercise for chronic non-specific low-back pain. *Cochrane Database Syst. Rev.* **2016**, *1*, cd012004. [CrossRef] [PubMed]
174. Bystrom, M.G.; Rasmussen-Barr, E.; Grooten, W.J. Motor control exercises reduces pain and disability in chronic and recurrent low back pain: a meta-analysis. *Spine* **2013**, *38*, E350–E358. [CrossRef] [PubMed]
175. Hodges, P. *Spinal Control: The Rehabilitation of Back Pain*, 1st ed.; Hodges, P., Cholewicki, J., van Dieen, J., Eds.; Churchill Livingston: Edinburgh, UK, 2013.
176. Van Dieen, J.H.; Reeves, N.P.; Kawchuk, G.; van Dillen, L.; Hodges, P.W. Analysis of Motor Control in Low-Back Pain Patients: A Key to Personalized Care? *J. Orthop. Sports Phys. Ther.* **2018**, *49*, 1–24. [CrossRef] [PubMed]
177. Hodges, P.W.; Barbe, M.F.; Loggia, M.L.; Nijs, J.; Stone, L.S. Diverse Role of Biological Plasticity in Low Back Pain and Its Impact on Sensorimotor Control of the Spine. *J. Orthop. Sports Phys. Ther.* **2019**, *49*, 389–401. [CrossRef] [PubMed]
178. Van Dieen, J.H.; Reeves, N.P.; Kawchuk, G.; van Dillen, L.R.; Hodges, P.W. Motor Control Changes in Low Back Pain: Divergence in Presentations and Mechanisms. *J. Orthop. Sports Phys. Ther.* **2019**, *49*, 370–379. [CrossRef] [PubMed]
179. Indahl, A.; Velund, L.; Reikeraas, O. Good prognosis for low back pain when left untampered. *Spine* **1995**, *20*, 473–477. [CrossRef]
180. Li, L.; Bombardier, C. Physical Therapy Management of Low Back Pain: An Expolratory Survey of Therapist Approaches. *Phys. Ther.* **2001**, *81*, 1018–1028.
181. Gracey, J.; McDonough, S.M.; Baxter, D.G. Physiotherapy Management of Low Back Pain. A Survey of Current Practice in Northern Ireland. *Spine* **2002**, *27*, 406–411. [CrossRef]

5

Are Mindful Exercises Safe and Beneficial for Treating Chronic Lower Back Pain?

Liye Zou [1,†], Yanjie Zhang [2,†], Lin Yang [3,4], Paul D. Loprinzi [5], Albert S. Yeung [6], Jian Kong [6], Kevin W Chen [1], Wook Song [2,7], Tao Xiao [8,*] and Hong Li [9,10,*]

1 Lifestyle (Mind-Body Movement) Research Center, College of Sports Science, Shenzhen University, Shenzhen 518060, China; liyezou123@gmail.com (L.Z.); Qigong4us@hotmail.com (K.W.C.)
2 Health and Exercise Science Laboratory, Institute of Sports Science, Seoul National University, Seoul 08826, Korea; elite_zhangyj@163.com (Y.Z.); songw3@snu.ac.kr (W.S.)
3 Cancer Epidemiology and Prevention Research, Alberta Health Services, Calgary, AB T2S 3C3, Canada; lin.yang@ahs.ca
4 Departments of Oncology and Community Health Sciences, Cumming School of Medicine, University of Calgary, Calgary, AB T2N 4Z6, Canada
5 Department of Health, Exercise Science and Recreation Management School of Applied Sciences, The University of Mississippi, Oxford, MS 36877, USA; pdloprin@olemiss.edu
6 Department of Psychiatry, Massachusetts General Hospital, Harvard Medical School, Boston, MA 02114, USA; ayeung@mgh.harvard.edu (A.S.Y.); JKONG2@mgh.harvard.edu (J.K.)
7 Institute on Aging, Seoul National University, Seoul 08826, Korea
8 College of Mathematics and Statistics, Shenzhen University, Shenzhen 518060, China
9 Shenzhen Key Laboratory of Affective and Social Cognitive Science, College of Psychology and Sociology, Shenzhen University, Shenzhen 518060, China
10 Shenzhen Institute of Neuroscience, Shenzhen 518057, China
* Correspondence: taoxiao@szu.edu.cn (T.X.); lihongszu@szu.edu.cn (H.L.)
† These authors contributed equally to this work.

Abstract: Background: Chronic low back pain (CLBP) is a common health issue worldwide. Tai Chi, Qigong, and Yoga, as the most widely practiced mindful exercises, have promising effects for CLBP-specific symptoms. Objective: We therefore conducted a comprehensive review investigating the effects of mindful exercises versus active and/or non-active controls while evaluating the safety and pain-related effects of mindful exercises in adults with CLBP. Methods: We searched five databases (MEDLINE, EMBASE, SCOPUS, Web of Science, and Cochrane Library) from inception to February 2019. Two investigators independently selected 17 eligible randomized controlled trials (RCT) against inclusion and exclusion criteria, followed by data extraction and study quality assessment. Standardized mean difference (SMD) was used to determine the magnitude of mindful exercises versus controls on pain- and disease-specific outcome measures. Results: As compared to control groups, we observed significantly favorable effects of mindful exercises on reducing pain intensity ($SMD = -0.37$, 95% CI −0.5 to −0.23, $p < 0.001$, $I^2 = 45.9$ %) and disability ($SMD = -0.39$, 95% CI −0.49 to −0.28, $p < 0.001$, $I^2 = 0$ %). When compared with active control alone, mindful exercises showed significantly reduced pain intensity ($SMD = -0.40$, $p < 0.001$). Furthermore, of the three mindful exercises, Tai Chi has a significantly superior effect on pain management ($SMD= -0.75$, 95% CI −1.05 to −0.46, $p < 0.001$), whereas Yoga-related adverse events were reported in five studies. Conclusion: Findings of our systematic review suggest that mindful exercises (Tai Chi and Qigong) may be beneficial for CLBP symptomatic management. In particular, Tai Chi appears to have a superior effect in reducing pain intensity irrespective of non-control comparison or active control comparison (conventional exercises, core training, and physical therapy programs). Importantly, training in these mindful exercises should be implemented with certified instructors to ensure quality of movement and injury prevention.

Keywords: Tai Chi; Yoga; Qigong; mind-body therapy; exercise; mind-body medicine; low back pain

---

1. Introduction

Low back pain is a common health issue worldwide, but notably, prevention and treatment of chronic low back pain (CLBP) is a major public health concern [1,2]. It has been widely recognized as the leading cause of disability, affecting work performance and general psychosomatic health and is associated with substantial economic and societal burden [2]. The estimated lifetime prevalence of CLBP is 12% to 33% in industrialized countries (period prevalence: 22% to 65% per year) [3]. The prevalence rate of CLBP is higher in adults than children and adolescents [4], particularly among the working population [5]. CLBP is widely treated with medications (e.g., nonsteroidal anti-inflammatory drug, analgesic, and muscle relaxant) to relieve pain, decrease inflammation, and reduce muscle tension [6]. However, these treatments may increase the likelihood of falls and drug-related side effects (e.g., mood disturbance, nausea, seizure, and/or tachycardia) among patients [6,7]. Furthermore, the long-term use of medications remains financially unaffordable in economically disadvantaged areas [7]. Other non-pharmacological treatments, such as physical therapy [8,9], spinal manipulation [10], and physical activity or exercise [11–13], have shown promising effects on improving CLBP-specific symptoms.

Tai Chi, Qigong (e.g., Baduanjin, Yijingjin, and Wuqinxi), and Yoga, also known as mindful exercises, are light-to-moderate intensity physical activities and have recently been popularized in both the fitness industry and clinical setting for disease prevention and symptomatic management [14–17]. Mindful exercises are typically performed at a slow pace, simultaneously integrated with mental focus on muscle and movement sense, rhythmic abdominal diaphragmatic breathing, and meditation [18–21]. These modalities may complement or act as an alternative practice to conventional rehabilitation programs [22–24]. Mindful exercises are beneficial for symptomatic management in a variety of diseases, such as multiple sclerosis [25,26], autism spectrum disorder [27], balance disorder [28,29], ankylosing spondylitis [30], mental illness [31,32], cerebrovascular disease [33], fibromyalgia [34], and knee osteoarthritis [35].

Recently, research has investigated the effects of mindful exercises in adults with CLBP. With the increasing number of experimental studies on this topic, two reviews were subsequently performed and published in 2013 [36,37]. Notably, these two systematic reviews only included eight to 10 randomized controlled trials (RCT) and focused on Yoga alone. Secondly, meta-analysis was only possible for the Yoga interventions versus non-active controls due to the small number of trials, lacking a direct comparison to active control conditions like conventional exercises or guideline-endorsed treatments. Thirdly, previous reviews simply evaluated the effectiveness of Yoga, but the safety of the broader mindful exercises in adults with CLBP still remains unknown. To fill these knowledge gaps, we therefore conducted an updated systematic review that includes all three most popular mindful exercises versus active and/or non-active controls while evaluating the safety and efficacy of mindful exercises in adults with CLBP.

2. Methods

2.1. Search Strategy

Two investigators independently searched five databases (MEDLINE, EMBASE, SCOPUS, Web of Science, and Cochrane library) from the inception to February 2019. We used two groups of keywords: (1) "Tai Chi" OR "Tai Chi Chuan" OR "Taiji" OR "Qigong" Or "Chi Kung" OR "Qi Gong" OR "Baduanjin" OR "Yijinjing" OR "Wuqinxi" OR "Yoga" OR "mind-body", OR "mindful exercise"; (2) "low back pain" OR "lower back pain" OR "back pain" OR "low back ache". Hand-searching was performed to identify relevant publications from the reference lists of eligible original articles and reviews. In addition to two separate investigators independently searching the five above-mentioned databases, these investigators also independently screened the titles and abstracts of the potentially eligible articles (described below). Full details on the search strategy and retrieval process are shown in Figure 1.

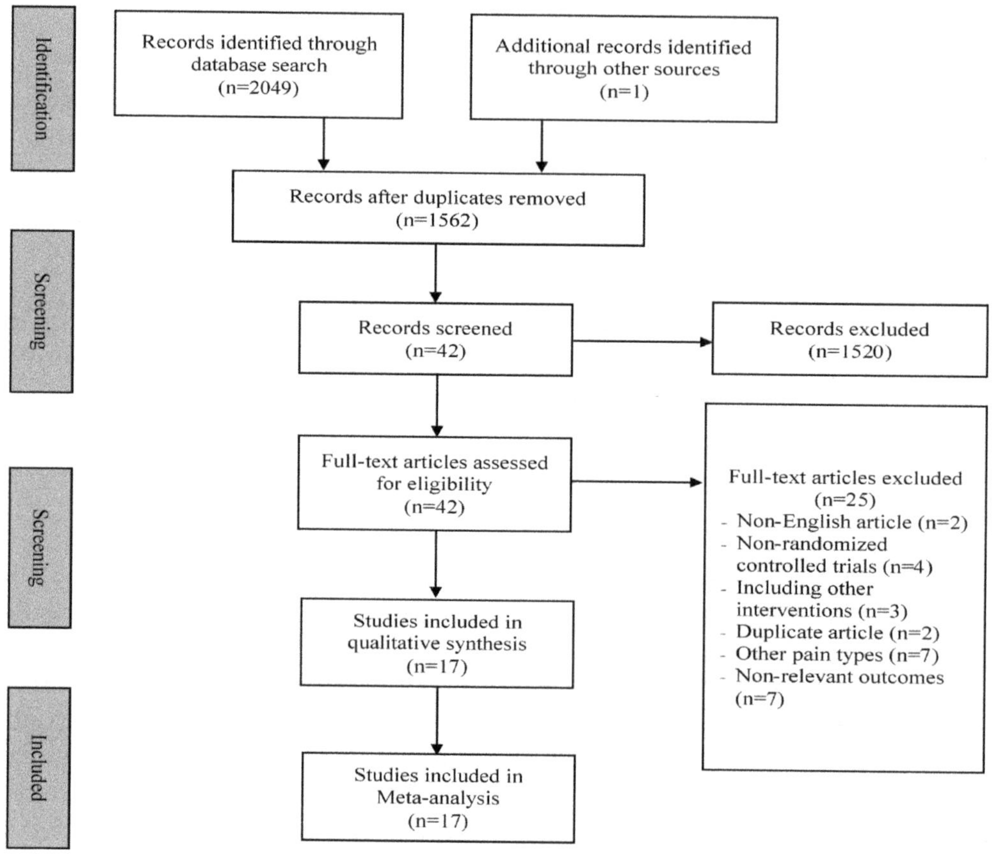

Figure 1. Flow chart of study searching.

2.2. *Inclusion and Exclusion Criteria*

In the present review, studies were only considered eligible if they: (1) were RCTs; (2) recruited adults diagnosed with CLBP (low back pain lasting or recurring for longer than 3 months [38]; (3) used at least one type of mindful exercise (e.g., Tai Chi, Qigong, and Yoga) or their combination as an intervention program; (4) included a control group using any form (e.g., aerobic exercise, self-care book, waitlist, or no treatment) other than mindful exercise; (5) reported at least one health outcome associated with disease-specific symptoms like pain, functional ability, or depression. Exclusion criteria were: (1) specific causes (e.g., spinal canal stenosis or herniated disc); (2) mindful exercise integrated with other treatments, like core training; (3) unobtainable data for calculating effect size (ES); (4) other types of publications, such as a case-study, observational study, or review articles.

2.3. *Data Extraction and Quality Assessment*

Detailed information of each included study were independently extracted by the two investigators and a third reviewer was consulted to reach consensus by discussion. Extracted information included the first author and year of publication, characteristics of participants (sample size and mean age), intervention protocol (mindful exercise, control type, and intervention duration), outcome measure (pain, disability, and/or depression), and reporting of an adverse event. In addition to descriptive information, the same investigators extracted the quantitative data for ES calculation.

Two investigators independently assessed methodological quality using the Physiotherapy Evidence Database (PEDro) scale. This scale consists of 11 items, including eligibility criteria, random allocation, allocation concealment, baseline equivalence, blinded assessor(s), blinded participants, blinded instructor, retention rate of ≥85%, intention-to-treat analysis (ITT), between group statistical comparisons, and point estimates of at least one set of outcome measures. One point is awarded for meeting each evaluation requirement. Since this review included all adults diagnosed with CLBP, the first eligibility criteria was not considered. Thus, each study could reach a maximum of 10 points: excellent (9–10 points), good (6–8 points), fair (4–5 points) and poor (less than 4 points) quality [39].

2.4. Statistical Analysis

The Comprehensive Meta-Analysis Software version 2.2 was employed to meta-analyze the extracted data. For each outcome, we used mean and standard deviations (SD) at baseline and post-intervention, along with the number of participants per group. If one study included two control groups, we halved the number of participants in the mindful exercise group with the two control groups, while mean and SD remained unchanged. We used random-effects model to calculate the pooled ES (standardized mean difference, SMD) to determine the magnitude of effect for mindful exercise intervention on two outcomes (pain and disability). Notably, we did not evaluate depression as an outcome variable, due to fewer than four studies evaluating this outcome [40]. Three levels of ES were adopted: small (0.2–0.49), moderate (0.50–0.79), and large (≥0.8) [40]. I^2 test was used to determine heterogeneity across included studies: $I^2 < 25\%$ (low), $I^2 < 50\%$ (moderate), and $I^2 > 75\%$ (high), respectively [40]. Furthermore, we performed sub-group analyses for categorical variables and meta-regression for continuous variables. The categorical variables included: (1) types of control condition (mindful exercise versus active control or non-active control), mindful exercise (Tai Chi, Yoga, and Qigong), and instrument; (2) use of allocation concealment. The continuous variables included mean age and total time spent over the entire intervention course (minutes). Finally, publication bias for each outcome was evaluated using the Egger's test and the visually-produced Funnel plot [40]. Subsequently, we removed studies that caused asymmetry.

3. Results

3.1. Search Results

Figure 1 describes the detailed search process of our meta-analysis. A total of 2049 potential studies were searched and 42 full-text publications were screened for further evaluation. After eliminating the irrelevant studies (n = 25), seventeen studies [41–57] were identified for data extraction and quality assessment.

3.2. Characteristics of Included Studies

Table 1 depicts the characteristics of the included studies, such as the sample size, age, intervention and control group details, and outcome measures. Seventeen studies [41–57] published in peer-review journals included a total of 2022 participants with CLBP. The mean age of participants ranged from 34 to 74 years. The sample size ranged from 20 to 320 per study. Intervention duration for the mindful exercise(s) lasted 1 to 24 weeks, with sessions occurring one to seven times per week (40 to 90 min per sessions). Control conditions varied greatly across the evaluated studies, including utilizing a self-care book, stretching exercise, and waitlist. Adverse events were reported in five Yoga intervention studies, including herniated discs (3.3% and 1.1%, respectively) [48,54,55], increased pain (2.6% and 14.1%, respectively) [53,54], and mild self-limited joint and back pain (7.1%) [56]. One study did not report an adverse event [57], while no adverse events were reported in the other mindful exercise intervention studies.

Table 1. Characteristics of randomized controlled trials in the meta-analysis.

Study	Participants		Intervention Protocol				Outcome Measured	Safety
	Sample Size	MA (years)	Mindful Exercise (Qualified Instructor)	Control	DR (wk)	Control Type	Pain and Disability	Adverse Events
Hall et al., (2011) [41]	160 CLBP TC = 80; C = 80	44	2 × 40 min/wk, TC	Wait-list	10	Passive	Pain intensity (NRS), disability (RMDQ)	No adverse event
Blödt et al., (2015) [42]	127 CLBP QG = 64; C = 63	47	1 × 90 min/wk, QG	1 × 60 min/wk Strengthening	12	Active	Pain intensity (VAS), disability (RMDQ)	No adverse event
Teut et al., (2016) [43]	176 CLBP QG = 58; YG = 61 C = 57	73	1 × 90 min/wk, QG; 2 × 45 min/wk, YG	Waitlist	12	Passive	Pain intensity (VAS)	No adverse event
Phattharasupharerk et al., (2018) [44]	72 CLBP QG = 36; C = 36	35	1 × 60 min/wk plus daily practice, YG	Waitlist	6	Passive	Pain intensity (VAS), disability (RMDQ)	No adverse event
Liu et al., (2019) [45]	43 CLBP TC = 15; C1 = 15; C2 = 13	74	3 × 60 min/wk, TC	C1: Core training C2: No intervention	12	C1: Active C2: Passive	Pain intensity (VAS)	No adverse event
Galantino et al., (2004) [46]	22 CLBP YG = 11; C = 11	30–65	2 × 60 min/wk plus 7 × 60 min/wk (home), YG	No treatment	6	Passive	disability (ODI) Depression (BDI)	No adverse event
Sherman et al., (2005) [47]	101 CLBP YG = 36; C1 = 35; C2 = 30	44	1 × 75 min/wk plus daily practice (home), YG	C1: 1 × 75min/wk + Daily practice, aerobic exercises and strength exercise C2: Self-care book	12	C1: Active C2: Passive	disability (RMDQ)	No adverse event
Williams et al., (2005) [48]	60 CLBP YG = 30; C = 30	48	1 × 90 min/wk plus 5 × 30 min/wk (home), YG	Newsletters on back pain	16	Passive	Pain intensity (VAS), disability (ODI)	1 participant diagnosed with a herniated disc in YG
Tekur et al., (2008) [49]	80 CLBP YG = 40; C = 40	48	7 × 120 min/wk, YG	Daily physical movements + education	1	Active	disability (ODI)	No adverse event
Williams et al., (2009) [50]	90 CLBP YG = 43; C = 47	48	2 × 90 min/wk plus 7 × 30 min/wk (home), YG	Waitlist	24	Passive	Pain intensity (VAS), disability (ODI)	No adverse event
Saper et al., (2009) [51]	30 CLBP YG = 15; C = 15	44	1 × 75 min/wk plus 7 × 30 min/wk (home), YG	Self-care book	12	Passive	Pain intensity (VAS), disability (RMDQ)	No adverse event
Cox et al., (2010) [52]	20 CLBP YG = 10; C = 10	45	1 × 75 min/wk plus home practice, YG	Self-care book	12	Passive	Pain intensity (ABPS), disability (RMDQ)	No adverse event
Tilbrook et al., (2011) [53]	313 CLBP YG = 156; C = 157	46	1 × 75min/wk plus 7 × 30 min/wk (home), YG	Self-care book	12	Passive	Pain intensity (ABPS), disability (RMDQ)	8 participants (increased pain) in YG
Sherman et al., (2011) [54]	228 CLBP YG = 92; C1 = 9 1; C2 = 45	48	1 × 75 min/wk plus 6 × 20 min/wk (home),YG	C1: 1 × 75min/wk + 20 min/wk (home) Stretching exercise C2: Self-care book	12	C1: Active C2: Passive	Pain intensity (NRS) disability (RMDQ)	13 participants (increased pain) and 1 herniated disc in yoga
Nambi et al., (2014) [55]	60 CLBP YG = 30; C = 30	44	1 × 60 min/wk plus 5 × 30 min/wk (home), YG	35days/wk, Exercise (strengthening and stretching)	4	Active	Pain intensity (VAS)	1 herniated disc in YG
Saper et al., (2017) [56]	320 CLBP YG = 127; C1 = 129; C2 = 64	46	1 × 75 min/wk plus 7 × 30 min/wk (home), YG	C1: 1 x 60min/wk, PT (stabilization and aerobic exercise) C2: Self-care book	12	C1: Active C2: Passive	Pain intensity (NRS) disability (RMDQ)	9 and 14 participants (mild self-limited joint and back pain) in YG and PT, respectively
Kuvačić et al., (2018) [57]	30 CLBP YG = 15; C = 15	34	2 × 75 min/wk, YG	Pamphlet program	8	Passive	Pain intensity (NRS), disability (ODI), depression (SDS)	Not reported

Note: TC = Tai Chi; YG = Yoga; QG = Qigong; PT = Physical therapy; = control group; MA = mean age; wk = week; DR = duration; CLBP = Chronic lower back pain; VAS = Visual Analog Scale; NRS = Numeric Rating Scale; ABPS = Aberdeen Back Pain Scale; ODI = Oswestry Disability Index; RMDQ = Roland–Morris Disability Questionnaire; Self-care book refers to reading *The Back Pain Book*, which emphasizing self-care management strategies for low back pain such as the causes of back pain and advice on exercising, appropriate lifestyle modification, and guidelines for managing flare-up; Pamphlet program refers to knowledge about vertebral spine and its biomechanical aspects; BDI = Beck depression inventory; SDS = Zung self-rating depression scale.

3.3. Study Quality Assessment

Study quality for each evaluated experiment is summarized in Table 2. Overall, the included studies demonstrated good quality (6–8 points). Notably, no studies implemented subject blinding or therapist blinding, and only one study [56] adopted assessor blinding. Concealed allocation was conducted in 40% of the studies, and four studies did not use intention-to-treat analysis [48–50,55].

Table 2. Methodological quality of the included studies (PEDro assessment).

Study	Score	Methodological Quality	PEDro Item Number										
			1	2	3	4	5	6	7	8	9	10	11
Hall et al., 2011 [41]	8	Good	✔	✔	✔	✔				✔	✔	✔	✔
Blödt et al., 2015 [42]	8	Good	✔	✔	✔	✔				✔	✔	✔	✔
Teut et al., 2016 [43]	8	Good	✔	✔	✔	✔				✔	✔	✔	✔
Phattharasupharerk et al., 2018 [44]	7	Good	✔	✔		✔				✔	✔	✔	✔
Liu et al., 2019 [45]	7	Good	✔	✔		✔				✔	✔	✔	✔
Galantino et al., 2004 [46]	7	Good	✔	✔		✔				✔	✔	✔	✔
Sherman et al., 2005 [47]	8	Good	✔	✔	✔	✔				✔	✔	✔	✔
Williams et al., 2005 [48]	6	Good	✔	✔		✔				✔		✔	✔
Tekur et al., 2008 [49]	7	Good	✔	✔	✔	✔				✔		✔	✔
Williams et al., 2009 [50]	6	Good	✔	✔		✔				✔		✔	✔
Saper et al., 2009 [51]	8	Good	✔	✔	✔	✔				✔	✔	✔	✔
Cox et al., 2010 [52]	8	Good	✔	✔	✔	✔				✔	✔	✔	✔
Tilbrook et al., 2011 [53]	8	Good	✔	✔	✔	✔				✔	✔	✔	✔
Sherman et al., 2011 [54]	8	Good	✔	✔	✔	✔				✔	✔	✔	✔
Nambi et al., 2014 [55]	6	Good	✔	✔		✔				✔		✔	✔
Saper et al., 2017 [56]	9	Excellent	✔	✔	✔	✔			✔	✔	✔	✔	✔
Kuvačić et al., 2018 [57]	7	Good	✔	✔		✔				✔	✔	✔	✔
Studies were classified as having excellent (9–10), good (6–8), fair (4–5) or poor (<4)													

Scale of item score: ✔, present. The PEDro scale criteria are (1) eligibility criteria; (2) random allocation; (3) concealed allocation; (4) similarity at baseline on key measures; (5) subject blinding; (6) therapist blinding; (7) assessor blinding; (8) more than 85% follow-up of at least one key outcome; (9) intention-to-treat analysis; (10) between-group statistical comparison for at least one key outcome; and (11) point estimates and measures of variability provided for at least one key outcome.

3.4. Meta-Analysis of Outcome Measured

3.4.1. Pain Intensity

There were 15 studies (18 pairs of intervention vs. control comparisons since three studies [43,54,56] included two control conditions) on pain intensity, measured by three different self-reported scales (Visual Analog Scale (VAS), Numeric Rating Scale (NRS), and Aberdeen Back Pain Scale (ABPS)). Based on the asymmetrical Funnel plot and the Egger's Regression test (Egger's regression intercept = −3.78, $p < 0.01$), we removed four comparisons [44,45,55,57] and the remaining studies showed a symmetrical Funnel plot (Figure 2) with Eggers test intercept = −1.54, $p = 0.16$. For the meta-analysis of 11 studies (14 comparisons), compared with the control groups, a significant benefit on reducing pain intensity was observed in favor of mindful exercises ($SMD = -0.37$, 95% CI −0.5 to −0.23, $p < 0.001$, $I^2 = 45.9\%$; Figure 3). Furthermore, we performed sub-group analyses and meta-regression for categorical variables (control type, type of mindful exercise, type of instrument, and use of allocation concealment) and continuous variables (mean age and total time). We observed significantly different effects on pain intensity across different types of mindful exercise ($Q = 8.46$, $p = 0.01$), with Tai Chi ($SMD = -0.75$, 95% CI −1.05 to −0.46, $p < 0.001$) and Yoga ($SMD = -0.33$, 95% CI −0.47 to −0.19, $p < 0.001$) showing significantly decreased pain intensity, but Qigong exercise did not demonstrate such an effect ($SMD = -0.21$, 95% CI −0.48 to 0.06, $p = 0.12$) (Table 3).

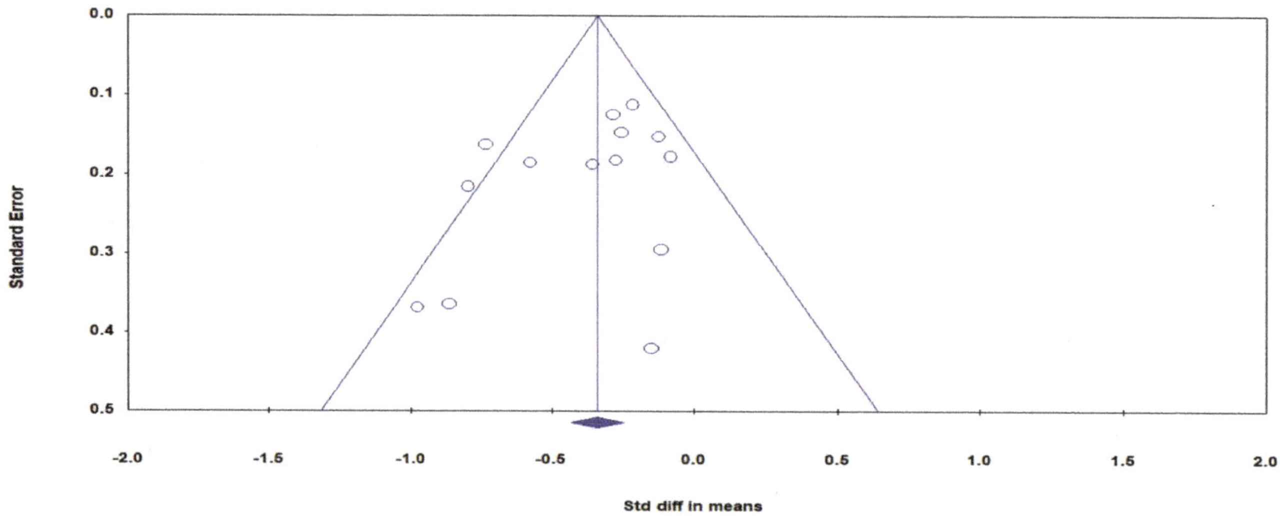

Figure 2. Funnel plot of publication bias for pain intensity.

Study name	Std diff in means	Standard error	Variance	Lower limit	Upper limit	Z-Value	p-Value
	Statistics for each study						
Teut 2016 YG vs WL	-0.27	0.18	0.03	-0.63	0.09	-1.49	0.14
Teut 2016 QG vs WL	-0.35	0.19	0.04	-0.72	0.01	-1.88	0.06
Liu 2019 TC vs CT	-0.86	0.36	0.13	-1.57	-0.15	-2.36	0.02
Saper 2009	-0.98	0.37	0.14	-1.70	-0.25	-2.65	0.01
Williams 2005	-0.11	0.30	0.09	-0.69	0.47	-0.38	0.70
Williams 2009	-0.80	0.22	0.05	-1.22	-0.37	-3.69	0.00
Hall 2011	-0.73	0.16	0.03	-1.05	-0.41	-4.51	0.00
Blodt 2015	-0.08	0.18	0.03	-0.43	0.27	-0.45	0.65
Saper 2017 YG vs PT	-0.28	0.12	0.02	-0.53	-0.04	-2.25	0.02
Saper 2017 YG vs SB	-0.12	0.15	0.02	-0.42	0.18	-0.79	0.43
Cox 2010	-0.15	0.42	0.18	-0.97	0.68	-0.35	0.73
Tilbrook 2011	-0.21	0.11	0.01	-0.43	0.01	-1.88	0.06
Sherman 2011 YG vs SB	-0.57	0.19	0.03	-0.94	-0.21	-3.10	0.00
Sherman 2011 YG vs SE	-0.25	0.15	0.02	-0.54	0.04	-1.70	0.09
	-0.37	0.07	0.00	-0.50	-0.23	-5.31	0.00

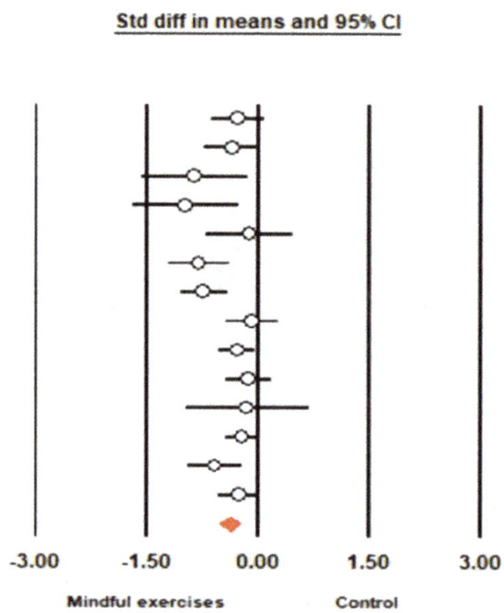

Figure 3. Effects of mindful exercises on pain intensity (YG = Yoga, WL = waitlist, TC = Tai Chi, CT = core training, QG = Qigong; PT = physical therapy, SB = self-care book; SE = stretching exercise). The red symbol represents the overall effect size in favor of mindful exercises.

3.4.2. Back-Specific Disability

Overall, there were 14 studies, including 17 pairs of mindful exercises vs. control comparisons (because three studies [47,54,56] included two control conditions, respectively), with disability measured by two different types of instruments (Roland–Morris Disability Questionnaire (RMDQ) and Oswestry Disability Index (ODI)). Based on the asymmetrical Funnel plot, we removed three outlying studies [47,49,51] and the remaining studies showed a symmetrical Funnel plot (Figure 4) with Eggers test intercept = –0.42, $p = 0.53$. For the meta-analysis in 12 studies (14 pairs of mindful exercises vs. control comparisons), compared with the control groups, the aggregated result showed a significant benefit in favor of mindful exercises on reducing disability (*SMD* = –0.39, 95% CI –0.49 to –0.28,

$p < 0.001$, $I^2 = 0\%$; Figure 5). We performed sub-group analyses and meta-regression for categorical variables (control type, type of mindful exercise, type of instrument, and use of allocation concealment) and continuous variables (mean age and total time) (Table 3). No significant differences were observed.

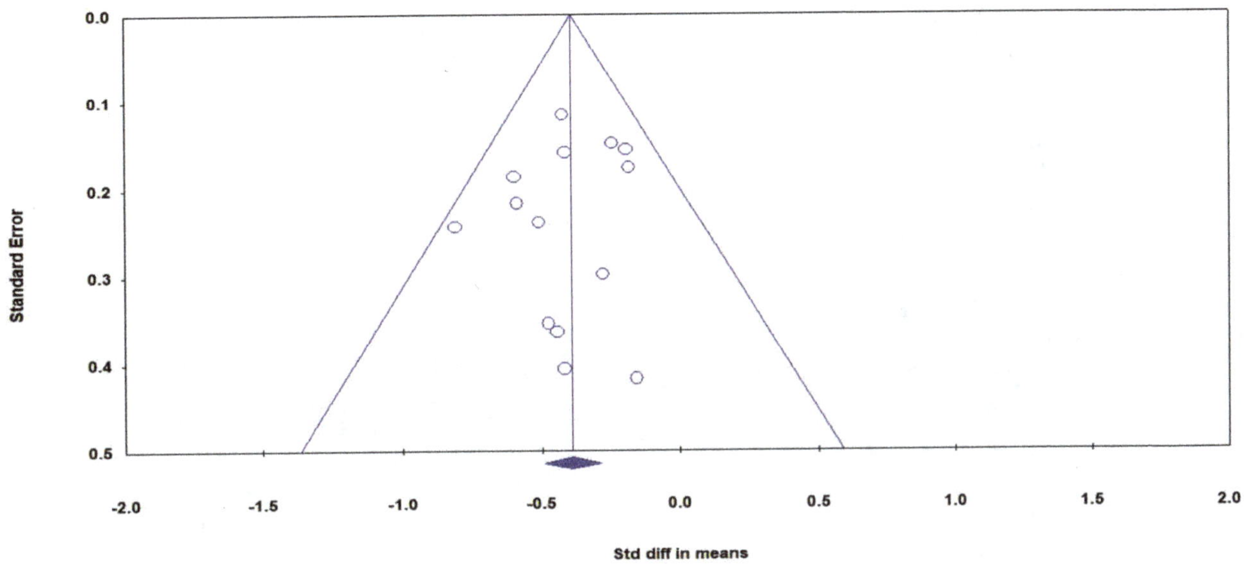

Figure 4. Funnel plot of publication bias for disability.

Study name	Std diff in means	Standard error	Variance	Lower limit	Upper limit	Z-Value	p-Value
Phattharasupharerk 2018	-0.81	0.24	0.06	-1.29	-0.33	-3.32	0.00
Hall 2011	-0.41	0.16	0.02	-0.72	-0.10	-2.61	0.01
Blodt 2015	-0.18	0.18	0.03	-0.52	0.16	-1.03	0.30
Cox 2010	-0.16	0.42	0.17	-0.97	0.66	-0.38	0.71
Sherman 2005 YG vs ASE	-0.51	0.24	0.06	-0.97	-0.04	-2.14	0.03
Tilbrook 2011	-0.42	0.11	0.01	-0.65	-0.20	-3.67	0.00
Saper 2009	-0.44	0.36	0.13	-1.15	0.27	-1.22	0.22
Saper 2017 YG vs SB	-0.19	0.16	0.02	-0.50	0.11	-1.23	0.22
Sherman 2011 YG vs SB	-0.24	0.15	0.02	-0.53	0.05	-1.64	0.10
Sherman 2011 YG vs SE	-0.60	0.19	0.03	-0.96	-0.23	-3.21	0.00
Galantino 2004	-0.42	0.41	0.16	-1.21	0.38	-1.02	0.31
Williams 2005	-0.27	0.30	0.09	-0.86	0.31	-0.92	0.36
Williams 2009	-0.59	0.22	0.05	-1.01	-0.16	-2.71	0.01
Kuvacic 2018	-0.47	0.35	0.13	-1.17	0.22	-1.34	0.18
	-0.39	0.05	0.00	-0.49	-0.28	-7.36	0.00

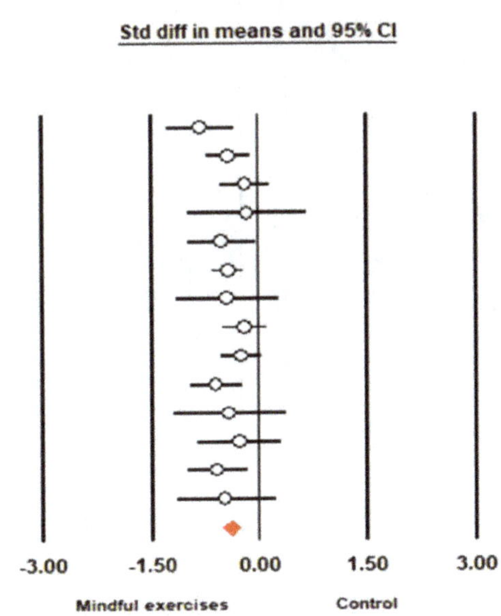

Figure 5. The effect of mindful exercises on disability (YG = Yoga, ASE = Aerobic and strength exercise, SB = self-care book, SE = stretching exercise).The red symbol below represents the overall effect size in favor of mindful exercises.

Table 3. The effect of mind-body exercise in moderator analysis.

Categorical Moderator	Outcome	Covariates	No. of Studies/Comparisons	SMD	95% Confidence Interval	I^2%	Test for Between-Group Hoterogeneity		
							Q-Value	df(*Q*)	*p*-Value
Control Type	Pain intensity	Active	7	−0.40	-0.48 to -0.20	53.2 %	0.08	1	0.78
		Passive	7	-0.35	−0.46 to −0.21	46.5%			
	Disability	Active	4	−0.28	−0.47 to −0.09	0%	1.62	1	0.20
		Passive	10	−0.43	−0.55 to −0.31	0%			
Mindful Type	Pain intensity	Yoga	10	−0.33	−0.47 to −0.19	33.7%	8.46	2	0.01*
		TC	2	−0.75	−1.05 to −0.46	0%			
		Qigong	2	−0.21	−0.48 to 0.06	10.0%			
	Disability	Yoga	11	−0.38	−0.50 to −0.26	0%	0.16	2	0.92
		TC	1	−0.41	−0.72 to −0.10	0%			
		Qigong	2	−0.47	−1.09 to 0.14	77.2%			
Instruments	Pain intensity	ABPS	2	−0.21	−0.42 to 0.01	0%	2.1	2	0.35
		VAS	7	−0.43	−0.68 to −0.18	50.5%			
		NRS	5	−0.38	−0.59 to −0.17	60.1%			
	Disability	RMDQ	10	−0.38	−0.49 to −0.27	0%	0.36	1	0.55
		ODI	4	−0.47	−0.76 to −0.18	0%			
Allocation Concealment	Pain intensity	Yes	11	−0.33	−0.46 to −0.19	39.5%	1.19	1	0.28
		No	3	−0.59	1.05 to −0.13	50.9%			
	Disability	Yes	9	−0.35	−0.46 to −0.24	0%	2.27	1	0.13
		No	5	−0.56	−0.80 to −0.31	0%			
Continuous moderator	**Outcome**	**No. of studies/comparisons**	β		**95% Confidence Interval**		***Q*-value**	**df(*Q*)**	***p*-value**
Age	Pain intensity	14	−0.00108		−0.01080 to 0.00865		0.05	1	0.83
	Disability	14	0.02454		−0.00706 to 0.05614		2.32	1	0.13
Total Time	Pain intensity	14	0.00002		−0.00007 to 0.00012		0.22	1	0.64
	Disability	14	−0.00002		−0.00012 to 0.00009		0.10	1	0.75

VAS = Visual Analog Scale; RMDQ = Roland-Morris Disability Questionnaire; SMD = Standardized Mean Difference; TC = Tai Chi; * $p < 0.01$.

4. Discussion

Mindful exercises are increasingly accepted by clinicians worldwide as an alternative therapy for chronic disease symptomatic management. To the best of our knowledge, this is the first systematic review to comprehensively evaluate the existing literature regarding the safety and pain- and disease-specific effects of three commonly practiced mindful exercises (Tai Chi, Qigong, and Yoga) among adults with CLBP. Our findings indicated that mindful exercises may be effective in reducing pain intensity and disability among CLBP patients. More importantly, the beneficial effects of mindful exercises were observed comparing to both non-active and active controls. Notably, several Yoga interventions induced varied adverse events (e.g., injury).

4.1. Pain Intensity

Overall, mindful exercises may be effective in reducing pain intensity level, with a small intervention effect ($SMD = -0.37$). However, we observed non-significant effects on this outcome in five comparisons [42,43,48,51,52] and marginally significant effects in three comparisons [43,47,53]. Such results may be attributed to inadequacy of weekly instructor-led training time (75 to 90 min) [42,43,47,53], relatively small sample size [48,51,52] (20 to 60 participants), and/or direct comparison to active controls (strengthening or stretching exercise) [42,47]. When compared with an active control alone, mindful exercises showed significantly reduced pain intensity ($SMD = -0.40$, $p < 0.001$). This suggests that mindful exercise may be more beneficial for pain management than conventional exercise (strengthening and/or stretching exercise) and guideline-endorsed (core training or physical therapy) programs. Furthermore, results from the sub-group analyses indicated that, when compared to Yoga and Qigong, Tai Chi appeared to have a superior effect on pain relief. Such positive intervention effects reached a moderate level ($SMD = -0.75$). Tai Chi emphasizes neutral spine or standing with upright posture during performance, providing an opportunity to strengthen core muscles (similar to a guideline-endorsed core training program) to reduce pain intensity. Additionally, a previous RCT by Hall [58] indicated that Tai Chi can reduce pain-catastrophizing, which partially mediates the effect of Tai Chi on pain intensity among adults with CLBP. Conversely, adverse events (increased pain, reduced range of motion at joints, and/or herniated disc) were reported in several Yoga intervention studies but not in Tai Chi studies. This is likely due to the Yoga routine, which involves movements of bending forward and backwards at the low back, which may initiate or exacerbate pain intensity. Taken together, Tai Chi may be a more suitable mindful exercise in rehabilitation programs for CLBP rather than Yoga.

4.2. Back-Specific Disability

In this meta-analysis, we observed a small overall positive effect (SMD = −0.39) of mindful exercise on disability. Of the 12 studies (including 14 comparisons), six comparisons (Qigong vs. waitlist, Tai Chi vs. waitlist, Yoga vs. aerobic plus strength exercises, Yoga vs. Waitlist, Yoga vs. self-care book, Yoga vs. stretching exercise, and Yoga vs. waitlist) [41,44,47,50,53,54] showed significant effects on CLBP-specific disability, whereas the other eight [42,46,48,51,52,54,56,57] demonstrated positive effects. Throughout the 12-week intervention period, weekly instructor-based training length ranged from 75 to 90 min in Qigong [42] and Yoga [54,56], which may not be sufficient to achieve significant reductions in disability risk. Notably, Neiyanggong, as one type of Qigong exercise, is not as popular as Baduanjin and Wuqinxi Qigong. Thus, it presumably takes beginners much longer to understand the principle and movement concepts, particularly during the initial stage of motor learning (cognitive stage) [59]. A 90-min session per week during a 12-week Neiyanggong intervention may not be sufficient to maximize the potential benefits of this modality of exercise. Likewise, movements in Yoga routine are relatively complex and require a certified instructor, and self-practice at home may lead to incorrect movement patterns, which may have contributed to the deterioration in disability or caused the observed adverse events (increased pain, herniated disc, and/or reduced range of motion at joints) reported in the five Yoga intervention studies [48,53–56]. Second, three studies included relatively small sample sizes of 20 [52], 30 [51] and 60 participants [48], which may have affected the power of detecting significant differences on disability risk.

4.3. Strengths and Limitations for Future Research

Strengths of this systematic review are as follows: (1) we provide a comprehensive review regarding the effectiveness of mindful exercises on CLBP disease-specific symptoms; (2) we were the first to include three popular mindful exercises; (3) we compared mindful exercises with active controls (conventional exercises and guideline-endorsed physical therapy); and (4) we evaluated the safety of mindful exercises in adults with CLBP [60,61]. Several limitations should be considered: (1) this review only included English-language studies, which possibly excluded Chinese-language journals that may be more likely to publish Tai Chi and Qigong studies; (2) we limited our meta-analysis to pain intensity and disability. We were not able to meta-analyze data on depressive symptomology (and other related outcomes) due to fewer than four studies reporting data on this outcome. Thus, future studies should include psychological outcome measures; (3) blinding of assessors was only used in one study (blinding of instructor and participants are, however, unrealistic), and it remains unclear whether greater expectations were associated with reduced pain intensity and disability in the mindful exercise groups; (4) some studies did not use "intention to treat analysis" and "allocation concealment", which possibly overestimated the pooled effect size; (5) none of studies used follow-up assessments, so it is difficult to determine how long the beneficial effects of mindful exercise interventions lasted in adults with CLBP; (6) previous studies suggest that different brain mechanisms are associated with different mindful exercises, thus, future studies should comparatively investigate different mind-body exercises as well as their underlying mechanisms [62,63].

5. Conclusions

Findings of our systematic review suggest that mindful exercises (Yoga, Tai Chi, and Qigong) may be beneficial for CLBP symptomatic management, irrespective of non-control comparison or active control comparison (conventional exercises, core training, and physical therapy programs). The potential of Tai Chi as a routine non-pharmacological approach for CLBP needs to be rigorously evaluated in future studies. Importantly, training in these mindful exercises should be implemented with certified instructors, to ensure quality of movement and injury prevention. Before definitive conclusions can be drawn, future work is needed that employs more robust study designs and implements long-term follow-up assessments.

Author Contributions: L.Z., Y.J.Z., A.Y., K.W.C., L.Y., P.D.L., T.X., and H.L. contributed to the conception and design of the review. Y.J.Z. and L.Z. applied the search strategy. L.Z. and Y.J.Z. applied the selection criteria. L.Z., Y.J.Z. and H.L. completed assessment of risk of bias. All authors analyzed and interpreted the data. All authors wrote this manuscript. All authors edited this manuscript. L.Z., Y.J.Z., T.X., and H.K. are responsible for the overall project.

Acknowledgments: The leading author would like to thank his family members (wife, son, daughter, and parents) for their consistent support.

References

1. Shmagel, A.; Foley, R.; Ibrahim, H. Epidemiology of chronic low back pain in US adults: Data from the 2009–2010 national health and nutrition examination survey. *Arthritis Care Res.* **2016**, *68*, 1688–1694. [CrossRef]
2. Murray, C.J.; Atkinson, C.; Bhalla, K.; Birbeck, G.; Burstein, R. The state of US health, 1990–2010: Burden of diseases, injuries, and risk factors. *JAMA* **2013**, *310*, 591–608. [CrossRef]

3. Taimela, S.; Kujala, U.M.; Salminen, J.J.; Viljanen, T. The prevalence of low back pain among children and adolescents: A nationwide, cohort-based questionnaire survey in Finland. *Spine* **1997**, *22*, 1132–1136. [CrossRef] [PubMed]
4. Balague, F.; Troussier, B.; Salminen, J.J. Non-specific low back pain in children and adolescents: Risk factors. *Eur. Spine J.* **1999**, *8*, 429–438. [CrossRef]
5. Richard, G.; David, W. The Adult Spine: Principles and Practice-Second Edition. *Neurosurgery* **1997**, *41*, 1208–1209. [CrossRef]
6. Enthoven, W.; Roelofs, P.; Deyo, R. Non-steroidal anti-inflammatory drugs for chronic low back pain. *Cochrane Database Syst. Rev.* **2016**, *2*, 012087. [CrossRef] [PubMed]
7. Marquardt, K.A.; Alsop, J.A.; Albertson, T.E. Tramadol exposures reported to statewide poison control system. *Ann. Pharmacother.* **2005**, *39*, 1039–1044. [CrossRef] [PubMed]
8. Shipton, E.A. Physical Therapy Approaches in the Treatment of Low Back Pain. *Pain Ther.* **2018**, *7*, 127–137. [CrossRef] [PubMed]
9. Burns, S.A.; Cleland, J.A.; Rivett, D.A.; Snodgrass, S.J. Effectiveness of physical therapy interventions for low back pain targeting the low back only or low back plus hips: A randomized controlled trial protocol. *Braz. J. Phys. Ther.* **2018**, *22*, 424–430. [CrossRef]
10. Cuenca-Martínez, F.; Cortés-Amador, S.; Espí-López, G.V. Effectiveness of classic physical therapy proposals for chronic non-specific low back pain: A literature review. *Phys. Ther. Res.* **2018**, *21*, 16–22. [CrossRef]
11. Searle, A.; Spink, M.; Ho, A.; Chuter, V. Exercise interventions for the treatment of chronic low back pain: A systematic review and meta-analysis of randomised controlled trials. *Clin. Rehabil.* **2015**, *29*, 1155–1167. [CrossRef] [PubMed]
12. Gordon, R.; Bloxham, S. A Systematic Review of the Effects of Exercise and Physical Activity on Non-Specific Chronic Low Back Pain. *Healthcare* **2016**, *4*, 22. [CrossRef]
13. Miyamoto, G.C.; Lin, C.C.; Cabral, C.M.; Van-Dongen, J.M.; Van-Tulder, M.W. Costeffectiveness of exercise therapy in the treatment of non-specific neck pain and low back pain: A systematic review with meta-analysis. *Br. J. Sports Med.* **2019**, *53*, 172–181. [CrossRef] [PubMed]
14. Zhou, S.; Zhang, Y.; Kong, Z.; Loprinzi, P.D.; Hu, Y.; Ye, J.; Liu, S.; Yu, J.J.; Zou, L. The Effects of tai chi on markers of atherosclerosis, lower-limb physical function, and cognitive ability in adults aged over 60: A randomized controlled trial. *Int. J. Environ. Res. Public Health* **2019**, *16*, 753. [CrossRef] [PubMed]
15. Zou, L.; Zeng, N.; Huang, T.; Yeung, A.S.; Wei, G.X.; Liu, S.J.; Zhou, J.; Hu, R.; Hui, S.S. The Beneficial Effects of Mind-body Exercises for People with Mild Cognitive Impairment: A Systematic Review with Meta-Analysis. *Arch. Phys. Med. Rehabil.* **2019**, in press. [CrossRef] [PubMed]
16. Zou, L.; Sasaki, J.E.; Wei, G.-X.; Huang, T.; Yeung, A.S.; Neto, O.B.; Chen, K.W.; Hui, S.C. Effects of mind–body exercises (Tai Chi/Yoga) on heart rate variability parameters and perceived stress: A systematic review with meta-analysis of randomized controlled trials. *J. Clin. Med.* **2018**, *7*, 404. [CrossRef] [PubMed]
17. Zou, L.; Yeung, A.; Li, C.; Wei, G.; Chen, K.; Kinser, P.; Chan, J.; Ren, Z. Effects of meditative movements on major depressive disorder: A systematic Review and meta-analysis of randomized controlled trials. *J. Clin. Med.* **2018**, *7*, 195. [CrossRef] [PubMed]
18. Zou, L.; Han, J.; Tsang, W.; Yeung, A. Effects of Tai Chi on lower limb proprioception in adults aged over 55: A systematic review ad meta-analysis. *Arch. Phys. Med. Rehabil.* **2018**, in press. [CrossRef]
19. Zou, L.; Sasaki, J.; Zeng, N.; Wang, C.; Sun, L.A. Systematic Review with Meta-Analysis of Mindful Exercises on Rehabilitative Outcomes among post-stroke patients. *Arch. Phys. Med. Rehabil.* **2018**, *9*, 2355–2364. [CrossRef] [PubMed]
20. Zou, L.; Yeung, A.; Li, C.; Chiou, S.; Zeng, N.; Tzeng, H. Effects of mind-body movement on balance function in stroke survivors: A meta-analysis of randomized controlled trials. *Int. J. Environ. Res. Public Health* **2018**, *15*, 1292. [CrossRef]
21. Zou, L.; Yeung, A.; Zeng, N.; Wang, C.; Sun, L.; Thomas, G.; Wang, H. Effects of Mind-Body Exercises for Mood and Functional Capabilities in Post-Stroke Patients: An Analytical Review of Randomized Controlled Trials. *Int. J. Environ. Res. Public Health* **2018**, *15*, 721. [CrossRef]
22. Zou, L.; Wang, C.; Tian, Z.; Wang, H.; Shu, Y. Effect of Yang-Style Tai Chi on Gait Parameters and Musculoskeletal Flexibility in Healthy Chinese Older Women. *Sports* **2017**, *5*, 52. [CrossRef]

23. Zhang, Y.; Loprinzi, P.D.; Yang, L.; Liu, J.; Liu, S.; Zou, L. The Beneficial Effects of Traditional Chinese Exercises for Adults with Low Back Pain: A Meta-Analysis of Randomized Controlled Trials. *Medicina* **2019**, *55*, 118. [CrossRef] [PubMed]
24. Zou, L.; Albert, Y.; Quan, X.; Wang, H. A Systematic review and meta-analysis of mindfulness-based (Baduanjin) exercise for alleviating musculoskeletal pain and improving sleep quality in people with chronic diseases. *Int. J. Environ. Res. Public Health* **2018**, *15*, 206. [CrossRef] [PubMed]
25. Zou, L.; SasaKi, J.; Wang, H.; Xiao, Z.; Fang, Q.; Zhang, M. A Systematic Review and Meta-Analysis Baduanjin Qigong for Health Benefits: Randomized Controlled Trials. *Evid. Based Complement. Altern. Med.* **2017**, *2017*. [CrossRef] [PubMed]
26. Zou, L.; Wang, H.; Xiao, Z.; Fang, Q.; Zhang, M.; Li, T. Tai chi for health benefits in patients with multiple sclerosis: A systematic review. *PLoS ONE* **2017**, *12*, e0170212. [CrossRef] [PubMed]
27. Zou, L.; Xiao, Z.; Wang, H.; Wang, C.; Hu, X.; Shu, Y. Asian martial arts for Children with Autism Spectrum Disorder: A Systematic Review. *Arch. Budo* **2017**, *13*, 79–92.
28. Zou, L.; Wang, H.; Yu, D. Effect of a long-term modified Tai Chi-based intervention in attenuating bone mineral density in postmenopausal women in southeast China: Study protocol for a randomized controlled trial. *Clin. Trials Degener. Dis.* **2017**, *2*, 46–52.
29. Zou, L.; Wang, C.; Chen, K.; Shu, Y.; Chen, X.; Luo, L.; Zhao, X. The effect of Taichi practice on attenuating bone mineral density loss: A systematic review and meta-analysis of randomized controlled trials. *Int. J. Environ. Res. Public Health* **2017**, *14*, 1000. [CrossRef]
30. Zou, L.; Wang, H.; Li, T.; Lu, L. Effect of traditional Chinese mind-body exercise on disease activity, spinal mobility, and quality of life in patients with ankylosing spondylitis. *Trav. Hum.* **2017**, *80*, 1585–1597.
31. Zou, L.; Wang, C.; Yeung, A.; Liu, Y.; Pan, Z. A Review Study on the beneficial effects of baduanjin. *J. Altern. Complement. Med.* **2018**, *24*, 324–335. [CrossRef] [PubMed]
32. Zou, L.; Yeung, A.; Quan, X. Mindfulness-based baduanjin exercise for depression and anxiety in people with physical or mental illnesses: A systematic review and meta-analysis of randomized controlled trials. *Int. J. Environ. Res. Public Health* **2018**, *15*, 321. [CrossRef]
33. Zou, L.; Wang, C.; Chen, X.; Wang, H. Baduanjin Exercise for Stroke Rehabilitation: A Systematic Review with Meta-Analysis of Randomized Controlled Trials. *Int. J. Environ. Res. Public Health* **2018**, *15*, 600. [CrossRef] [PubMed]
34. Theadom, A.; Cropley, M.; Smith, H.E.; Feigin, V.L.; Mcpherson, K. Mind and body therapy for fibromyalgia. *Cocrane Database Syst. Rev.* **2015**, *9*, CD001980. [CrossRef] [PubMed]
35. Selfe, T.K.; Innes, K.E. Mind-body therapies and osteoarthritis of the knee. *Curr. Rheumatol. Rev.* **2009**, *5*, 204–211. [CrossRef]
36. Holtzman, S.; Beggs, R.T. Yoga for chronic low back pain: A meta-analysis of randomized controlled trials. *Pain Res. Manag.* **2013**, *18*, 267–272. [CrossRef]
37. Cramer, H.; Lauche, R.; Haller, H.; Dobos, G. A systematic review and meta-analysis of yoga for low back pain. *Clin. J. Pain* **2013**, *29*, 450–460. [CrossRef]
38. Treede, R.D.; Rief, W.; Barke, A.; Aziz, Q.; Bennett, M.; Benoliel, R.; Wang, S.J. Chronic pain as a symptom or a disease: The IASP classification of chronic pain for the international classification of disease (ICD-11). *Pain* **2019**, *160*, 19–27. [CrossRef]
39. Maher, C.; Sherrington, C.; Herbert, R.; Moseley, A.; Elkins, M. Reliability of the PEDro scale for rating quality of randomized controlled trials. *Phys. Ther.* **2003**, *83*, 713–721. [CrossRef] [PubMed]
40. Higgins, J.P.; Green, S. *Cochrane Handbook for Systematic Reviews of Interventions*; John Wiley & Sons: New York, NY, USA, 2011; ISBN 9780470057964.
41. Hall, A.M.; Maher, C.G.; Lam, P.; Ferreira, M.; Latimer, J. Tai chi exercise for treatment of pain and disability in people with persistent low back pain: A randomized controlled trial. *Arthritis Care Res.* **2011**, *63*, 1576–1583. [CrossRef]
42. Blödt, S.; Pach, D.; Kaster, T.; Lüdtke, R.; Icke, K.; Reisshauer, A.; Witt, C.M. Qigong versus exercise therapy for chronic low back pain in adults—A randomized controlled non-inferiority trial. *Eur. J. Pain (UK)* **2015**, *19*, 123–131. [CrossRef]
43. Teut, M.; Knilli, J.; Daus, D.; Roll, S.; Witt, C.M. Qigong or Yoga Versus No Intervention in Older Adults with Chronic Low Back Pain—A Randomized Controlled Trial. *J. Pain* **2016**, *17*, 796–805. [CrossRef]

44. Phattharasupharerk, S.; Purepong, N.; Eksakulkla, S.; Siriphorn, A. Effects of Qigong practice in office workers with chronic non-specific low back pain: A randomized control trial. *J. Bodyw. Mov. Ther.* **2018**. [CrossRef]
45. Liu, J.; Yeung, A.; Xiao, T.; Tian, X.; Kong, Z.; Zou, L.; Wang, X. Chen-Style Tai Chi for Individuals (Aged 50 Years Old or Above) with Chronic Non-Specific Low Back Pain: A Randomized Controlled Trial. *Int. J. Environ. Res. Public Health* **2019**, *16*, 517. [CrossRef]
46. Galantino, M.L.; Bzdewka, T.M.; Eissler-Russo, J.L.; Holbrook, M.L.; Mogck, E.P.; Geigle, P.; Farrar, J.T. The impact of modified hatha yoga on chronic low back pain: A pilot study. *Altern. Ther. Health Med.* **2004**, *10*, 56–59. [CrossRef]
47. Sherman, K.J.; Cherkin, D.C.; Erro, J.; Miglioretti, D.L.; Deyo, R.A. Comparing yoga, exercise, and a self-care book for chronic low back pain: A randomized, controlled trial. *Ann. Intern. Med.* **2005**, *143*, 849–856. [CrossRef] [PubMed]
48. Williams, K.A.; Petronis, J.; Smith, D.; Goodrich, D.; Wu, J.; Ravi, N.; Doyle, E.J.; Juckett, R.G.; Kolar, M.M.; Gross, R. Effect of Iyengar yoga therapy for chronic low back pain. *Pain* **2005**, *115*, 107–117. [CrossRef]
49. Tekur, P.; Singphow, C.; Nagendra, H.R.; Raghuram, N. Effect of Short-Term Intensive Yoga Program on Pain, Functional Disability and Spinal Flexibility in Chronic Low Back Pain: A Randomized Control Study. *J. Altern. Complement. Med.* **2008**, *14*, 637–644. [CrossRef]
50. Williams, K.; Ph, D.; Abildso, C.; Ph, D.; Steinberg, L.; Ph, D.; Doyle, E.; Epstein, B.; Pt, M.D.; Smith, D. Evaluation of the effectiveness and efficacy of Iyengar Yoga Therapy on Chronic Low Back Pain. *Spine* **2009**, *34*, 2066–2076. [CrossRef] [PubMed]
51. Saper, R.B.; Sherman, K.J.; Cullum-Dugan, D.; Davis, R.B.; Phillips, R.S.; Culpepper, L. Yoga for chronic low back pain in a predominantly minority population: A pilot randomized controlled trial. *Altern. Ther. Health Med.* **2009**, *15*, 18–27. [CrossRef]
52. Cox, H.; Torgerson, D.; Semlyen, A.; Tilbrook, H.; Watt, I.; Aplin, J.; Trewhela, A. A randomised controlled trial of yoga for the treatment of chronic low back pain: Results of a pilot study. *Complement. Ther. Clin. Pract.* **2010**, *16*, 187–193. [CrossRef]
53. Tilbrook, H.E.; Cox, H.; Hewitt, C.E.; Kangombe, A.R.; Chuang, L.H.; Jayakody, S.; Aplin, J.D. Yoga for Chronic Low Back Pain. *Ann. Intern. Med.* **2011**, *155*, 569–578. [CrossRef]
54. Sherman, K.J.; Cherkin, D.C.; Wellman, R.D.; Cook, A.J.; Hawkes, R.J.; Delaney, K.; Deyo, R.A. A randomized trial comparing yoga, stretching, and a self-care book for chronic low back pain. *Arch. Intern. Med.* **2011**, *171*, 2019–2026. [CrossRef] [PubMed]
55. Nambi, G.S.; Inbasekaran, D.; Khuman, R.; Devi, S. Changes in pain intensity and health related quality of life with Iyengar yoga in nonspecific chronic low back pain: A randomized controlled study. *Int. J. Yoga* **2014**, *7*, 48–53. [CrossRef] [PubMed]
56. Saper, R.B.; Lemaster, C.; Delitto, A.; Sherman, K.J.; Herman, P.M.; Sadikova, E.; Stevans, J.; Keosaian, J.E.; Cerrada, C.J.; Femia, A.L. Yoga, Physical Therapy, or Education for Chronic Low Back Pain. *Ann. Intern. Med.* **2017**, *167*, 85. [CrossRef] [PubMed]
57. Kuvačić, G.; Fratini, P.; Padulo, J.; Antonio, D.I.; De Giorgio, A. Effectiveness of yoga and educational intervention on disability, anxiety, depression, and pain in people with CLBP: A randomized controlled trial. *Complement. Ther. Clin. Pract.* **2018**, *31*, 262–267. [CrossRef]
58. Hall, A.M.; Kamper, S.J.; Emsley, R.; Maher, C.G. Does pain-catestrophising mediate the effects of tai Chi on treatment outcomes ofr people with low back pain? *Complement. Ther. Med.* **2016**, *25*, 61–66. [CrossRef] [PubMed]
59. Enghauser, R. Motor learning and the dance technique class: Science, tradition and pedagogy. *J. Dance Educ.* **2003**, *3*, 87–95. [CrossRef]
60. Wayne, P.M.; Berkowitz, D.L.; Litrownik, D.E.; Buring, J.E.; Yeh, G.Y. What do we really know about the safety of tai chi? A systematic review of adverse event reports in randomized trials. *Arch. Phys. Med. Rehabil.* **2014**, *95*, 2470–2483. [CrossRef]
61. Zou, L.; Zhang, Y.; Liu, Y.; Tian, X.; Xiao, T.; Liu, X.; Yeung, A.S.; Liu, J.; Wang, X. The effects of tai chi chuan versus core stability training on lower-limb neuromuscular function in aging individuals with non-specific chronic lower back pain. *Medicina* **2019**, *55*, 60. [CrossRef] [PubMed]

62. Liu, J.; Tao, J.; Liu, W.; Huang, J.; Xue, X.; Li, M.; Yang, M.; Zhu, J.; Lang, C.; Park, J.; et al. Different modulation effects of tai chi chuan and baduanjin on resting state functional connectivity of the default mode network in older adults. *Soc. Cogn. Affect. Neurosci.* **2019**, *14*, 217–224. [CrossRef] [PubMed]
63. Tao, J.; Chen, X.; Liu, J.; Egorova, N.; Xue, X.; Liu, W.; Zheng, G.; Li, M.; Wu, J.; Hu, K.; et al. Tai Chi Chuan and Baduanjin mind-body training changes resting-state low-frequency fluctuations in the frontal lobe of older adults: A resting-state fmri study. *Front. Hum. Neurosci.* **2017**, *11*, 514. [CrossRef] [PubMed]

6

Supporting Teens with Chronic Pain to Obtain High School Credits: Chronic Pain 35 in Alberta

Kathy Reid [1,2,*], Mark Simmonds [1,2], Michelle Verrier [2] and Bruce Dick [1,2]

1 Stollery Children's Hospital, Alberta Health Services, Edmonton, AB T6G 2B7, Canada; mark.simmonds@ualberta.ca (M.S.); bruce.dick@ualberta.ca (B.D.)
2 Department of Anaesthesiology and Pain Medicine, University of Alberta, Edmonton, AB T6G 2R3, Canada; mrheault@ualberta.ca
* Correspondence: Kathy.Reid@ahs.ca

Academic Editor: Carl L. von Baeyer

Abstract: Chronic pain is a significant problem in children and teens, and adolescents with chronic pain often struggle to attend school on a regular basis. We present in this article a novel program we developed that integrates attendance at a group cognitive-behavioural chronic pain self-management program with earning high school credits. We collaborated with Alberta Education in the development of this course, Chronic Pain 35. Adolescents who choose to enroll are invited to demonstrate their scientific knowledge related to pain, understanding of and engagement with treatment homework, and demonstrate their creativity by completing a project, which demonstrates at least one concept. Integrating Chronic Pain 35 into an adolescent's academic achievements is a creative strategy that facilitates the engagement of adolescents in learning and adopting pain coping techniques. It also helps teens to advocate for themselves in the school environment and improve their parents' and teachers' understanding of adolescent chronic pain. This is one of the first successful collaborations between a pediatric health program and provincial education leaders, aimed at integrating learning and obtaining school credit for learning about and engaging in health self-management for teens. The authors hope this paper serves as an effective reference model for any future collaborating programs aimed at supporting teens with chronic pain to obtain high school credits.

Keywords: chronic pain; adolescent; school; cognitive-behavioural therapy

1. Introduction

Chronic pain is a significant problem in the pediatric population. Chronic pain is defined as any prolonged pain that lasts longer than the expected healing time or any recurrent pain that occurs at least three times during a three-month period [1,2]. Common pain diagnoses in children and adolescents include headaches, chronic abdominal pain, back pain, and musculoskeletal pain [3]. The pain may result from a disease, injury, a trauma, or surgery. For a significant number of children, there are no identifiable causes for the reported pain. Increasingly, this type of pain is discussed as a result of neurobiological changes that result in pain syndromes including pain centralization and pain amplification [4,5]. Population studies demonstrate that 20%–35% of children and adolescents report symptoms meeting research definitions of chronic pain [1,2,6]. It is estimated that between 5%–8% of children with chronic pain will develop significant pain-related disability [7,8]. This pain-related disability is known to affect children's functioning including their ability to attend school on a regular basis [9]. These children often require an interdisciplinary team to help manage chronic pain and pain-related disability.

Research has demonstrated that adolescents with chronic pain report being less socially developed than their peers [10] and that they may avoid social situations with peers [11]. Lower social functioning can contribute to school impairment, and therefore having children socially connected to their peers can limit the detrimental effects on school functioning [12].

As mentioned, evidence demonstrates that children and adolescents with chronic pain often struggle to attend school on a regular basis [9]. In one study, 44% of students with chronic pain missed at least 25% of school days, and 20% missed more than one half of school days [13]. In addition, 44% of the students reported a decline in grades. A study comparing school absences of children with functional abdominal pain (FAP), inflammatory bowel disease (IBD), and healthy controls found that children with both IBD and FAP missed significantly more school than healthy controls [14]. In the Pediatric Pain Program at the Stollery Children's Hospital (Edmonton, AB, Canada), our records suggest that a majority of individuals presenting with chronic pain miss at least one half to two days per week on average, and approximately 15%–20% of adolescents are either no longer attending school on a regular basis or have stopped attending in person and complete their studies in a correspondence program. In addition, chronic pain is shown to affect children's cognitive function, but more research is required to determine the long-term effects of this cognitive dysfunction on the developmental trajectory of young people with chronic pain [15].

Given the prevalence of chronic pain, and the magnitude of its effects on adolescents' social development and school functioning, it is critical that teens be provided with the opportunity to continue to learn. Additionally, young people in our program report that it is important to their mental health and self-concept to make progress in their educational programming and pursuit of their school and life goals, despite experiencing ongoing pain. It is also important to maintain contact with a peer group, in order to support normal social adolescent development.

2. Managing Chronic Pain: Biopsychosocial Approach

Adolescents with chronic pain benefit from multimodal approaches to improve their function and return to regular activities, including school. Interventions that include the 3Ps—physical, psychological and pharmacological approaches—are more likely to be successful than single interventions. One of the most effective treatments for chronic pain is cognitive-behavioural therapy (CBT), which has been shown to be effective in managing headache, recurrent and functional abdominal pain in children [16], sickle cell disease [17], and juvenile fibromyalgia [18]. CBT strategies for chronic pain management address pain education, and teach active coping strategies such as relaxation and imagery, stress management, cognitive restructuring, goal setting, and relapse prevention [19]. Treatment approaches that enhance self-efficacy, or increase confidence to function despite pain, have been suggested as helpful for youth with headaches [20,21].

A group intervention for adolescents with chronic pain (n = 40) and their parents, called "Coping with Pain School" in Boston, MA, USA, by Logan and Simons [22] provided either four sessions of CBT or a day long CBT session aimed at improving school function. The study found the program was feasible, families who participated were satisfied with the program and school attendance improved after completion of the sessions; however, enrollment challenges were a significant problem identified by the authors in the study. They recommended the need to develop treatments focusing on school functioning and involving school personnel in future studies.

3. The Stollery Experience

The Pediatric Chronic Pain Program at the Stollery Children's Hospital opened in 2008, to provide treatment for children and adolescents with chronic, difficult to manage pain. The large geographical catchment area includes northern Alberta, the Northwest Territories, and North Eastern British Columbia. Children from Saskatchewan and Manitoba have also been included. All patients must be referred to the clinic by a physician or nurse practitioner and must meet the clinic's referral criteria (tab:children-03-00031-t001).

Table 1. Stollery Chronic Pain Clinic referral criteria.

Request for Consultation: Referral by Physician/Nurse Practitioner only	The goal of this service is to treat and care for children 17 years and under who are experiencing chronic, difficult-to-manage pain. Children should always have been seen and assessed first by the appropriate pediatric services prior to being referred to the Pediatric Chronic Pain Clinic.
Inclusion criteria	• 0–17 years, 11 months • chronic pain of at least three months' duration • chronic pain as primary complaint • chronic pain which impacts activities of daily living, school attendance, sleep, quality of life or family functioning

The family attends an intake appointment in person with the full interdisciplinary team to share their pain experience. The team consists of a chronic pain physician, a nurse practitioner, a physiotherapist and a psychologist. The initial appointment takes up to two hours to complete a comprehensive physical and psychosocial history, physical examination and development of a treatment plan with input from the child and family. For many of the children, participation in group cognitive behavioural therapy becomes part of the treatment plan. This program, called Pain 101, consists of 10 sessions, provided jointly by the psychologist and nurse practitioner. Pain 101 is a treatment program provided by our clinic to children 12–18 years old. Although the treatment is offered for a broad range of ages, due to the careful screening process that takes place prior to Pain 101 admission, we have yet to experience significant issues associated with developmental differences in participant responses.

Participants are invited to attend the sessions in person or by telehealth (secure videoconferencing). Given the large catchment area of our program, telehealth is offered to children who reside outside of the city, which makes attending the program much more feasible, especially to children whose school has access to this secure videoconference service. Pain 101 classes take place in the afternoon to best accommodate high school students who can set their schedule to avoid missing core classes. Group sizes for the class range from 5–15 participants for each 10-session block. Teens who participate are expected to attend all sessions and complete the homework as outlined. In addition to the classes for teens, sessions for parents are offered and provided by the nurse practitioner. The purpose of these sessions is to help parents understand the science of chronic pain, factors that exacerbate pain, and self-management techniques aimed at promoting increased function, mental health, coping, self-efficacy, mindfulness, acceptance, and self-compassion. Attendance for these sessions is encouraged but not required for the program, and consequently attendance of the parent session varies. However, since implementing a parallel course, Chronic Pain 35 (see Section 4), we have noted an increase in the number of parents who attend, as well as requests for additional sessions to be held. For parents, sessions aim to teach them appropriate developmental expectations, strategies to facilitate children's self-management and parent coping all with a global aim help their child function despite pain. It is important that parental behaviours, especially protectiveness [23] and parent pain–related fear [24], be addressed in order to facilitate the return to school for the small but significant number of students who miss extensive amounts of school.

3.1. Pain 101 Session Content

3.1.1. Pain Education

The biopsychosocial model of chronic pain is introduced (Figure 1), and this model is reviewed throughout Pain 101. Pain pathways in the body are reviewed, including how pain messages are sent from the periphery and received by the brain. Participants learn how chronic pain differs from acute pain. The Gate Control Theory of Pain is introduced and up-to-date scientific information on our understanding of this theory is discussed. For homework, participants are asked to complete specific questionnaires.

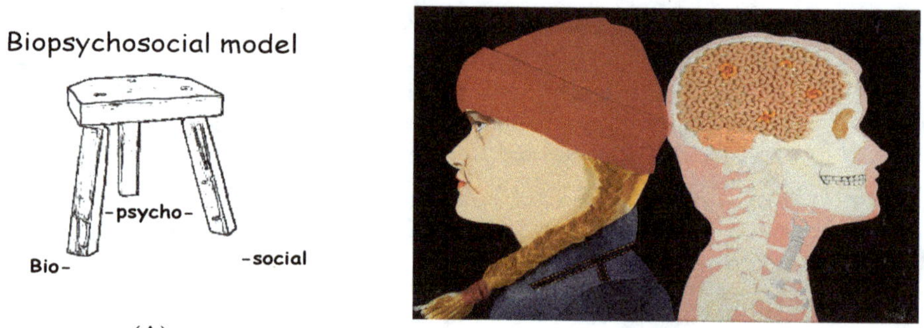

(A) (B)

Figure 1. (**A**) Biopsychosocial model—the example of a three-legged stool is often used to discuss this topic with the participants, focusing on the concept that all three legs are needed to be able to sit on the stool; (**B**) this image, created by a student of the Pain 101 course entitled "Untitled", is often used to assist in the explanation of the biopsychosocial model, in order to explain pain locations in the brain to participants.

3.1.2. Tension and Relaxation

Participants learn how tension opens pain gates and thereby increases pain and how relaxation strategies have the potential to modify the pain experience. Relaxation exercises including progressive muscle relaxation, guided imagery and diaphragmatic breathing are taught and practiced with the group. For homework, participants are asked to complete relaxation diaries and practice the techniques daily.

3.1.3. Pacing

Participants learn how activity avoidance and activity cycling can open pain gates and lead to disability in chronic pain. Methods to break this downward cycle are reviewed. Participants are expected to complete activity goals for themselves. The goals are broken down from long-term goals to intermediate goals to mini goals. Activity tolerance times are calculated, and then, from this time, baseline activity times are calculated. Participants are then expected to meet their baseline activity goals on a daily basis. For homework, participants are asked to develop a specific, measurable, achievable, relevant and time dependent (S.M.A.R.T.) goal and determine tolerance and baseline for individual activities.

3.1.4. Dealing with Negative Thoughts

Participants learn how living with chronic pain can be associated with negative thoughts and negative moods, including sadness or being overwhelmed, and may even contribute to depression or unhealthy, negative coping behaviours. Methods to challenge these negative thoughts are reviewed including active and positive coping strategies, reframing thoughts, recognition of feelings and challenging unhelpful thoughts. For homework, participants are asked to complete the daily thought diary.

3.1.5. Mindfulness

Participants review the theory of mindfulness-based stress reduction. Practice activities for mindfulness are completed in class. Participants are encouraged to practice various daily activities in a mindful way, such as taking the bus, exercising, and completing chores. For homework, participants are asked to complete one mindfulness activity daily.

3.1.6. Sleep and Nutrition

Participants review the importance of sleep in managing chronic pain and closing pain gates. Healthy sleep practice strategies that support restorative sleep are reviewed, including cognitive, behavioural, and environment modification sleep practices. Dietary habits that affect pain and sleep, including caffeine and energy drinks are also reviewed. For homework, participants are asked to perform a practical application of sleep hygiene strategies and a minimum of one dietary change.

3.1.7. Stress and Anxiety

In this session, we discuss how stress and anxiety lead to biological responses that affect pain gates, mood, and sleep, thereby exacerbating pain. Participants review stressors, such as school, homework, dealing with others, and chores. Fear of pain and how that fear contributes to disability are also reviewed. Recognizing the physical effects of stress and anxiety, including physical reactions (fight or flight response) and emotional reactions are discussed. Additionally, methods to decrease stress and anxiety are reviewed, such as recognition and coping strategies that include relaxation and pacing activities. For homework, participants are asked to recognize personal stressors and find coping strategies.

3.1.8. Communication

Pain behaviours and communication are reviewed. Participants learn about both verbal and non-verbal communication messages and discuss how the messages may be interpreted by others. This session includes a video demonstrating how society sees what they are conditioned to see. Discussion takes place regarding how strategies can be practically applied to teach family, friends, and others about pain. For homework, participants are asked to complete a communication diary.

3.1.9. Setback Planning (Relapse Prevention)

Participants learn how to develop their own personal setback plan to be utilized whenever they have a flare in their pain. This plan includes recognizing the flare early, implementing the various strategies reviewed through the course—relaxation, pacing, thoughts, sleep, stress, and communication. For homework, participants are asked to complete their setback plan worksheet.

3.1.10. Life with Pain

This final session includes strategies to live life to the fullest despite having pain. Concrete methods include simplifying activities of daily living such as school work and activities, chores, work, social activities, and other activities of daily living. We review how strategies that have previously been covered in Pain 101 can be applied to each of these life activities, structuring activities to allow for breaks while still meeting goals. Individual setback plans are reviewed and participants are asked to provide a copy of their set-back plan to the pain clinic staff. For homework, participants are asked to submit the written set-back plan, along with submission of their Chronic Pain 35 project for those who are registered in the parallel course. An example of participant work from this session can be seen in Figure 2.

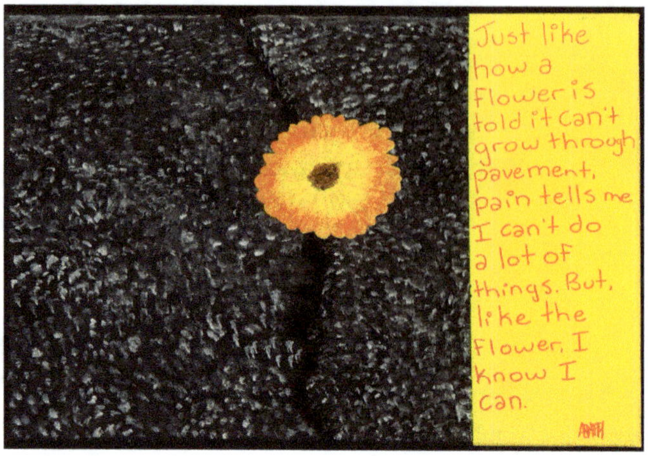
Just like how a Flower is told it can't grow through pavement, pain tells me I can't do a lot of things. But, like the Flower, I know I can.

Figure 2. "A flower can grow" created by a Pain 101 participant, A.F.H.

3.2. Participant Measures

All participants who attend Pain 101 are requested to complete questionnaires (tab:children-03-00031-t002) as per the Pediatric Initiative on Methods, Measurement, and Pain Assessment in Clinical Trials (PedIMMPACT) recommendations [25]. These data are used for the establishment of a clinical baseline, monitoring, and, for those who consent, research. The two primary findings from our analyses that have been continually replicated are significant reductions in pain-related disability ($p < 0.001$) and anxiety ($p < 0.005$).

Table 2. Questionnaire measurements.

Pain History and Demographics	Details including age, school grade, gender and school absences are recorded. Additionally, information on pain experience, chronicity, frequency, location and intensity are entered.
Visual Analogue Scale	The child is instructed to illustrate, by drawing a line on a scale from 0–10 (0 = no pain, 10 = worst possible pain), the intensity of pain felt in the past week [26].
Pediatric Quality of Life Inventory	Participants are asked to report how their pain has impacted their quality of life, including their activities, feelings, social interactions and school performance. Parents are asked to fill out the parent version of this scale which includes the same questions, but reporting their observations of their child's quality of life [27].
Children's Sleep Habits Questionnaire	The child is asked 26 questions about own bedtime habits, sleep behaviour and daytime sleepiness. The parent form is constructed of 33 questions on child's bedtime habits, sleep behaviour, waking during the night, morning waking, and daytime sleepiness [28].
Functional Disability Index	Child and parent(s) are asked to report the child's level of physical trouble or difficulty when performing various tasks [29].
Tampa Scale of Kinesiophobia for Children	A self-report form asking the child to identify how they cope with pain. This measure records the child's somatic focus and activity avoidance [30].
Revised Child Anxiety and Depression Scale	This 47-item self-report measure assesses the symptoms of separation anxiety, general anxiety, panic, social phobia, obsession/compulsion, and depression. The child is asked to report the frequency (from 'never' to 'always') of various worrying and sad thoughts [31].
The Children's Chronic Pain Stigma Scale (CCPSS)	This scale is also currently being developed and validated in our program based on the adult Chronic Pain Stigma Scale [32]. This measure explores perceived stigma from physicians, family members and the general public associated with chronic pain.

3.3. Session Completion

The questionnaire measurements are completed prior to the start of Pain 101, at the end of Pain 101 (three months later), and again at the six- and 12-month post-group completion milestones, and then annually at the five-year mark, post-group completion. Additionally, we have begun tracking education outcomes and the number of school days missed in comparison to pre- and post-completion of Pain 101.

4. Chronic Pain 35

In 2010, our healthcare team from the pediatric chronic pain clinic, along with several teens, started to work on ways to consistently obtain high school credits for completing the program and demonstrating their learning. Prior to that point, some students had been granted high school credit for completing Pain 101, but the number of credits granted and the categorization of those credits was highly variable between students. It was up to each student to advocate for themselves at their local school, with support from our team, to obtain credits. Several students were able to obtain between one and three credits, but we lacked consistency at a local or provincial level. In 2014, we approached Alberta Education, which is the provincial government agency responsible for public education in Alberta. We explained the program that we were providing and shared samples of the projects completed by students for successful credits at their local school. Together with educational consultants at Alberta Education and the Alberta Distance Learning program (a provincial online school), we developed the course syllabus. This course syllabus included specific learner outcomes for each of the classes that must be demonstrated for successful completion of the course. Examples of outcomes include: Pain Education—identify two methods by which pain gates in the body are opened; Pacing—develop a S.M.A.R.T. goal for a physical activity and demonstrate following through on that goal; Negative Thoughts—identify at least one cognitive distortion and modify negative thoughts associated with the noted distortion. The course was submitted to the Alberta Education curriculum board, and, in February 2015, it was approved as a locally developed course called Chronic Pain 35. Students who successfully complete the course obtain three credits at the Grade 12 (senior year) level in Alberta. In order to obtain a high school diploma in Alberta, students must complete courses which total 100 credits.

Participants attending Pain 101, enrolled in Grades 10–12 (ages 14–18 years old) are eligible to enroll for the course Chronic Pain 35, in order to earn high school credits. Although junior high school students are allowed to attend Pain 101, there is not a credit program in Alberta for grades 7–9, and therefore the Chronic Pain 35 course is restricted to high school students only. The course is only open to students who are followed in our clinic, as parallel attendance in Pain 101 is required. Not all teens who attend Pain 101 register for Chronic Pain 35, since many teens do not need the credits, live outside of Alberta, or are younger than high school age. Enrollment requires completion of the Alberta Distance Learning (ADL) registration form and written consent of a parent/guardian. Prior to registering, we provide the family with a written outline of the course and completion requirements. Additionally, before registration, teens and their parents choosing to enroll are informed that credits for the course "Chronic Pain 35" will appear on their official transcripts. Any ethical concerns expressed regarding this are discussed with the teen and family directly prior to enrollment. To date, only one student expressed concern over the course name appearing on the transcripts, although the student chose to continue and receive credits.

Students who enroll are required to attend all Pain 101 sessions, submit weekly homework assignments, including completion of relaxation diaries, thought challenging worksheets, development of S.M.A.R.T. goals, and a written setback plan for managing pain flares. Any missed sessions must be made up. Additionally, students must complete a project that demonstrates their learning of at least one concept related to the sessions. Projects have been produced using a variety of media, including written work such as essays, personal reflections and poetry. Other projects have used visual arts, such as collages, story boards, paintings, sculptures, and a host of other genres. A small number of students have composed and produced various forms of music. The course mark is 20% for attendance, participation and homework, and 80% for completion of the project. A certified teacher in the province of Alberta has been assigned to the program and grades all course projects. The teacher attends several sessions to meet the students and answer any questions they may have related to the planned project. She is also available via the online distance learning site to discuss projects with the students.

As of July 2016, 35 students have enrolled in Chronic Pain 35. Of these, 32 students have completed the course and received school credits, since three students completed Pain 101, but chose not to complete the course requirements for Chronic Pain 35. Samples of the participant's work can be found in the Supplementary Material. Feedback from students thus far has been very positive, and attendance and homework completion consistency have markedly risen since the formalization of Chronic Pain 35. To quote one of the 17-year-old student participants: "Without this class I would be short credits to graduate. I used to miss a few days of school each week, but now I barely miss any." In addition to obtaining school credits, several students have discussed the importance of having the opportunity to meet and learn with other students who have chronic pain, and to be with others who understand what it is like to live with chronic pain. These students motivate each other to incorporate the strategies into their own lives and help support each other in achieving goals. These students have reported that one of the most important aspects of the group work is the opportunity to continue to meet with other teens who "get them"; who truly understand what it is like to live with chronic pain. As demonstrated by Forgeron [33], the majority of students who attend group CBT for chronic pain self-management are interested in friendships with their class peers for emotional support.

5. Discussion

This paper highlights our unique program that incorporates attendance at a group CBT program for chronic pain and the provision of high school credits for the completion of a course that is provided in a health care setting. Our CBT program includes many recommendations from previous research studies that have addressed multiple facets of the chronic pain experience while helping young people return to school. School avoidance and absences arise from multiple personal and psychosocial factors. Addressing these factors in a group setting can help youth return to school and thereby improve school performance. In a study of 349 youth treated in a chronic pain clinic, Khan et al. [34] found that anxiety played an important role in both school attendance and function while at school. Addressing anxiety, enhancing self-confidence and self-efficacy, and assisting teens in developing methods to manage anxiety using CBT, are all pillars of practice that are incorporated into our program. Additionally, in a study of 47 adolescents with chronic headache, Claar et al. [35] suggest that having the health care team address methods to return to school can help decrease the frequency and duration of headaches. In several sessions of our program, teens are taught concrete techniques to return to function, such as pacing and goal setting. Additionally, by receiving school credits for completion, the student is increasingly empowered to continue to attend school.

In a study by Logan and Curran [36], 38 teachers were interviewed about their needs when dealing with an adolescent with chronic pain. The study revealed that teachers needed to further understand chronic pain and how to manage pain-related behaviours. In our program, we offer a specific class in which we discuss ways to communicate and how to ask others to help in managing pain, including school personnel. Teachers are further supported by the Alberta Education Chronic Pain 35 curriculum guide, in which teachers can access the relevant information on our program and learn how it can help students succeed. Therefore, the completion of Chronic Pain 35 has opened communication with teachers and school administrators that may not have otherwise occurred. Having a certified teacher involved in the program, who is available to intervene with the teens at a school level, also serves to increase understanding of chronic pain in schools across the province.

As identified by Boutilier and King [37], school sites have been undervalued in helping children with chronic pain management, along with the inherent additional challenges. They recommended increased interdisciplinary collaboration between schools and health care teams. Our program directly meets this recommendation by working with Alberta Education at a local and provincial level to best meet the needs of our students. The program has been endorsed by both the Alberta provincial Education Minister and Health Minister.

Future Directions

Given that up to 50% of adolescents with chronic pain miss several school opportunities, days of classes, and social involvement with peers, it is essential that programs providing services to these children incorporate school functioning efforts into their treatment plans. As recommended by Gorodzinsky et al. [38], measurement of school functioning should include the assessment of absenteeism, academic performance, and cognitive function within a developmental framework. Our program will continue to use outcome measures to determine both short-term and long-term results in adolescents who complete Chronic Pain 35, including tracking school absences and school functioning. We will continue to request permission from the students to share their projects which demonstrate their learning. It is hoped that other jurisdictions can work with their educational boards at a local, provincial (or other) level to develop similar programs. Most importantly, we will continue to advocate for students to be able to return to the classroom and continue with their education, and we encourage other programs to contact us if they are interested in modeling our program or learning more about our work. Children are the future of our societies and children with chronic pain require unique support from teams, including the collaboration of health care providers and teachers, to meet their goals of learning, graduating, gaining fulfilling employment, and contributing to society.

Acknowledgments: We would like to thank the students who have granted us permission to share their Chronic Pain 35 projects. We would like to acknowledge Karen Campbell, certified teacher at the Alberta Distance Learning Center, who marked the students' projects for credit. Photo credit Mathew Martin, Alberta Health Services. We received no research funding for this program.

Author Contributions: K.R., M.V., M.S. and B.D. all contributed significantly in the conceptualization, writing, and editing of this article.

References

1. American Pain Society Assessment and Management of Children with Chronic Pain: A Position Statement from the American Pain Society. 2012. Available online: http://americanpainsociety.org/uploads/get-involved/pediatric-chronic-pain-statement.pdf (accessed on 26 July 2016).
2. Van Der Kerkhof, E.; van Dijk, A. Prevalence of Chronic Pain Disorders in Children. In *Encyclopaedia Reference of Pain*; Schmidt, R.F., Willis, W.D., Eds.; Springer: Heidelberg, Germany, 2006; pp. 1972–1974.
3. King, S.; Chambers, C.T.; Huguet, A.; MacNevin, R.C.; McGrath, P.J.; Parker, L.; MacDonald, A.J. The epidemiology of chronic pain in children and adolescents revisited; a systematic review. *Pain* **2011**, *152*, 2729–2738. [CrossRef] [PubMed]
4. Latremoliere, A.; Woolf, C.J. Central Sensitization: A generator of pain hypersensitivity by central neural plasticity. *J. Pain* **2009**, *10*, 895–926. [CrossRef] [PubMed]
5. Woolf, C.J. Cenrtal sensitization: Implications for the diagnosis and treatment of pain. *Pain* **2011**, *152*, S2–S15. [CrossRef] [PubMed]
6. Von Baeyer, C. Interpreting the high prevalence of pediatric chronic pain revealed in community surveys. *Pain* **2011**, *152*, 2683–2684. [CrossRef] [PubMed]
7. Gauntlett-Gilbert, J.; Eccleston, C. Disability in adolescents with chronic pain: Patterns and predictors across different domains of functioning. *Pain* **2007**, *131*, 132–141. [CrossRef] [PubMed]
8. Huguet, A.; Miró, J. The severity of chronic pediatric pain: An epidemiological study. *J. Pain* **2008**, *9*, 226–236. [CrossRef] [PubMed]
9. Logan, D.; Simons, L.; Stein, M.J.; Chastain, L. School impairment in adolescents with chronic pain. *J. Pain* **2008**, *9*, 407–416. [CrossRef] [PubMed]

10. Eccleston, C.; Wastel, S.; Crombez, G.; Jordan, A. Adolescent social development and chronic pain. *Eur. J. Pain* **2007**, *12*, 765–774. [CrossRef] [PubMed]
11. Forgeron, P.; McGrath, P.; Stevens, B.; Evans, J.; Dick, B.; Finley, A.G.; Carlson, T. Social information processing in adolescents with chronic pain; my friends don't really understand me. *Pain* **2011**, *152*, 2773–2780. [CrossRef] [PubMed]
12. Simons, L.; Logan, D.; Chastain, L.; Stein, M. The relation of social functioning to school impairment among adolescents with chronic pain. *Clin. J. Pain* **2009**, *26*, 16–22. [CrossRef] [PubMed]
13. Eccleston, C. Managing chronic pain in children; the challenge of delivering chronic care in a 'modernising' health care system. *Arch. Dis. Child* **2005**, *90*, 332–333. [CrossRef] [PubMed]
14. Assa, A.; Ish-Tov, A.; Rinawi, F.; Shamir, R. School attendance in children with functional abdominal pain and inflammatory bowel diseases. *JPGN* **2015**, *61*, 553–557. [CrossRef] [PubMed]
15. Dick, B.; Pillai-Riddell, R. Cognitive and school functioning in children and adolescents with chronic pain: A critical review. *Pain Res. Manag.* **2010**, *15*, 238–244. [CrossRef] [PubMed]
16. Eccleston, C.; Palermo, T.; de C Williams, A.C.; Lewandowski, A.; Morley, S.; Fisher, E.; Law, E. Psychological therapies for the management of current and chronic pain in children and adolescents (review). *Cochrane Libr.* **2014**. [CrossRef]
17. Anie, K.A.; Green, J. Psychological therapies for sickle cell disease and pain. *Cochrane Database Syst. Rev.* **2015**. [CrossRef]
18. Kashikar-Zuck, S.; Ting, T.V.; Arnold, L.M.; Bean, J.; Powers, S.W.; Graham, T.B.; Passo, M.H.; Schikler, K.N.; Hashkes, P.J.; Spalding, S.; et al. Cognitive-behavioral therapy for the treatment of juvenile fibromyalgia: A multisite, single- blinded, randomized control trial. *Arth. Rheum.* **2012**, *64*, 297–305. [CrossRef] [PubMed]
19. Palermo, T.; Law, E. *Managing Your Child's Chronic Pain*; Oxford University Press: New York, NY, USA, 2015; pp. 1–3, 11–13.
20. Carpino, E.; Segal, S.; Logan, D.; Lebel, A.; Simons, L.E. The interplay of pain-related self-efficacy and fear on functional outcomes among youth with headache. *J. Pain* **2014**, *15*, 527–534. [CrossRef] [PubMed]
21. Kalapurakkel, S.; Carpino, E.; Lebel, A.; Simons, L.E. "Pain can't stop me": Examining pain self-efficacy and acceptance as resilience processes among youth with chronic headache. *J. Pediatr. Psychol.* **2014**, *40*, 926–933. [CrossRef] [PubMed]
22. Logan, D.; Simons, L. Development of a group intervention to improve school functioning in adolescents with chronic pain and depressive symptoms; a study of feasibility and preliminary efficacy. *J. Pediatr. Psychol.* **2010**, *35*, 823–836. [CrossRef] [PubMed]
23. Logan, D.; Simons, S.; Carpino, E.A. Too sick for school? Parent influences on school functioning among children with chronic pain. *Pain* **2012**, *153*, 437–443. [CrossRef] [PubMed]
24. Chow, E.T.; Otis, J.D.; Simons, L.E. The longitudinal impact of parent distress and behavior on functional outcomes among youth with chronic pain. *J. Pain* **2016**, *17*, 729–738. [CrossRef] [PubMed]
25. McGrath, P.J.; Walco, G.A.; Turk, D.C.; Dworkin, R.H.; Brown, M.T.; Davidson, K.; Eccleston, C.; Finley, G.A.; Goldschneider, K.; Haverkos, L.; et al. Core outcome domains and measures for pediatric acute and chronic/recurrent pain clinical trials: PedIMMPACT recommendations. *J. Pain* **2008**, *9*, 771–783. [CrossRef] [PubMed]
26. McGrath, P.A.; Seifert, C.E.; Speechley, K.N.; Booth, J.C.; Stitt, L.; Gibson, M.C. A new analogue scale for assessing children's pain: An initial validation study. *Pain* **1996**, *64*, 435–443. [CrossRef]
27. Varni, J.W.; Seid, M.; Rode, C.A. The PedsQL: Measurement model for the pediatric quality of life inventory. *Med. Care* **1999**, *37*, 126–139. [CrossRef] [PubMed]
28. Owens, J.A.; Spirito, C.E.; McGuinn, M. The childrens' sleep habits questionnaire (CSHQ); psychometric properties of a survey instrument for school-aged children. *Sleep* **2000**, *23*, 1043–1051. [PubMed]
29. Walker, L.S.; Greene, W. The functional disability inventory: Measuring a neglected dimension of child health status. *J. Pediatr. Psychol.* **1991**, *16*, 39–58. [CrossRef] [PubMed]
30. Miller, R.P.; Kori, S.; Todd, D. The Tampa scale; a measure of kinesiophobia. *Clin. J. Pain* **1991**, *7*, 51–52. [CrossRef]
31. Chorpita, B.F.; Moffitt, C.E.; Gray, J. Psychometric properties of the Revised Child Anxiety and Depression Scale in a clinic sample. *Behav. Res. Ther.* **2005**, *43*, 309–322. [CrossRef] [PubMed]

32. Vallab, P.K.; Rashiq, S.; Verrier, M.J.; Baker, G.; Sanderman, B.; Dick, B.D. The effect of a cognitive-behavioral therapy chronic pain management program on perceived stigma: A clinical controlled trial. *J. Pain Manag.* **2015**, *7*, 291–299.
33. Forgeron, P.; Chorney, J.; Carlson, T.E.; Dick, B.D.; Plante, E. To befriend or not; naturally developing friendships amongst a clinical group of adolescents with chronic pain. *Pain Manag. Nurs.* **2015**, *16*, 721–723. [CrossRef] [PubMed]
34. Khan, K.; Tran, S.; Mano, K.E.J.; Simpson, P.M.; Cao, Y.; Hainsworth, K.R. Predicting multiple facets of school functioning in pediatric chronic pain: Examining the direct impact of anxiety. *Clin. J. Pain* **2015**, *31*, 867–875. [CrossRef] [PubMed]
35. Claar, R.; Kaczynski, K.; Minster, A.; McDonald-Nolan, L.; LeBel, A.A. School functioning and chronic tension headaches in adolescents: Improvement only after multidisciplinary evaluation. *JCN* **2012**, *28*, 719–724. [CrossRef] [PubMed]
36. Logan, D.; Curran, J. Adolescent chronic pain problems in the school setting: Exploring the experiences and beliefs of selected school personnel through focus group methodology. *J. Adolesc. Health* **2005**, *37*, 281–288. [CrossRef] [PubMed]
37. Boutilier, J.; King, S. Missed opportunities: School as an undervalued site for effective pain management. *Pediatr. Pain Lett.* **2013**, *15*, 9–15.
38. Gorodzinsky, A.; Hainsworth, K.; Weisman, S.J. School functioning and chronic pain: A review of methods. *J. Pediatr. Psychol.* **2011**, *36*, 991–1002. [CrossRef] [PubMed]

7

Moderate and Stable Pain Reductions as a Result of Interdisciplinary Pain Rehabilitation: A Cohort Study from the Swedish Quality Registry for Pain Rehabilitation (SQRP)

Åsa Ringqvist [1], Elena Dragioti [2], Mathilda Björk [3], Britt Larsson [2] and Björn Gerdle [2,*]

1 Department of Neurosurgery and Pain Rehabilitation, Skåne University Hospital, SE-221 85 Lund, Sweden; asa.ringqvist@skane.se

2 Pain and Rehabilitation Centre, and Department of Medical and Health Sciences, Linköping University, SE-581 85 Linköping, Sweden; elena.dragioti@liu.se (E.D.); britt.larsson@liu.se (B.L.)

3 Department of Social and Welfare Studies, Linköping University, SE-602 21 Norrköping, Sweden; mathilda.bjork@liu.se

* Correspondence: bjorn.gerdle@liu.se

Abstract: Few studies have investigated the real-life outcomes of interdisciplinary multimodal pain rehabilitation programs (IMMRP) for chronic pain. This study has four aims: investigate effect sizes (ES); analyse correlation patterns of outcome changes; define a multivariate outcome measure; and investigate whether the clinical self-reported presentation pre-IMMRP predicts the multivariate outcome. To this end, this study analysed chronic pain patients in specialist care included in the Swedish Quality Registry for Pain Rehabilitation for 22 outcomes (pain, psychological distress, participation, and health) on three occasions: pre-IMMRP, post-IMMRP, and 12-month follow-up. Moderate stable ES were demonstrated for pain intensity, interference in daily life, vitality, and health; most other outcomes showed small ES. Using a Multivariate Improvement Score (MIS), we identified three clusters. Cluster 1 had marked positive MIS and was associated with the overall worst situation pre-IMMRP. However, the pre-IMMRP situation could only predict 8% of the variation in MIS. Specialist care IMPRPs showed moderate ES for pain, interference, vitality, and health. Outcomes were best for patients with the worst clinical presentation pre-IMMRP. It was not possible to predict who would clinically benefit most from IMMRP.

Keywords: chronic pain; musculoskeletal pain; patient care team; rehabilitation; treatment outcome

---

1. Introduction

Pain is an unpleasant experience with complex interactions between sensorimotoric, affective, and cognitive brain networks. As such, pain, especially chronic pain, is influenced by and interacts with physical, psychological, social, and contextual factors [1–3]. One-fifth of the European population has moderate to severe chronic pain conditions [4]. These conditions are associated with psychological distress, low health, sick leave, and high socioeconomic costs [5]. Therefore, a biopsychosocial (BPS) framework should be considered in clinical practice [6–8].

Unlike single/unimodal interventions, interdisciplinary multimodal pain rehabilitation programs (IMMRPs) for chronic pain—an interdisciplinary treatment according to the International Association for the Study of Pain (IASP)—distinguish themselves as well-coordinated complex interventions. Typically, IMMRPs are based on cognitive behavioural therapy (CBT) models (including Acceptance Commitment Therapy, ACT) and are administered over several weeks to months [9–12]. The Swedish programs generally include group activities such as pain education, supervised physical activity, training in simulated environments, and CBT coordinated by an interdisciplinary team (e.g., physician, occupational therapist, physiotherapist, psychologist, and social worker) based on a BPS framework [9–12]. The components of IMMRP are most often chosen based on the available evidence for unimodal interventions for chronic pain, for example, with respect to education, exercise, psychological interventions, and interventions for return to work. The core goals of rehabilitation programs in general [13] and especially for patients with chronic pain [14] are broad and multifactorial in combination with the individualised goals of the patient. These include increased ability to participate in valued activities such as work. Hence, IMMRP is a complex intervention [13,15] and, unlike pharmacological intervention, focusses on the whole person rather than just biochemical processes, implying complex patient conditions matched with complex IMMRPs [16,17]. The components of IMMRP can be active independently or interdependently [15], resulting in a combination of effects explained by known and unknown mechanisms. The effects are assumed to be greater than the sum of its components [18].

Systematic reviews (SRs) have generally reported higher efficacy both on a general level and for specific outcomes of IMMRP compared with single-treatment or treatment-as-usual programs [10,12,19–23]. SRs and Randomised Controlled Trials (RCTs) may be associated with risk for bias resulting from, for example, an unrepresentative selection of patients and researcher allegiance [24–26]. Thus, it is necessary to investigate whether the evidence obtained from SRs and RCTs can be replicated within a consecutive non-selected flow of patients in practice settings using prospective observational cohort study designs such as practice-based evidence (PBE). PBE has also been applied in the field of rehabilitation research [27]. The importance of such an approach is also emphasised in the real-effectiveness medicine framework [28]. IMMRPs are time consuming and expensive, even when most of the activities are group-based. From an ethical, individual, and socioeconomic perspective, it is indeed remarkable to note the lack of studies investigating effect sizes (ES) in patient populations in real-life practice settings. A recent study from two Swedish university clinics reported effect sizes of 0.51–0.61 (i.e., moderate ES) for two pain intensity variables at 12-month follow-up [29]. These effect sizes should be confirmed in larger studies based not only on patients at university hospitals, but also on specialist units in general. It would be motivating for patients to endure increases in pain, which is often observed in clinical practise during the start-up period of rehabilitation characterised by an increase in activity levels, if it were known that the long-term effects include the reduction of pain levels.

Complex interventions such as IMMRP should have several outcomes measured at multiple levels and strategies for handling multiple outcomes [17,30]. IMMRPs are evaluated using many outcomes. For example, one SR including 46 RCTs reported nine outcomes per RCT (median) [10]. However, outcomes are not usually divided into primary and secondary outcomes [10]. In addition, although it is most likely that changes in several of the selected outcomes are correlated, most SRs of IMMRPs evaluate the outcomes as independent from each other. Patterns of potential correlations (i.e., multivariate correlation patterns) are mainly unknown/uninvestigated, even though they could give valuable information regarding how to optimise IMMRPs. Hence, there is a need to develop clinically applicable ways to evaluate the multiple outcomes of MMPRs both for individual patients and within research studies.

The above knowledge gaps motivated this PBE study of chronic pain patients based on patient reported outcome measures (PROMs) from the Swedish Quality Registry for Pain Rehabilitation (SQRP) [31]. This registry offers an opportunity to investigate clinical outcomes and patterns of change, since all the relevant specialist care units throughout Sweden deliver data to SQRP. Hence, this PBE study has the general aim of investigating the effects of IMMRP in specialist care in Sweden considering the multivariate complexity of outcomes. We hypothesised that IMMRP in special care is associated with small-to-medium ES, that changes in outcomes generally are intercorrelated, and that the baseline situation (pre-IMMRP) can predict the multivariate outcomes. More specifically, we defined the following four aims:

- To investigate the outcome effect sizes of IMMRP immediately post-IMMRP and at 12-month follow-up.
- To analyse the multivariate correlation patterns of changes in outcomes of IMMRP: pre-IMMRP versus post IMMRP and pre-IMMRP versus 12-month follow-up.
- To define a multivariate outcome measure of IMMRP.
- To investigate if the clinical self-reported presentation pre-IMMRP can predict the multivariate outcome measure.

2. Materials and Methods

2.1. The Swedish Quality Registry for Pain Rehabilitation (SQRP)

The SQRP, recognised by the Swedish Association of Local Authorities and Regions, receives data from all specialist care units in Sweden [31]. The SQRP is based on PROM questionnaires that capture biopsychosocial data such as the patient's background, pain distribution and intensity, pain-related cognitions, and psychological distress symptoms (e.g., depression and anxiety), as well as activity/participation aspects and health-related quality of life variables. Patients complete the PROM questionnaires on up to three occasions: (1) during assessment at the first visit to the unit (pre-IMMRP); (2) immediately after the IMMRP (post-IMMRP); and (3) at the 12-month follow-up (FU) after IMMRP discharge (12-month FU).

2.2. Subjects

This study included SQRP data from women and men ≥18 years old with complex chronic (≥3 months) non-malignant pain who were referred to specialist pain and rehabilitation units (i.e., specialist care centres) between 2008–2016. These patients can be characterised as complex, as their health profiles included psychiatric comorbidities such as depression and anxiety, low levels of acceptance, high levels of kinesiophobia, decreased working life and participation in social activities, and/or did not respond to routine pharmacological/physiotherapeutic treatments delivered in a monodisciplinary fashion. Strict inclusion and exclusion criteria for inclusion in the registry is not available, since this is a registry study of patients with complex chronic pain conditions referred from mainly the primary care to specialist care in Sweden. A minority of patients were referred from other specialist clinics e.g., orthopedic and rheumatology clinics. The following general inclusion criteria for IMMRP were used: (i) disabling chronic pain (on sick leave or experiencing major interference in daily life due to chronic pain); (ii) age 18 years and above; (iii) no further medical investigations needed; and (iv) written consent to participate and attend IMMRP. General exclusion criteria for IMMRP included severe psychiatric morbidity, abuse of alcohol and/or drugs, diseases that did not allow physical exercise, and specific pain conditions with other treatment options available (i.e., red flags).

The proportions of patients within primary health care with chronic pain conditions are not exactly known, but 10–20% are estimates [32,33]. Furthermore, the proportion of chronic pain patients within primary health care that are referred to specialist clinics is not known.

The study was conducted in accordance with the Helsinki Declaration and Good Clinical Practice and approved by the Ethical Review Board in Linköping (Dnr: 2015/108-31). All the participants received written information about the study and gave their written consent.

2.3. Variables

Background variables that were collected pre-IMMRP and symptom-related self-reported variables that were collected at all three times (pre, post, and 12-month FU) were used in the analyses. The variables and instruments used are mandatory for the units registering their data with the SQRP.

Background Variables

The following background variables were collected: age (years), gender (man or woman), education level, and country of birth. Education level was dichotomised into university and the other alternatives (i.e., upper secondary school, elementary school, or other); this variable was labelled as University. Country of birth was dichotomised as from Europe and outside Europe and labelled as Outside-Europe. In addition, self-reported pain duration (days), persistent pain duration (days), and number of days off work (Days no work) were obtained.

Pain distribution was registered using 36 predefined anatomical areas (18 on the front and 18 on the back of the body) and the patients registered the areas with pain: (1) head/face, (2) neck, (3) shoulder, (4) upper arm, (5) elbow, (6) forearm, (7) hand, (8) anterior aspect of chest, (9) lateral aspect of chest, (10) belly, (11) sexual organs, (12) upper back, (13) low back, (14) hip/gluteal area, (15) thigh, (16) knee, (17) shank, and (18) foot. The number of areas with pain (range: 1–36) were summed, and the obtained variable was denoted as the Pain Region Index (PRI).

2.4. *Repeated Self-Reported Measures*

For reports of the psychometric aspects of the self-reported measures, the reader is referred to other studies summarising these [7,34–36].

2.4.1. Pain Aspects

Pain intensity average during the previous seven days was registered using a 0–10 (0 = no pain and 10 = worst possible pain) numeric rating scale (NRS)—NRS-7days.

2.4.2. The Multidimensional Pain Inventory (MPI)

MPI is a 61-item self-report questionnaire that measures the psychosocial, cognitive, and behavioural effects of chronic pain [37,38]. Part 1 consists of five scales: Pain severity—measuring several aspects of the pain experience (MPI-Pain-severity); Interference—pain-related interference in everyday life (MPI-Pain-interfer); Perceived Life Control (MPI-LifeCon); the level of affective distress (MPI-Distress); and Social Support—perceived support from a spouse or significant others (MPI-SocSupp). Part 2 assesses the perception of responses to displays of pain and suffering from significant others and consists of three scales: Punishing Responses (MPI-Punish); Solicitous Responses (MPI-Solict); and Distracting Responses (MPI-Distract). Part 3 measures to what extent the patients participate in various activities using four scales. These scales can be combined into a composite scale—the General Activity Index (MPI-GAI)—which was used in the present study [39].

2.4.3. Psychological Distress Variables

Symptoms of anxiety and depression were registered using the Hospital Anxiety and Depression Scale (HADS) [40,41]. This instrument comprises seven items in each of two subscales: depression (HADS-D) and anxiety (HADS-A) symptoms. Both subscale scores have a range of 0 to 21. A score of 7 or less in each subscale indicates a non-case, a score of 8–10 indicates a possible case, and a score of 11 or more indicates an almost definite case [40].

2.4.4. The Short Form Health Survey (SF36)

The Short Form Health Survey (SF36) attempts to represent multidimensional health concepts and measurements of the full range of health states, including levels of well-being and personal evaluations of health [42]. Scores are standardised into eight dimensions with a scale from 0 to 100 where higher scores indicate a better perception of health [42]: (1) physical functioning (sf36-pf), physical activity level including activities of daily living; (2) role limitations due to physical functioning (sf36-rp), to what extent physical health limits the performance of work and other regular activities; (3) bodily pain (sf36-bp), pain and related disability; (4) general health (sf36-gh), evaluation of health situation;

(5) vitality (sf36-vt), how rested and energetic; (6) social functioning (sf36-sf), disturbances of social life due to physical or mental illness; (7) role limitations due to emotional problems (sf36-re), difficulties in performing work or other regular activities due to emotional problems; and (8) mental health (sf36-mh), anxiety and depressive symptoms. Based on the eight scales, a physical summary component and a mental (psychological) summary component can be calculated, but these two summary component variables were not used in the present study.

2.4.5. The European Quality of Life Instrument (EQ-5D)

The European Quality of Life Instrument (EQ-5D) captures a patient's perceived state of health [43–45]. The first part of the instrument defines five dimensions: mobility, self-care, usual activities, pain/discomfort, and anxiety/depression. Each of these were measured at three levels. An EQ-5D-index is derived by applying a formula that essentially attaches values (weights) to each of the levels in each dimension. The collection of index values (weights) for all the possible EQ-5D states is called a value set. Most EQ-5D value sets have been obtained from a standardised valuation exercise where a representative sample of the general population in a country/region is asked to place a value on EQ-5D health states. The EQ5D also measures the self-estimation of today's health according to a 100-point scale, which is a thermometer-like scale (EQ-VAS) with defined end points (high values indicate good health and low values indicate bad health).

2.4.6. Estimations of Changes in Pain and in Life Situation

The patients post-IMMRP and at the 12-month FU estimated the degree of positive change in pain (Change-pain) and in their ability to handle life situations in general (Change-life situation). The Change-pain item was rated on a five-point Likert scale from markedly increased pain (0) to markedly decreased pain (4). The Change-life situation item was rated on a five-point Likert scale from markedly worsened (0) to markedly improved (4).

2.5. Statistics

All the statistics were performed using the statistical package IBM SPSS Statistics (version 24.0) and SIMCA-P+ (version 15.0; Umetrics Inc., Umeå, Sweden). A probability of <0.001 (two-tailed) was accepted as the criteria for significance due to the large number of subjects.

The text and tables generally report the mean value ± one standard deviation (±1 SD) together with a median and range of continuous variables. Percentages (%) are reported for categorical variables. The detailed analyses also report 95% confidence intervals (95% CI). SQRP uses predetermined rules when handling single missing items of a scale or a subscale; details about this have been reported elsewhere [29]. To compare groups, we used Student´s *t*-test for unpaired observations, analysis of variance (ANOVA with post hoc test if significant difference), and Chi square test. Effect sizes (ES; Cohen's d) for within-group analysis were computed using a calculator when appropriate (https://webpower.psychstat.org/models/means01/effectsize.php). Hedges' g, which provides a measure of effect size weighted according to the relative size of each sample, was used for between ES using a calculator (https://www.socscistatistics.com/effectsize/default3.aspx). The absolute effect size was considered very large for values ≥ 1.3, large for values between 0.80–1.29, moderate for values between 0.50–0.79, small for values between 0.20–0.49, and insignificant for values < 0.20 [46].

Common methods such as logistic regression (LR) and multiple linear regression (MLR) can quantify the level of relations of individual factors but disregard interrelationships among different factors and thereby ignore system-wide aspects [47]. Moreover, such methods assume variable independence when interpreting results [48], and there are several risks when considering one variable at a time [49]. To account for our aims, the problems related to handling missing data (see below), and the risks associated with multicollinearity problems (see above), we used advanced multivariate analyses (MVDA).

Hence, using SIMCA-P+, we applied advanced Principal Component Analysis (PCA) for the multivariate correlation analyses of all investigated variables and Orthogonal Partial Least Square Regressions (OPLS) for the multivariate regressions. These techniques do not require normal distributions of the included variables [50]. Note that the PCA of SIMCA-P+ differs considerably from the simpler version implemented (e.g., the version used in SPSS).

PCA extracts and displays systematic variation in the data matrix. All the variables were log transformed before the statistical analyses if data were skewed. Using PCA, we analysed the multivariate correlation pattern for the changes in the 22 outcome variables for all the subjects. Note that changes in outcomes are calculated so that a positive value indicates an improvement. A cross-validation technique was used to identify nontrivial components (p). Variables loading on the same component p were correlated, and variables with high loadings but with opposing signs were negatively correlated. Variables with high absolute loadings were considered significant. The obtained components are per definition not correlated and are arranged in decreasing order with respect to explained variation. The loading plot reports the multivariate relationships between variables. A corresponding plot reporting the relationships between subjects (i.e., *t*-scores) can also be used (score plot), and each subject receives a score (*t*) for each of the significant components. The *t*-score was used to calculate a Multivariate Improvement Score (MIS). R^2 describes the goodness of fit—the fraction of sum of squares of all the variables explained by a principal component [51]. Q^2 describes the goodness of prediction—the fraction of the total variation of the variables that can be predicted using principal component cross-validation methods [51]. Outliers were identified using two methods: score plots in combination with Hotelling's T^2 and distance to model in the X-space. No extreme outliers were detected.

OPLS was used for the longitudinal multivariate regression analyses of the *t*-scores of the PCA mentioned above using pre-IMMRP data (i.e., baseline data) [51]. The variable influence on projection (VIP) indicates the relevance of each X-variable pooled over all dimensions and Y-variables—the group of variables that best explain Y. VIP $\geq$ 1.0 was considered significant if VIP had a 95% jack-knife uncertainty confidence interval non-equal to zero. p(corr) was used to note the direction of the relationship (positive or negative). This is the loading of each variable scaled as a correlation coefficient, and thus standardising the range from -1 to $+1$. [50] p(corr) is stable during iterative variable selection and comparable between models [50]. Thus, a variable/regressor was considered significant when VIP > 1.0. For each regression, we report R^2, Q^2, and the *p*-value of a cross-validated analysis of variance (CV-ANOVA). SIMCA-P+ uses the Non-linear Iterative Partial Least Squares (NIPALS) algorithm to handle missing data: maximum 50% missing data for variables/scales and maximum 50% missing data for subjects.

To identify clusters based on the *t*-scores of the PCA mentioned above, we performed hierarchical clustering analysis (HCA). Based on the identified clusters (subgroups) defined by HCA, we performed partial least squares discriminant analysis (PLS-DA). In addition, we applied a bottom–up HCA to the principal component score vectors using the default Ward linkage criterion to identify relevant subgroups of patients. HCA can find subtle clusters in the multivariate space. In the resulting dendrogram, clusters were identified and, based on these groups, we performed PLS-DA using group belonging as the Y-variable and the psychometric data as predictors (X-variables). The PLS-DA model was computed to identify associations between the X-variables and the subgroups. Based on the HCA defined clusters, traditional inferential statistics (ANOVA including post hoc tests when appropriate) were computed using SPSS.

3. Results

3.1. Background Data

There were 14,666 chronic pain patients registered in the SQRP that fulfilled the inclusion criteria: chronic pain; >18 years of age; and completed the SQRP questionnaire before and on at least one of the two time points after the IMMRP. More than half (60%) of the patients answering the questionnaires pre-IMMRP and post-IMMRP also answered the questionnaires at 12-m FU. Most of the patients (76.3%) were women, 25.2% had studied at university, and 10.4% were born outside of Europe. More men were born outside Europe (men: 13.4% versus women: 9.5%; $Chi^2 = 43.437$, $p < 0.001$), and fewer men had university education (men: 18.0% versus women: 27.4%; $Chi^2 = 123.672$; $p < 0.001$). Continuous background variables are shown in Table 1. Women were slightly younger than men (42.9 ± 10.7 versus 44.5 ± 10.7; $p < 0.001$) and reported more spreading of pain according to PRI (15.4 ± 8.8 versus 10.8 ± 7.0; $p < 0.001$). The other variables in Table 2 were not affected by gender.

Table 1. Continuous background variables; mean ± SD and 95% confidence intervals (95% CI).

Variables	Mean ± SD	95% CI Lower Bound	95% CI Upper Bound
Age (years)	43.2 ± 10.7	43.3	43.9
Days no work	1055 ± 2461	968	1095
Pain duration	3057 ± 3341	2970	3170
Persistent pain duration	2368 ± 2980	2239	2414
PRI	15.4 ± 8.6	15.1	15.6

Notes: SD = standard deviation; CI = confidence intervals; PRI = Pain Region Index.

Table 2. Outcome variables at baseline (pre-IMMRP) and immediately after IMMRP (post-IMMRP). Statistical comparisons are presented furthest to the right together with effects sizes (i.e., Cohen's d). Effect sizes in bold were moderate, i.e., Cohen's d ≥ 0.50. IMMRP: interdisciplinary multimodal pain rehabilitation programs.

Baseline vs. After IMMRP		Pre-IMMRP		Post-IMMRP			
	N	Mean	SD	Mean	SD	*p*-Value	Cohen's d
NRS-7days	14,146	6.86	1.72	5.95	2.09	<0.001	0.45
HADS-A	14,774	9.00	4.76	7.78	4.55	<0.001	0.32
HADS-D	14,772	8.49	4.44	6.70	4.31	<0.001	0.47
MPI-Pain-severity	14,692	4.39	0.93	3.87	1.16	<0.001	**0.52**
MPI-Pain-interfer	14,552	4.38	1.02	3.94	1.19	<0.001	0.49
MPI-LifeCon	14,687	2.72	1.10	3.30	1.18	<0.001	0.47
MPI-Distress	14,697	3.46	1.26	2.89	1.38	<0.001	0.42
MPI-Socsupp	14,618	4.16	1.34	3.95	1.35	<0.001	0.21
MPI-punish	13,054	1.74	1.36	1.72	1.33	0.037	0.02
MPI-protect	12,999	2.98	1.40	2.85	1.38	<0.001	0.12
MPI-distract	13,048	2.54	1.19	2.56	1.17	0.043	0.02
MPI-GAI	14,676	2.44	0.84	2.63	0.82	<0.001	0.26
EQ-5D-index	13,989	0.26	0.31	0.39	0.33	<0.001	0.40
EQ-VAS	13,777	41.22	19.09	50.99	21.38	<0.001	0.44
sf36-pf	14,253	52.76	20.58	57.67	21.17	<0.001	0.30
sf36-rp	13,945	12.53	24.40	22.46	33.12	<0.001	0.30
sf36-bp	14,268	24.36	14.49	32.96	17.41	<0.001	**0.52**
sf36-gh	13,988	41.70	20.22	46.69	21.88	<0.001	0.29
sf36-vt	14,206	23.95	18.48	35.67	22.76	<0.001	**0.54**
sf36-sf	14,229	47.29	25.19	54.93	25.91	<0.001	0.30
sf36-re	13,701	42.77	42.92	51.15	43.48	<0.001	0.18
sf36-mh	14,194	55.03	21.35	62.55	21.55	<0.001	0.38

NRS-7days = Pain intensity as measured by a numeric rating scale for the previous seven days; HADS = Hospital Anxiety and Depression Scale; MPI = Multidimensional Pain Inventory; EQ-5D-index = The index of the European quality of life instrument; EQ-VAS = The European quality of life instrument thermometer-like scale; sf36 = The Short Form (36) Health Survey. For explanations of the subscale abbreviations, see Methods.

3.2. *Pairwise Comparisons of Repeated Measures*

The results for pre-IMMRP and post-IMMRP are shown in Table 2. Significant improvements were generally found except for two of the three scales of the second part of the MPI. In addition, the comparisons between pre-IMMRP and the 12-month FU generally revealed significant improvements except for one of the scales on the second part of the MPI (Table 3). Some outcomes were associated with moderate effect sizes. For the pre-IMMRP versus post-IMMRP comparisons, three variables had moderate effects sizes: MPI-pain-severity, sf36-bp, and sf36-vt (Table 2). At the 12-month FU, MPI-pain-severity and sf36-bp were associated with moderate effect sizes; this was also the case for MPI-pain-interference and EQ5d-index (Table 3). However, generally small effect sizes were found for the significant improvements (Tables 2 and 3). The variables of the second part of the MPI had insignificant effect sizes both post-IMMRP and 12-month FU.

Table 3. Outcome variables at baseline (pre-IMMRP) and at the 12-month follow-up (FU). Statistical comparisons are presented furthest to the right together with effects sizes (i.e., Cohen's d). Effect sizes in bold were moderate (i.e., Cohen's d ≥ 0.50).

Baseline vs. 12-Month Follow-Up		Pre IMMRP		12-Month FU			
	N	Mean	SD	Mean	SD	*p*-Value	Cohen's d
NRS-7days	8568	6.84	1.72	5.78	2.32	<0.001	0.47
HADS-A	8865	8.73	4.69	7.38	4.70	<0.001	0.33
HADS-D	8865	8.18	4.37	6.74	4.66	<0.001	0.35
MPI-Pain-severity	8904	4.36	0.91	3.71	1.33	<0.001	**0.56**
MPI-Pain-interfer	8829	4.34	1.02	3.73	1.37	<0.001	**0.54**
MPI-LifeCon	8871	2.77	1.10	3.28	1.27	<0.001	0.40
MPI-Distress	8889	3.42	1.27	2.92	1.45	<0.001	0.35
MPI-Socsupp	8830	4.17	1.33	3.77	1.42	<0.001	0.35
MPI-punish	7824	1.69	1.34	1.69	1.35	0.676	0.01
MPI-protect	7784	2.96	1.39	2.78	1.40	<0.001	0.16
MPI-distract	7811	2.52	1.17	2.45	1.17	<0.001	0.06
MPI-GAI	8859	2.47	0.83	2.64	0.86	<0.001	0.20
EQ-5D-index	8844	0.27	0.31	0.44	0.34	<0.001	**0.50**
EQ-VAS	8607	41.90	19.29	52.96	22.87	<0.001	0.46
sf36-pf	8459	53.07	20.30	59.73	22.57	<0.001	0.36
sf36-rp	8301	13.07	24.91	27.74	36.32	<0.001	0.39
sf36-bp	8458	24.60	14.11	35.41	20.05	<0.001	**0.56**
sf36-gh	8342	42.59	20.49	47.35	23.52	<0.001	0.25
sf36-vt	8441	24.96	18.79	34.41	23.85	<0.001	0.41
sf36-sf	8459	48.95	25.50	57.66	27.05	<0.001	0.32
sf36-re	8159	44.69	43.17	55.60	43.53	<0.001	0.22
sf36-mh	8435	56.34	21.15	62.70	22.53	<0.001	0.30

NRS-7days = Pain intensity as measured by a numeric rating scale for the previous seven days; HADS = Hospital Anxiety and Depression Scale; MPI = Multidimensional Pain Inventory; EQ-5D-index = The index of the European quality of life instrument; EQ-VAS = The European quality of life instrument thermometer-like scale; sf36 = The Short Form (36); Health Survey; FU = Follow-up. For explanations of the subscale abbreviations see Methods.

3.3. *Patients Not Participating in the 12-Month FU*

There were only small differences between those reporting PROM data at the 12-month FU and those not reporting their situation pre-IMMRP (Supplementary Table S1). Although those not reporting had a somewhat worse situation for most of the PROM variables, the differences were of no clinical importance.

3.4. *Estimations of Changes in Pain and in Life Situation*

At both post-IMMRP and 12-month FU, most patients reported that their pain situation had improved as well as their ability to handle their life situation (Table 4).

Table 4. Estimations of pain situation (Change-pain) and in the ability to handle life situation in general (Change-life situation) made immediately after IMMRP (post-IMMRP) and at the 12-month FU.

Change-Pain		Post-IMMRP		12-Month FU
	n	%	*n*	%
0. Markedly increased pain	447	3.2	225	2.6
1. Partially increased pain	1517	11	590	6.9
2. No change	4008	29.1	2905	34
3. Partially diminished pain	6178	44.9	3662	42.8
4. Markedly diminished pain	1607	11.7	1174	13.7
Total	13 757	100	8 556	100
Change-Life situation		**Post-IMMRP**		**12-Month FU**
	n	%	*n*	%
0. Markedly deteriorated	74	0.5	108	1.3
1. Partially deteriorated	248	1.8	282	3.3
2. No change	1923	13.9	1615	18.8
3. Partially improved	8412	60.9	4628	54
4. Markedly improved	3161	22.9	1937	22.6
Total	13 818	100	8 570	100

FU = Follow-up.

3.5. *Multivariate Correlation Pattern of Changes in Outcomes*

PCAs of the changes (i.e., the difference) were performed for pre-IMMRP versus post-IMMRP and pre-IMMRP versus 12-month FU. Significant models were achieved for both analyses (Table 5). Similar patterns were obtained for the first significant component of the two PCAs (Table 5). The first component of both analyses, reflecting the most important variations, showed that changes in HAD-D, MPI-pain-severity, MPI-pain interference, MPI-control, MPI-distress, sf-36-bp, sf-36-vt, sf-36-sf, and sf36-mh were most important and intercorrelated significantly. Hence, it was obvious that the changes in outcome variables are intercorrelated. That is, rather than representing 22 independent variables, the multivariate analyses show that most changes in these variables are highly intercorrelated.

At 12-month FU, the PCA also identified two additional components (Table 5). The second component mainly reflected the intercorrelation pattern between the social support scale of the MPI and the scales of part 2 of the MPI. A third significant component only explaining 6% of the variation in the dataset was also obtained in the analysis of changes at the 12-month follow-up versus baseline (Table 5).

The loading plot (i.e., the intercorrelations between variables of the two most important components for the changes pre IMMRP versus 12-month FU) is shown in Figure 1 (Figure 1a is a graphic presentation of the first two components reported in Table 5). Figure 1b shows the corresponding score plot (i.e., the relationships between subjects/patients). Each patient can be described with a score (*t*-score) for each significant component. Patients with high positive *t*-scores on the first component show prominent changes in the important variables constituting the first component, whereas patients near zero do not benefit, and patients with negative *t*-scores (located to the left in the score plot) deteriorate in the multivariate context. Hence, the *t*-score of the first component of both analyses can be considered as a Multivariate Improvement Score, in the following denoted MIS-post-IMMRP and MIS-12-month FU.

Table 5. Principal component analysis (PCA) of changes pre-IMMRP vs. post-IMMRP (left part) and pre-IMMRP vs. 12-month FU (right part). The significant components (p) are shown. Absolute loadings ≥ 0.25 are shown in bold to facilitate interpretation. Changes in outcomes are calculated so that a positive value indicates an improvement.

	Changes Pre-IMMRP vs. Post-IMMRP	**Changes Pre-IMMRP vs. 12-Month FU**		
	p[1]	p[1]	p[2]	p[3]
diff-NRS-7days	0.23	0.23	−0.15	**0.29**
diff-HADS-A	0.23	0.22	0.19	**−0.33**
diff-HADS-D	**0.26**	**0.25**	0.17	−0.24
diff-MPI-Pain-sever	**0.27**	**0.27**	−0.16	0.26
diff-MPI-Pain-interfer	**0.26**	**0.28**	−0.11	0.10
diff-MPI-LifeCon	**0.26**	**0.25**	0.09	−0.05
diff-MPI-distress	**0.27**	**0.26**	0.13	−0.21
diff-MPI-SOCsupp	−0.03	−0.07	**0.41**	0.21
diff-MPI-punish	0.07	0.08	**0.32**	0.11
diff-MPI-protect	−0.02	−0.02	**0.51**	**0.33**
diff-MPI-distract	0.01	0.00	**0.45**	**0.36**
diff-MPI-GAI	0.12	0.15	0.00	0.07
diff-EQ-5D-index	0.22	0.22	−0.07	0.12
diff-EQ-VAS	0.22	0.23	−0.03	0.09
diff-sf36-pf	0.20	0.21	−0.14	0.20
diff-sf36-rp	0.19	0.21	−0.10	0.17
diff-sf36-bp	**0.26**	**0.27**	−0.15	**0.25**
diff-sf36-gh	0.21	0.21	0.02	0.02
diff-sf36-vt	**0.27**	**0.26**	0.03	−0.03
diff-sf36-sf	**0.25**	0.24	0.05	−0.09
diff-sf36-re	0.18	0.17	0.13	**−0.26**
diff-sf36-mh	**0.27**	**0.25**	0.21	**−0.30**
R^2	0.31	0.36	0.10	0.06
Q^2	0.25	0.31	0.04	0.02
N	14,666	8851		

diff = change in a certain variable; *p* = principal component; NRS-7days = Pain intensity as measured by a numeric rating scale for the previous seven days; HADS = Hospital Anxiety and Depression Scale; MPI = Multidimensional Pain Inventory; EQ-5D-index = The index of the European quality of life instrument; EQ-VAS = The European quality of life instrument thermometer-like scale; sf36 = The Short Form (36) Health Survey; FU = Follow-up. For explanations of the subscale abbreviations see Methods.

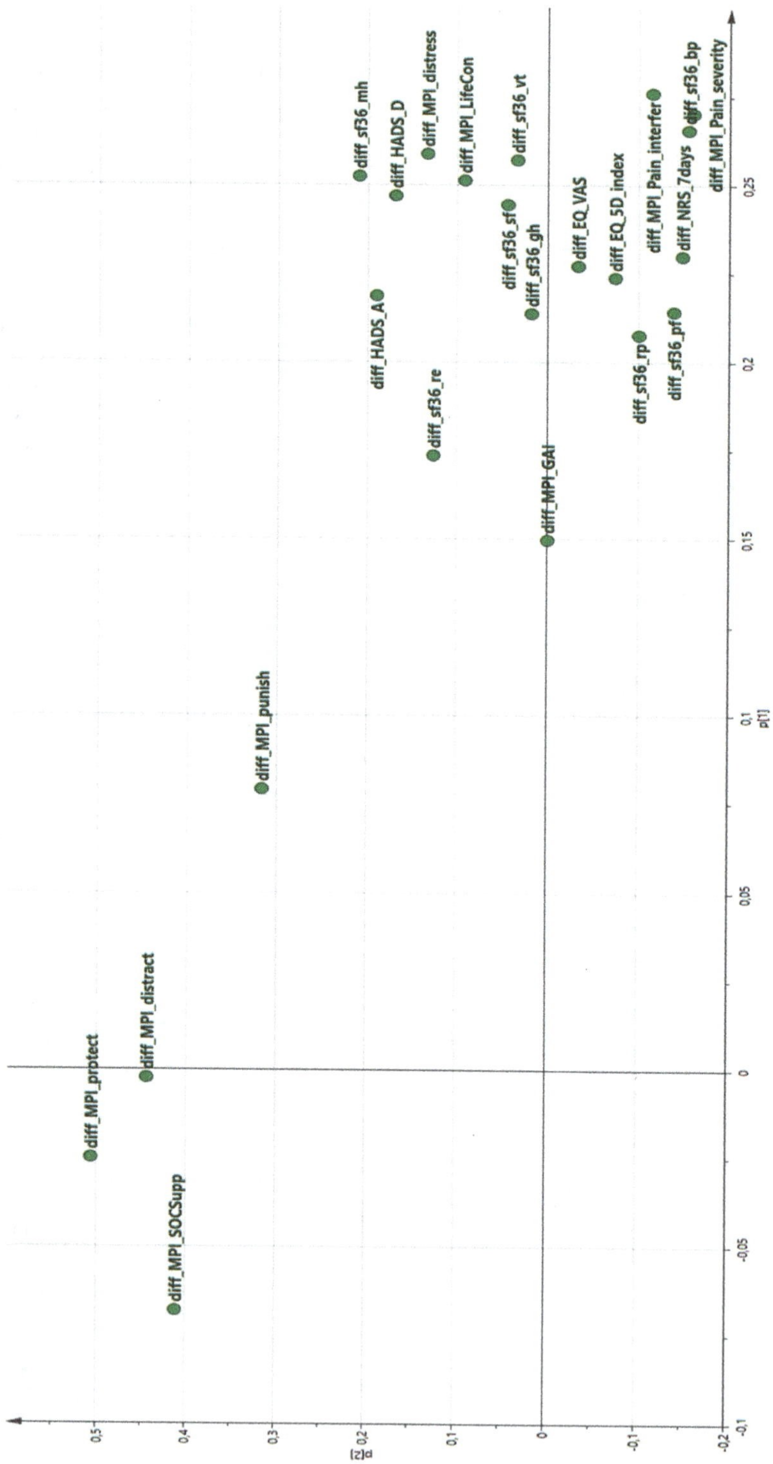

(a)

Figure 1. *Cont.*

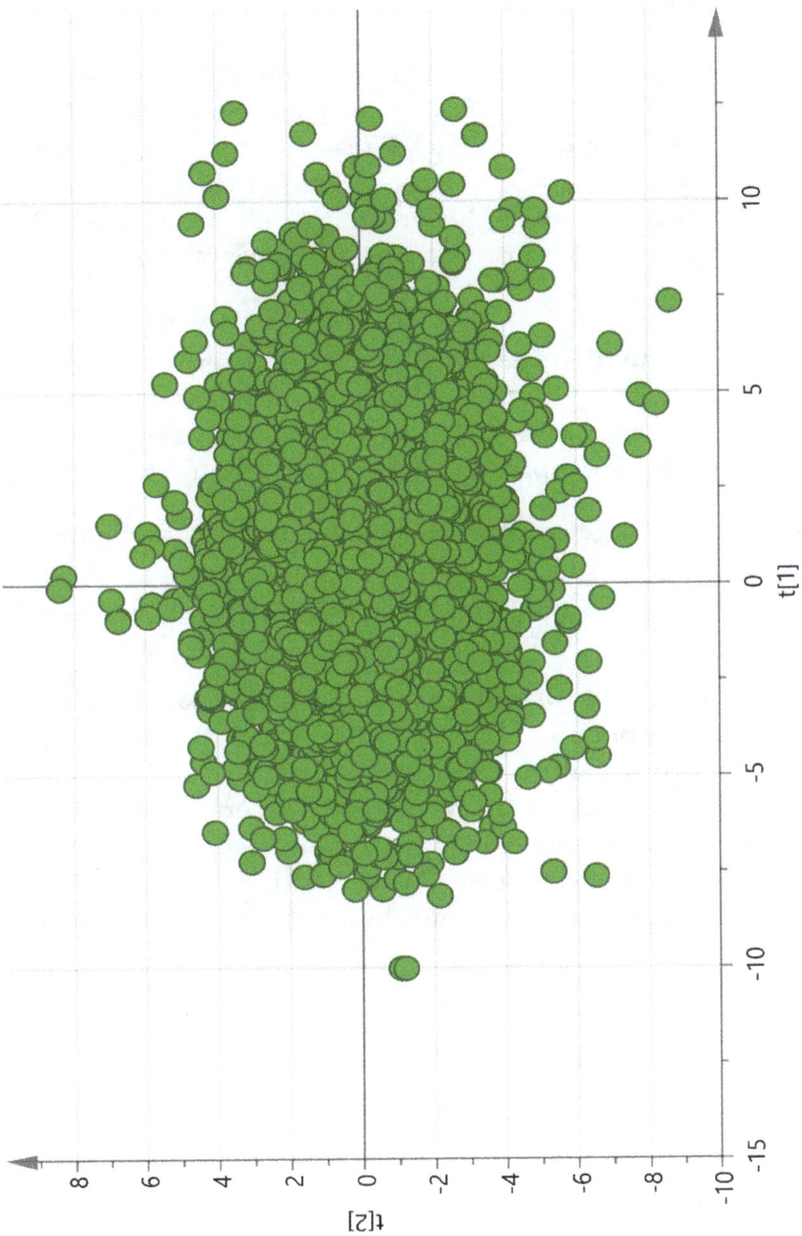

(b)

Figure 1. Loading plot of changes (pre-IMMRP vs. 12-month follow-up) in the 22 outcome variables—i.e., the relationships between the changes (**a**) and score plot ((**b**); the relationships between the patients). diff = change in a certain variable; NRS-7days = Pain intensity as measured by a numeric rating scale for the previous seven days; HADS = Hospital Anxiety and Depression Scale; MPI = Multidimensional Pain Inventory; EQ-5D-index = The index of the European quality of life instrument; EQ-VAS = The European quality of life instrument thermometer-like scale; sf36 = The Short Form (36) Health Survey; For explanations of the subscale abbreviations, see Methods.

3.6. *Identification of Subgroups Based on the Multivariate Improvement Scores (MIS)*

An HCA based on MIS-post-IMMRP was performed. Three subgroups/clusters were identified. Based on the HCA, a PLS-DA model with two predictive components was obtained with group belonging as the Y-variable (R^2 = 0.35; Q^2 = 0.35; CV-ANOVA $p < 0.001$; n = 14,666). Using a similar approach, we performed an HCA based on MIS-12-month FU. This analysis identified three subgroups/clusters. Based on the HCA, a PLS-DA model with two predictive components was obtained with group belonging as the Y-variable (R^2 = 0.37; Q^2 = 0.37; CV-ANOVA $p < 0.001$; n = 8851).

The MIS (i.e., *t*-score) showed clear positive values (i.e., improvements) for cluster 1 and negative scores (i.e., deterioration) for cluster 3 (Tables 6 and 7). Cluster 2 was an intermediary cluster with overall slightly positive improvements. Prominent effect sizes in the pairwise comparisons were observed post-IMMRP: cluster 1 versus cluster 2 = 3.33; cluster 1 versus cluster 3 = 5.36; and cluster 2 versus cluster 3 = 2.77; 12-month FU: cluster 1 versus cluster 2 = 2.92; cluster 1 versus cluster 3 = 4.99; and cluster 2 versus cluster 3 = 2.34. Thus, distinct differences in improvement levels were detected between the three clusters.

To facilitate the understanding of the identified clusters, the clusters were compared for the variables in each PCA (Tables 6 and 7). The three clusters differed significantly for all changes according to the ANOVAs performed. The post hoc tests showed that 20 of the 22 changes post-IMMRP differed significantly between all three clusters. The corresponding figure at 12-month FU was 21 of 22 changes.

The estimations of changes in pain (Change-pain) and in management of life (Change-life situation) were not included in the PCAs and thus not included in the calculations of MIS. However, these estimations showed a similar pattern: the most prominent positive changes were in cluster 1, and the least positive changes were in cluster 3 (Tables 6 and 7).

In the next step, the identified three clusters of both analyses were compared for their pre-IMMRP values (Tables 8 and 9). For the clusters obtained post-IMMRP (Table 8), small irrelevant cluster differences existed for age. The proportion with university education was significantly highest in cluster 1 and lowest in cluster 3, although the differences were small. Generally, cluster 1 was associated with the worst situation for the most variables followed longitudinally except for social support, two of the scales of Section 2 of the MPI, and sf36-pf. In contrast, cluster 3 had the best situation, and cluster 2 was intermediate (Table 8). A very similar pattern was found when using the clusters obtained from the 12-month FU (Table 9).

Table 6. Clusters from hierarchical clustering analysis (HCA) based on Multivariate Improvement Score (MIS) (*t*-scores) of the first component of the PCA for the changes in outcomes from pre-IMMRP to post-IMMRP (denoted ***MIS post-IMMRP***). To facilitate understanding, the changes for all the outcomes are shown (mean, SD, and 95% confidence interval). The two bottom rows show the estimations of changes (not included in PCA and the calculation of MIS).

	Cluster 1 (15.0%)					Cluster 2 (54.1%)					Cluster 3 (30.8%)						
	N	Mean	SD	95% CI		*N*	Mean	SD	95% CI		*N*	Mean	SD	95% CI		ANOVA	
Variables				LB	UB				LB	UB				LB	UB	*p*-Value	Post Hoc
MIS post-IMMRP	**2205**	***4.37***	***1.61***	***4.31***	***4.44***	***7938***	***0.33***	***1.08***	***0.30***	***0.35***	***4523***	**−2.74**	***1.16***	**−2.78**	**−2.71**	**<0.001**	***all different***
diff-NRS-7days	2086	3.04	2.05	2.95	3.13	7511	1.01	1.69	0.97	1.04	4267	−0.28	1.58	−0.32	−0.23	<0.001	all different
diff-HADS-A	2191	5.12	3.72	4.96	5.28	7873	1.59	3.08	1.52	1.66	4458	−1.30	3.24	−1.39	−1.20	<0.001	all different
diff-HADS-D	2188	5.93	3.55	5.78	6.08	7869	2.24	2.95	2.17	2.30	4462	−0.96	3.04	−1.05	−0.87	<0.001	all different
diff-MPI-Pain-severity	2185	1.77	1.02	1.73	1.82	7874	0.56	0.74	0.54	0.58	4500	−0.17	0.69	−0.19	−0.15	<0.001	all different
diff-MPI-Pain-interfer	2173	1.53	0.99	1.49	1.57	7811	0.50	0.70	0.48	0.51	4453	−0.17	0.66	−0.18	−0.15	<0.001	all different
diff-MPI-LideCon	2189	1.94	1.05	1.89	1.98	7861	0.71	0.96	0.69	0.73	4491	−0.33	0.99	−0.36	−0.30	<0.001	all different
diff-MPI-distress	2187	2.18	1.17	2.13	2.23	7869	0.71	1.02	0.69	0.73	4487	−0.46	1.05	−0.49	−0.43	<0.001	all different
diff-MPI-SOCsupp	2180	−0.34	1.12	−0.39	−0.30	7828	−0.24	0.98	−0.26	−0.21	4462	−0.11	0.98	−0.14	−0.08	<0.001	all different
diff-MPI-punish	1991	0.39	1.20	0.34	0.45	7016	0.04	1.12	0.02	0.07	4008	−0.20	1.15	−0.24	−0.17	<0.001	all different
diff-MPI-protect	1988	−0.18	1.17	−0.23	−0.13	6984	−0.14	1.00	−0.17	−0.12	3989	−0.05	1.05	−0.09	−0.02	<0.001	cl1 NE cl2, cl2 NE cl3
diff-MPI-distract	1992	0.11	1.10	0.06	0.16	7012	0.00	0.96	−0.03	0.02	4006	0.01	1.03	−0.02	0.04	<0.001	cl1 NE cl2, cl3
diff-MPI-GAI	2187	0.57	0.82	0.53	0.60	7866	0.23	0.68	0.21	0.24	4489	−0.06	0.69	−0.08	−0.03	<0.001	all different
diff-EQ-5D-index	2105	0.44	0.30	0.43	0.45	7494	0.16	0.28	0.15	0.17	4205	−0.07	0.28	−0.08	−0.06	<0.001	all different
diff-EQ-VAS	2068	30.51	19.66	29.66	31.36	7409	11.61	18.58	11.19	12.03	4126	−3.84	19.15	−4.42	−3.25	<0.001	all different
diff-sf36-pf	2147	18.74	16.97	18.02	19.46	7644	6.02	13.63	5.72	6.33	4324	−3.83	14.22	−4.25	−3.40	<0.001	all different
diff-sf36-rp	2110	39.93	39.28	38.25	41.60	7513	10.46	29.70	9.79	11.13	4215	−5.96	25.56	−6.74	−5.19	<0.001	all different
diff-sf36-bp	2146	28.04	16.27	27.35	28.73	7663	9.72	12.96	9.43	10.01	4323	−2.93	12.38	−3.30	−2.56	<0.001	all different
diff-sf36-gh	2126	21.06	17.59	20.31	21.81	7529	6.05	14.51	5.72	6.37	4235	−4.89	14.57	−5.33	−4.45	<0.001	all different
diff-sf36-vt	2139	37.45	18.74	36.65	38.24	7626	13.58	17.26	13.19	13.96	4311	−4.20	16.16	−4.69	−3.72	<0.001	all different
diff-sf36-sf	2146	34.26	22.17	33.32	35.20	7652	10.12	20.39	9.66	10.58	4324	−9.86	21.10	−10.49	−9.23	<0.001	all different
diff-sf36-re	2087	43.52	44.58	41.60	45.43	7390	11.98	43.21	11.00	12.97	4121	−15.81	42.02	−17.09	−14.52	<0.001	all different
diff-sf36-mh	2139	29.61	17.48	28.86	30.35	7620	10.12	14.90	9.78	10.45	4307	−8.01	15.89	−8.49	−7.54	<0.001	all different
Change-Pain	2059	3.28	0.69	3.25	3.31	7280	2.53	0.87	2.51	2.55	4015	2.08	0.93	2.05	2.11	<0.001	all different
Change-Life situation	2067	3.51	0.58	3.48	3.53	7315	3.07	0.63	3.05	3.08	4032	2.76	0.72	2.74	2.79	<0.001	all different

LB = Lower Bound; UB = Upper Bound; diff = change in a certain variable; NRS-7days = Pain intensity as measured by a numeric rating scale for the previous seven days; HADS = Hospital Anxiety and Depression Scale; MPI = Multidimensional Pain Inventory; EQ-5D-index = The index of the European quality of life instrument; EQ-VAS = The European quality of life instrument thermometer-like scale; sf36 = The Short Form (36) Health Survey. For explanations of the subscale abbreviations, see Methods.

Table 7. Clusters from HCA based on MIS (*t*-scores) of the first component of the PCA for the changes in outcomes from pre-IMMRP to 12-month FU (denoted as ***MIS 12-m FU***). To facilitate understanding, the changes for all the outcomes are shown (mean, SD, and 95% confidence interval). The two bottom rows show the estimations of changes (not included in PCA and the calculation of MIS).

	Cluster 1 (12.4%)					Cluster 2 (46.6%)					Cluster 3 (41.0%)						
	N	Mean	SD	95% CI		*N*	Mean	SD	95% CI		*N*	Mean	SD	95% CI		ANOVA	
Variables				LB	UB				LB	UB				LB	UB	*p*-Value	Post Hoc
MIS -12-m FU	***1099***	***5.01***	***1.78***	***4.90***	***5.11***	***4123***	***0.78***	***1.35***	***0.74***	***0.82***	***3629***	***−2.43***	***1.39***	***−2.47***	***−2.38***	***<0.001***	***all different***
diff-NRS-7days	1031	3.67	2.15	3.54	3.80	3876	1.46	1.89	1.40	1.52	3435	−0.16	1.66	−0.21	−0.10	<0.001	all different
diff-HADS-A	1095	5.72	3.84	5.49	5.95	4087	2.06	3.34	1.96	2.16	3588	−0.80	3.53	−0.91	−0.68	<0.001	all different
diff-HADS-D	1096	6.13	3.75	5.90	6.35	4086	2.39	3.13	2.29	2.48	3588	−1.05	3.39	−1.16	−0.94	<0.001	all different
diff-MPI-Pain-severity	1092	2.30	1.14	2.24	2.37	4108	0.88	0.90	0.85	0.91	3619	−0.09	0.76	−0.12	−0.07	<0.001	all different
diff-MPI-Pain-interfer	1092	2.30	1.14	2.24	2.37	4108	0.88	0.90	0.85	0.91	3589	−0.14	0.74	−0.17	−0.12	<0.001	all different
diff-MPI-LifeCon	1086	2.27	1.10	2.21	2.34	4076	0.83	0.85	0.81	0.86	3604	−0.25	1.05	−0.28	−0.21	<0.001	all different
diff-MPI-distress	1091	2.10	1.10	2.03	2.16	4095	0.75	1.00	0.71	0.78	3618	−0.38	1.13	−0.41	−0.34	<0.001	all different
diff-MPI-SOCsupp	1086	−0.69	1.25	−0.77	−0.62	4081	−0.60	1.16	−0.64	−0.57	3583	−0.10	1.04	−0.13	−0.07	<0.001	all different
diff-MPI-punish	979	0.57	1.19	0.50	0.65	3633	−0.02	1.22	−0.06	0.02	3194	−0.13	1.22	−0.18	−0.09	<0.001	all different
diff-MPI-protect	980	−0.23	1.24	−0.31	−0.15	3616	−0.35	1.20	−0.39	−0.31	3173	0.03	1.09	−0.01	0.06	<0.001	all different
diff-MPI-distract	981	0.02	1.15	−0.05	0.10	3627	−0.22	1.09	−0.25	−0.18	3188	0.08	1.02	0.04	0.11	<0.001	CL NE cl3, cl2 NE cl3
diff-MPI-GAI	1090	0.76	0.95	0.70	0.82	4094	0.26	0.73	0.23	0.28	3613	−0.11	0.73	−0.14	−0.09	<0.001	all different
diff-EQ-5D-index	1048	0.53	0.30	0.51	0.55	3886	0.25	0.30	0.24	0.26	3351	−0.04	0.30	−0.05	−0.03	<0.001	all different
diff-EQ-VAS	1022	36.06	20.47	34.80	37.32	3833	16.27	19.82	15.64	16.89	3316	−3.31	19.66	−3.98	−2.64	<0.001	all different
diff-sf36-pf	1054	26.77	19.09	25.61	27.92	3953	10.00	15.13	9.53	10.47	3445	−3.31	15.24	−3.81	−2.80	<0.001	all different
diff-sf36-rp	1043	57.34	39.51	54.94	59.74	3889	19.15	34.30	18.07	20.22	3365	−3.69	27.14	−4.60	−2.77	<0.001	all different
diff-sf36-bp	1054	37.44	19.56	36.26	38.63	3954	14.29	14.79	13.83	14.75	3444	−1.33	13.03	−1.76	−0.89	<0.001	all different
diff-sf36-gh	1044	25.26	19.09	24.10	26.42	3908	7.78	16.33	7.26	8.29	3388	−5.04	15.87	−5.57	−4.50	<0.001	all different
diff-sf36-vt	1054	40.71	19.72	39.52	41.91	3951	13.32	17.83	12.77	13.88	3433	−4.60	16.67	−5.16	−4.05	<0.001	all different
diff-sf36-sf	1053	40.73	23.26	39.32	42.14	3958	14.43	21.21	13.77	15.09	3445	−7.66	22.38	−8.40	−6.91	<0.001	all different
diff-sf36-re	1031	53.10	44.27	50.40	55.81	3849	17.22	45.08	15.79	18.64	3277	−9.79	45.59	11.35	−8.22	<0.001	all different
diff-sf36-mh	1054	32.77	18.81	31.64	33.91	3948	10.62	16.33	10.11	11.13	3430	−6.66	17.25	−7.24	−6.09	<0.001	all different
Change-Pain	1049	3.32	0.74	3.28	3.37	3887	2.72	0.81	2.69	2.75	3373	2.20	0.85	2.17	2.22	<0.001	all different
Change-Life situation	1049	3.52	0.64	3.48	3.56	3901	3.05	0.70	3.03	3.08	3375	2.62	0.83	2.59	2.65	<0.001	all different

LB = Lower Bound; UB = Upper Bound; diff = change in a certain variable; NRS-7days = Pain intensity as measured by a numeric rating scale for the previous seven days; HADS = Hospital Anxiety and Depression Scale; MPI = Multidimensional Pain Inventory; EQ-5D-index = The index of the European quality of life instrument; EQ-VAS = The European quality of life instrument thermometer-like scale; sf36 = The Short Form (36) Health Survey. For explanations of the subscale abbreviations, see Methods.

Table 8. Pre-IMMRP values for the three clusters based on MIS obtained post-IMMRP.

	Cluster 1					Cluster 2					Cluster 3						
Baseline	*N*	Mean	SD	95% CI		*N*	Mean	SD	95% CI		*N*	Mean	SD	95% CI		ANOVA	
Variables				LB	UB				LB	UB				LB	UB	*p*-Value	Post Hoc
Gender	2205	0.22	0.41	0.20	0.23	7938	0.24	0.43	0.23	0.25	4523	0.25	0.43	0.24	0.26	0.014	NA
Age	2205	42.7	11.2	42.2	43.2	7938	43.5	10.7	43.3	43.8	4523	43.0	10.6	42.7	43.3	0.001	cl1 NE cl3, cl2 NE cl3
Outside-Europe	2185	0.11	0.31	0.09	0.12	7877	0.10	0.30	0.09	0.10	4484	0.11	0.32	0.10	0.12	0.011	NA
University	2168	0.28	0.45	0.26	0.29	7826	0.26	0.44	0.25	0.27	4445	0.23	0.42	0.22	0.24	0.000	cl1 NE cl2, cl2 NE cl3
Days no work	716	889	2912	675	1102	2976	1037	2311	954	1120	1774	1152	2502	1036	1269	0.045	NA
PRI	2205	13.8	8.3	13.4	14.1	7938	14.4	8.3	14.2	14.6	4523	14.5	8.3	14.3	14.7	0.002	NA
NRS-7days	2158	7.1	1.7	7.0	7.2	7801	6.9	1.7	6.8	6.9	4440	6.7	1.7	6.7	6.8	0.000	all different
HADS-A	2199	10.4	4.7	10.2	10.6	7891	9.0	4.7	8.9	9.1	4494	8.2	4.6	8.1	8.4	0.000	all different
HADS-D	2197	9.6	4.4	9.4	9.8	7892	8.6	4.4	8.5	8.7	4494	7.7	4.3	7.6	7.9	0.000	all different
MPI-Pain-severity	2193	4.5	0.9	4.5	4.6	7895	4.4	0.9	4.4	4.4	4510	4.3	0.9	4.3	4.3	0.000	all different
MPI-Pain-interfer	2187	4.6	1.0	4.6	4.6	7853	4.4	1.0	4.4	4.4	4485	4.3	1.0	4.2	4.3	0.000	all different
MPI-LifeCon	2195	2.4	1.1	2.4	2.5	7880	2.7	1.1	2.7	2.7	4502	2.9	1.1	2.9	3.0	0.000	all different
MPI-Distress	2191	3.9	1.2	3.9	4.0	7891	3.5	1.3	3.5	3.5	4502	3.2	1.3	3.1	3.2	0.000	all different
MPI-Socsupp	2190	4.2	1.4	4.2	4.3	7861	4.2	1.3	4.1	4.2	4488	4.1	1.4	4.1	4.2	0.005	NA
MPI-punish	2069	1.9	1.5	1.8	1.9	7319	1.8	1.4	1.7	1.8	4169	1.7	1.3	1.6	1.7	0.000	all different
MPI-protect	2065	3.0	1.5	2.9	3.1	7295	2.9	1.4	2.9	3.0	4158	3.0	1.4	2.9	3.0	0.136	NA
MPI-distract	2069	2.6	1.2	2.5	2.6	7312	2.5	1.2	2.5	2.5	4168	2.5	1.2	2.5	2.6	0.075	NA
MPI-GAI	2193	2.4	0.8	2.4	2.4	7885	2.4	0.8	2.4	2.5	4500	2.5	0.8	2.5	2.5	0.000	cl1 NE cl2, cl2 NE cl3
EQ-5D-index	2126	0.2	0.3	0.2	0.2	7587	0.3	0.3	0.2	0.3	4277	0.3	0.3	0.3	0.3	0.000	all different
EQ-VAS	2097	38.0	18.2	37.2	38.8	7529	40.7	19.0	40.3	41.1	4224	43.9	19.4	43.3	44.5	0.000	all different
sf36-pf	2151	52.1	21.0	51.2	52.9	7683	52.8	20.6	52.3	53.2	4349	53.2	20.2	52.6	53.8	0.119	NA
sf36-rp	2139	9.0	19.8	8.2	9.9	7629	11.8	23.8	11.3	12.4	4283	15.3	26.8	14.5	16.1	0.000	all different
sf36-bp	2151	21.1	13.8	20.5	21.7	7694	24.1	14.3	23.8	24.4	4347	26.4	14.6	26.0	26.8	0.000	all different
sf36-gh	2139	39.8	20.0	38.9	40.6	7610	41.4	20.1	41.0	41.9	4299	43.3	20.4	42.7	43.9	0.000	all different
sf36-vt	2151	19.7	16.6	19.0	20.4	7679	23.3	18.4	22.9	23.7	4347	27.3	19.0	26.7	27.8	0.000	all different
sf36-sf	2151	40.0	23.7	39.0	41.0	7690	46.6	24.9	46.1	47.2	4348	52.1	25.3	51.4	52.9	0.000	all different
sf36-re	2126	30.6	39.6	28.9	32.2	7549	41.6	42.6	40.7	42.6	4220	50.6	43.6	49.3	51.9	0.000	all different
sf36-mh	2151	47.3	20.7	46.5	48.2	7672	54.5	21.2	54.0	54.9	4343	60.1	20.5	59.4	60.7	0.000	all different

LB = Lower Bound; UB = Upper Bound; NA = not applicable; NRS-7days = Pain intensity as measured by a numeric rating scale for the previous seven days; HADS = Hospital Anxiety and Depression Scale; MPI = Multidimensional Pain Inventory; EQ-5D-index = The index of the European quality of life instrument; EQ-VAS = The European quality of life instrument thermometer-like scale; sf36 = The Short Form (36) Health Survey; PRI = Pain Region Index. For explanations of the subscale abbreviations, see Methods.

Table 9. Pre-IMMRP values for the three clusters based on MIS obtained at 12-month FU.

	Cluster 1					Cluster 2					Cluster 3						
Baseline	*N*	Mean	SD	95% CI		*N*	Mean	SD	95% CI		*N*	Mean	SD	95% CI		ANOVA	
Variables				LB	UB				LB	UB				LB	UB	*p*-Value	Post Hoc
Gender	1099	0.24	0.43	0.21	0.26	4123	0.21	0.41	0.20	0.22	3629	0.25	0.43	0.24	0.27	<0.001	all different
Age	1099	41.9	11.1	41.2	42.5	4123	43.7	11.1	43.4	44.0	3629	44.2	10.4	43.8	44.5	<0.001	all different
Outside-Europe	1088	0.09	0.29	0.07	0.11	4091	0.08	0.28	0.08	0.09	3606	0.10	0.30	0.09	0.11	0.012	NA
University	1079	0.29	0.45	0.26	0.31	4060	0.27	0.45	0.26	0.29	3567	0.23	0.42	0.21	0.24	<0.001	all different except cl2 vs. cl3
Days no work	358	661	2587	392	930	1409	1046	2339	923	1168	1323	1270	2604	1130	1411	<0.001	all different
PRI	1099	12.8	8.0	12.3	13.2	4123	14.2	8.3	14.0	14.5	3629	14.8	8.3	14.5	15.1	<0.001	all different
NRS-7days	1071	7.0	1.7	6.9	7.1	4049	6.8	1.7	6.8	6.9	3574	6.8	1.7	6.8	6.9	0.049	NA
HADS-A	1096	9.7	4.7	9.4	10.0	4101	8.7	4.7	8.6	8.9	3606	8.4	4.6	8.3	8.6	<0.001	all different
HADS-D	1096	8.8	4.4	8.6	9.1	4102	8.2	4.3	8.1	8.3	3606	8.0	4.4	7.9	8.1	<0.001	all different
MPI-Pain-severity	1094	4.5	0.9	4.4	4.5	4114	4.4	0.9	4.3	4.4	3625	4.3	0.9	4.3	4.4	<0.001	cl1NE cl2, cl2 NE cl1, cl3
MPI-Pain-interfer	1093	4.5	0.9	4.5	4.6	4101	4.4	1.0	4.3	4.4	3609	4.3	1.0	4.2	4.3	<0.001	all different
MPI-LifeCon	1096	2.5	1.1	2.5	2.6	4113	2.8	1.1	2.7	2.8	3614	2.9	1.1	2.8	2.9	<0.001	all different
MPI-Distress	1095	3.8	1.2	3.8	3.9	4114	3.4	1.3	3.4	3.5	3621	3.3	1.3	3.2	3.3	<0.001	all different
MPI-Socsupp	1090	4.3	1.3	4.2	4.4	4097	4.2	1.3	4.2	4.3	3604	4.1	1.4	4.1	4.1	<0.001	all different
MPI-punish	1036	1.8	1.4	1.7	1.9	3833	1.7	1.3	1.6	1.7	3355	1.7	1.3	1.7	1.8	0.047	NA
IMP-protect	1038	3.0	1.4	2.9	3.1	3824	2.9	1.4	2.9	3.0	3341	2.9	1.4	2.9	3.0	0.583	NA
MPI-distract	1039	2.6	1.2	2.5	2.6	3831	2.6	1.2	2.5	2.6	3352	2.5	1.2	2.4	2.5	0.003	NA
MPI -GAI	1094	2.4	0.9	2.4	2.5	4108	2.5	0.8	2.5	2.5	3623	2.5	0.8	2.5	2.5	0.071	NA
EQ-5D-index	1058	0.2	0.3	0.2	0.2	3935	0.3	0.3	0.3	0.3	3407	0.3	0.3	0.3	0.3	<0.001	all different
EQ-VAS	1037	39.2	18.2	38.1	40.3	3905	41.3	19.2	40.7	42.0	3389	43.1	19.6	42.4	43.7	<0.001	all different
sf36-pf	1056	51.9	20.4	50.7	53.1	3969	53.0	20.4	52.4	53.7	3459	53.4	20.1	52.7	54.1	0.120	NA
sf36-rp	1053	8.5	20.6	7.2	9.7	3938	12.4	24.1	11.6	13.1	3417	15.3	26.9	14.4	16.2	<0.001	all different
sf36-bp	1058	21.5	13.3	20.7	22.3	3974	24.4	14.2	23.9	24.8	3461	25.9	14.0	25.4	26.3	<0.001	all different
sf36-gh	1052	43.1	21.0	41.8	44.4	3944	42.6	20.5	42.0	43.2	3424	42.3	20.3	41.7	43.0	0.556	NA
sf36-vt	1058	21.4	17.8	20.3	22.5	3972	24.7	19.1	24.1	25.3	3452	26.3	18.6	25.7	26.9	<0.001	all different
sf36-sf	1056	42.4	24.2	40.9	43.9	3976	48.2	25.6	47.4	49.0	3458	51.9	25.2	51.0	52.7	<0.001	all different
sf36-re	1046	32.1	40.3	29.7	34.5	3906	44.0	43.2	42.7	45.4	3363	49.1	43.2	47.6	50.5	<0.001	all different
sf36-mh	1058	49.6	20.9	48.3	50.9	3970	56.0	21.0	55.3	56.7	3451	58.7	20.9	58.0	59.4	<0.001	all different

LB = Lower Bound; UB = Upper Bound; NA = not applicable; NRS-7days = Pain intensity as measured by a numeric rating scale for the previous seven days; HADS = Hospital Anxiety and Depression Scale; MPI = Multidimensional Pain Inventory; EQ-5D-index = The index of the European quality of life instrument; EQ-VAS = The European quality of life instrument thermometer-like scale; sf36 = The Short Form (36) Health Survey; PRI = Pain Region Index. For explanations of the subscale abbreviations, see Methods.

3.7. Longitudinal Regression of MIS Using Baseline Data

The outcome data at baseline (pre-IMMRP) together with the background variables were used to regress MIS-post-IMMRP and MIS-12-month FU (Table 10). For both MIS, psychological distress variables were the most important regressors, but life impact variables, pain aspects, and health and vitality aspects contributed significantly. The directions of the correlations revealed that a more severe clinical situation (e.g., psychological distress, lack of control, low vitality and health, pain interference, and high pain intensity) were associated with high MIS (i.e., multivariate improvements). Although the obtained regressions were highly significant according to the CV-ANOVA, the explained variations in MIS were less than 10% ($R^2 = 0.08$ in both analyses). Hence, most of the variations in the two MIS were not possible to predict.

Similar analyses for each of the clusters (Supplementary Tables S2 and S3) revealed that regressions were highly significant, but only explained a minority of the variations in MIS. Although the relative importance of the variables pre-IMMRP differed somewhat between the three clusters, no marked differences existed; that is, psychological distress aspects were the most important post-IMMRP (Supplementary Table S2). For the 12-month FU, somewhat more pronounced differences existed between the clusters: in cluster 2, the pain intensity aspects were the most important for MIS, and in cluster 1 and cluster 3, psychological distress variables together with pain interference were the most important for MIS.

Table 10. Orthogonal Partial Least Square Regressions (OPLS) regressions of MIS post-IMMRP (left part) and at 12-month FU (right part) using the variables pre-IMMRP as regressors. Variables in bold type are significant regressors.

Post-IMMRP	VIP	p(corr)	12-Month FU	VIP	p(corr)
Variables Pre-IMMRP			Variables Pre-IMMRP		
sf36-mh	**1.80**	**−0.80**	**sf36-mh**	**1.63**	**−0.62**
MPI-Distress	**1.72**	**0.76**	**MPI-Distress**	**1.59**	**0.61**
HADS-D	**1.56**	**0.68**	**sf36-sf**	**1.44**	**−0.53**
MPI-LifeCon	**1.48**	**−0.65**	**sf36-re**	**1.39**	**−0.54**
HADS-A	**1.48**	**0.65**	**MPI-LifeCon**	**1.35**	**−0.49**
sf36-sf	**1.47**	**−0.63**	**HADS-D**	**1.34**	**0.46**
sf36-re	**1.43**	**−0.64**	**HADS-A**	**1.28**	**0.46**
sf36-vt	**1.27**	**−0.54**	**MPI-Pain-interfer**	**1.26**	**0.39**
MPI-Pain-interfer	**1.26**	**0.45**	**Persistent-Pain-duration**	**1.16**	**−0.46**
EQ-5D-index	**1.12**	**−0.41**	**Pain duration**	**1.15**	**−0.45**
sf36-bp	**1.07**	**−0.35**	**EQ-5D-index**	**1.14**	**−0.37**
MPI-Pain-severity	**1.05**	**0.28**	**sf36-bp**	**1.11**	**−0.35**
EQ-VAS	**1.04**	**−0.39**	**sf36-vt**	**1.11**	**−0.36**
sf36-gh	0.95	−0.30	MPI-Pain-severity	0.99	0.21
NRS-7days	0.88	0.20	EQ-VAS	0.97	−0.28
sf36-pf	0.87	−0.07	sf36-rp	0.96	−0.37
sf36-rp	0.80	−0.33	PRI	0.95	−0.26
PRI	0.72	−0.09	sf36-gh	0.87	−0.10
MPI-GAI	0.68	−0.20	NRS-7days	0.81	0.11
MPI-punish	0.59	0.25	Days no work	0.80	-0.31
Outside-Europe	0.45	−0.01	sf36-pf	0.76	−0.05
Days no work	0.44	−0.16	Age	0.75	−0.30
University	0.43	0.12	MPI-GAI	0.72	−0.22
Persistent Pain duration	0.42	−0.16	University	0.54	0.18
MPI-protect	0.41	−0.04	MPI-punish	0.43	0.12
Pain duration	0.38	−0.15	Outside-Europe	0.39	−0.03
MPI-Socsupp	0.32	−0.05	MPI-protect	0.31	0.03
MPI-distract	0.29	−0.01	MPI-distract	0.26	0.06
Age	0.23	−0.10	MPI-Socsupp	0.22	0.07
Gender	0.04	−0.01	Gender	0.10	−0.04

Table 10. *Cont.*

Post-IMMRP Variables Pre-IMMRP	VIP	p(corr)	12-Month FU Variables Pre-IMMRP	VIP	p(corr)
R^2	0.08		R^2	0.08	
Q^2	0.08		Q^2	0.07	
n	14 657		*n*	7 976	
CV-ANOVA *p*-value	<0.001		CV-ANOVA *p*-value	<0.001	

VIP (VIP > 1.0 is significant) and p (corr) are reported for each regressor. The sign of p (corr) indicates the direction of the correlation with the dependent variable (+ = positive correlation; − = negative correlation). The four bottom rows of each regression report R^2, Q^2, and *p*-value of the CV-ANOVA and number of patients included in the regression (*n*). NRS-7days = Pain intensity as measured by a numeric rating scale for the previous seven days; HADS = Hospital Anxiety and Depression Scale; MPI = Multidimensional Pain Inventory EQ-5D-index = The index of the European quality of life instrument; EQ-VAS = The European quality of life instrument thermometer-like scale; sf36 = The Short Form (36) Health Survey; PRI = Pain Region Index. For explanations of the subscale abbreviations see Methods.

4. Discussions

The major findings of the present large PROM study from SQRP are listed below:

- Moderate long-term ES were found for pain intensity (MPI Pain severity and SF-36 bodily pain), interference in daily life (MPI Interference), and state of health (EQ-5D-index); most other variables showed small ES. Vitality also displayed moderate effect sizes immediately after IMMRP but fell slightly under cut-off for moderate change at 12-month follow-up. The majority of the 22 investigated outcomes were significantly improved.
- Significant intercorrelations between changes in pain intensity, interference, control, psychological distress, and mental health were confirmed. The changes in 22 outcomes reflected one (pre-IMMRP versus post-IMMRP) or three (pre-IMMRP versus 12-month follow-up) latent components (groups of variables).
- The outcomes were best for patients with the worst self-reported clinical presentation pre-IMMRP. Based on a defined multivariate improvement score (MIS), three clusters were identified. Cluster 1—overall, the worst situation pre-IMMRP—showed positive multivariate improvements in outcomes. Cluster 3—deteriorated—showed negative scores. Cluster 2, the intermediate cluster, was associated with overall slightly positive multivariate improvements.
- Certain variables (especially psychological distress and life impact variables, pain, and health and vitality aspects) pre-IMMRP were associated with improvements according to MIS both post-IMMRP and at 12-month FU. However statistically significant, the pre-IMMRP situation could only explain a small part of the variation in MIS (8%); therefore, for clinical use, it was not possible to predict those who would benefit most from IMMRP.

The outcome variables mandatory in SQRP and presented in the present study are in good agreement with the BSP model of chronic pain and the outcome domains presented by the Initiative on Methods, Measurement, and Pain Assessment in Clinical Trials (IMMPACT) [7,52] and the Validation and Application of a patient-relevant core set of outcome domains to assess multimodal PAIN therapy (VAPAIN) [14] initiatives.

The present study was not primarily designed to evaluate the efficacy of IMMRP, which requires RCTs and SRs/meta-analyses. However, our results for the repeated measurements (Tables 2 and 3) of chronic pain patients in real-life practice settings are in agreement with the positive evidence for IMMRPs reported in SRs [10–12] and in other studies [22,23,53]. As such, the small to moderate ES are noteworthy as these patients, who receive pain rehabilitation in specialist care centres, often have tried other treatments for their chronic pain with no or little effect. That is, these patients have severe problems and relative treatment resistance. Interestingly, the changes in outcomes with moderate ES are broad and not limited to a single outcome domain, and the most stable moderate ES were demonstrated for pain intensity aspects with moderate improvement both immediately after

IMMRPs and at 12-month follow-up. Pain interference demonstrated moderate ES improvement at 12-month follow-up, and vitality was moderately improved immediately after IMMRPs. Both objective registrations (e.g., sick-leave registrations and actigraphic recordings [54]) and subjective PROM data may be important for understanding the efficacy of IMMRPs. Very recently, a SQRP study using a subgroup of the same cohort of patients reported that sick leave benefits according to the Swedish Social Insurance Agency decreased as a consequence of IMMRP [55]. Hence, both PROM data and objective sick leave data indicate clinically important positive changes in response to IMMRPs for patients in real-life practice settings. As a comparison, SRs conclude that common pharmacological treatments—e.g., paracetamol, non-steroidal anti-inflammatory drugs, and opioids—for patients with chronic pain have no effects, small effects, and/or lack of long-term follow-up effects [56–58].

The present study reported medium ES for two of three pain intensity variables both post-IMMRP and at 12-month FU (i.e., for MPI-pain-severity and sf36-bp); the third pain intensity variable had effect sizes near medium ES. These results contrasted some SRs reporting of no evidence for efficacy with respect to pain intensity [10,11]. However, not all RCTs of IMMRP included pain intensity outcomes, since the interventions are not focused on the pain itself but rather on its consequences [10,11]. Obviously, many pain patients consider pain intensity improvement to be the most important aspect of treatments [59]. However, changing this perspective is considered important in IMMPRs, since focusing on pain reduction in many cases leads to short-sighted attempts to control pain, and this may, when not successful, lead to increased physical and psychological disability and reduced life quality [60,61]. Thus, specialist care IMMRPs in Sweden have largely adopted the idea of introducing acceptance as a cornerstone of the psychological component of IMMRP (i.e., the willingness to have the experiences of pain as it is and to encourage patients to set up activity-related rehabilitation goals and risk initial pain flare-ups). This also means that patients are advised against establishing pain reduction goals. Thus, it could be considered problematic to communicate the present results showing medium effect sizes in real-world practice settings on pain. On the other hand, it may also be ethically problematic if both clinical practice and research ignore the reports and wishes of the patients regarding pain intensity. However, health care providers should not underestimate their patients' ability to grasp, once explained, the complex pain experience. Therefore, health care providers should emphasise pain education, including descriptions of the affective and cognitive elements of pain as rational for the different components of IMMRPs, and stress the need to experiment with new behaviours and risk short-term pain flare-ups. Since the results are obtained in this context, no change in clinical practise as far as pain communication is called for.

SRs of IMMRP report that it is an effective intervention with small to moderate effects for patients with chronic pain conditions [11,12,62,63]. The present results concerning ES agree with most SRs of IMMRP, but it may also be appropriate to compare with ES results reported in other clinical studies. The moderate ES for two of the pain intensity variables agree with studies in clinical routine care (n = 65–395), and therefore, for long-term follow-up (6–12 months), such studies report small (Cohen's d: 0.20–0.33 [64,65]) to moderate (Cohen's d: 0.59–0.70 [26,66,67]) ES for pain intensity. For psychological distress variables, these studies agree with the present results: they generally found small ES for long-term follow-up (i.e., Cohen's d = 0–0.38 for depressive symptoms [26,64,65] and Cohen's d = 0.22–0.34 for anxiety) [26,65]. In a recent RCT comparing transdiagnostic emotion-focused exposure treatment (Hybrid) and Internet-delivered pain management treatment (ICBT) for chronic pain patients with comorbid anxiety and depression, we found that within group ES pre versus follow-up for pain interference were reported both for hybrid (ES = 1.17) and for ICBT (ES = 0.65) compared the present effect size of 0.49 [68]. However, the patients were not exclusively recruited from specialist care (i.e., clinical departments of pain rehabilitation); they were also recruited via advertisements in local newspapers and social media [68], and the numbers investigated were considerably smaller. An important observation from the present study is that moderate ES found at 12-month follow-up covered broad aspects (e.g., pain intensity, interference in daily life, and perceived health).

The number of outcomes in IMMRPs in RCTs are generally high, which reasonably reflects the broad goals of the complex intervention. The present study used 22 outcomes that are mandatory in SQRP measured on up to three occasions (i.e., pre-IMMRP, post-IMMRP, and 12-month follow-up). PCA was applied to handle the pattern of changes in potentially intercorrelated outcomes as suggested by the Medical Research Council of the United Kingdom [69]. From these analyses, it can be concluded that changes in pain intensity, pain interference, psychological distress, vitality, etc. were positively intercorrelated (Table 5). In fact, our study showed that the changes in the majority of the 22 outcomes are significantly intercorrelated. Hence, the changes in these variables cannot be considered independent of each other. As a consequence of this observation, the appropriateness to evaluate changes in outcomes separately, as done in a recent SR [70], must be questioned, since the treatment was not designed to target only a single outcome. Moreover, the ES must be seen in this complex context. Thus, small changes in many outcomes may be more important than one prominent change in a single or few outcomes. Furthermore, the Grading of Recommendations Assessment, Development and Evaluation (GRADE) used for evidence ratings in SRs may not adequately describe the evidence base of complex interventions [71]. Different definitions of positive outcomes of IMMRP interventions exist (e.g., the majority of outcomes had to be significantly better than for the control intervention) [10,11]. Another approach was that the authors of the SR predetermined primary and secondary outcomes and what was necessary to classify an intervention as positive before reviewing the RCTs [12].

The presented PCAs also highlight that it may be possible to reduce the number of outcome variables, since several of these appear to measure similar aspects of the chronic pain condition. The fact that 22 outcomes were analysed (Tables 2 and 3) may raise an issue of multiple comparisons. In such situations, Bonferroni corrections are frequently used [72,73]. This is a conservative approach when the number of tests increases [72,74,75], the chances to detect real treatment effects decrease, and corrections were designed for corrections of *independent* comparisons [74]. The latter is obviously not present for most changes in outcome variables according to the PCAs performed (Table 5). Hierarchal or 'gatekeeping' procedures do not require adjustment for multiplicity [73], but require a natural hierarchy of the outcomes, as such a hierarchy is not obvious for IMMRP, as discussed above. Another approach is that outcomes are combined into a single composite outcome (i.e., a composite outcome consists of two or more component outcomes) [76], but this may be problematic with respect to missing cases and when the components of the composite endpoint are measured on different scales (i.e., non-commensurate outcomes) [76]. However, some multivariate methods such as PCA and OPLS can handle non-commensurate outcomes [76]. We used advanced PCA, including the NIPALS algorithm, to handling missing data and non-commensurate outcomes. We calculated the *t*-scores for the most relevant latent factor (component). Hence, we defined an objective Multivariate Improvement Score (MIS; the *t*-score of the first PCA component), which on an individual patient level defines the multivariate improvement; a positive MIS indicates multivariate improvements because of IMMRP.

Three clearly separated clusters based on MIS were identified. On a group level, clusters 1 and 2 were associated with various degrees of improvements, whereas cluster 3 showed negative MIS, indicating deterioration. Although the greater improvement in cluster 1 can be interpreted as a sign of regression to the mean and that these patients did not benefit from IMMRP more than cluster 2, this cluster still improves from IMMRP at least as well as those with e.g., less severe psychological distress symptoms (clusters 2 and 3). This may seem unexpected, but it is important to recognise that addressing psychological symptoms with CBT is an important component of IMMRPs. The patients at post-IMMRP and 12-month follow-up estimated the degree of positive change in pain (i.e., Change-pain) and the ability to handle life situation in general (i.e., Change-life situation). Most patients reported improvements according to both the Change-pain and Change-life situations (Table 4). Relatively small proportions of the patients reported worse situations post-IMMRP and at the 12-month follow-up, which are results that agree with other studies [29,77,78]. These two variables have retrospective elements even though they are not explicitly expressed. There are several problems with such items in general—e.g., desirability and memory aspects, recall time [79–81], and in treatment context (e.g., overly optimistic assessments) [82]. However, on a general level, these estimations and the two MIS variables (Tables 6 and 7) agreed.

We found that cluster 1, which had high MIS values (i.e., prominent improvements), had a more severe clinical picture at baseline/pre-IMMRP than those with lower MIS (i.e., less improvements). These results agree with another SQRP study ($N > 35{,}000$) that identified clusters based on the clinical presentation at assessment (decision not taken about participation in IMMRP); the study found that patients with the most severe clinical situation who later participated in IMMRP had the most prominent improvements in six investigated outcomes [34]. Although IMMRP has been commended for its effectiveness ('of all approaches to the treatment of chronic pain, none has a stronger evidence basis for efficacy, cost-effectiveness, and lack of iatrogenic complications') [83], both this and our recent study [34] indicate that not all patients show important improvements in several domains of outcome after IMMRP. Both this and our previous study identified a large subgroup of patients that do not seem to significantly benefit from IMMRP. Presumably, these patients—in the present study, those with negative MIS (i.e., cluster 3)—need other interventions. In a relative context, they have a somewhat less complicated self-reported clinical picture pre-IMMRP than those in clusters 1 and 2, even though they are referred to specialist care and hence represent patients with complex needs.

The longitudinal regressions of MIS using background variables and pre-IMMRP data as regressors were significant (Table 10). A blend of variables was important; psychological distress variables were most important, but life impact variables, pain aspects, and health and vitality aspects contributed. Our results appear to be in line with a recent meta-analysis on prognostic factors for IMMRP outcome, demonstrating that both pre-treatment general emotional distress and pain-specific cognitive behavioural factors are related to worse long-term (>6 months) physical functioning [84]. Unfortunately, these regressions cannot be used clinically, since they only explained 8% of variations in MIS. Although the prediction does not work clinically, this and a previous study from our group give clear indications that patients with a severe clinical situation benefit from IMMRP [34].

4.1. Important Clinical Implications

Outcomes of IMMRP in real-life practice settings agree with the conclusions from SRs. Partly in contrast to SRs, this registry study of patients managed within specialist care found that pain intensity was positively affected because of IMMRP. It was also obvious that not all patients benefit from IMMRP. Hence, there is a need to develop better matching between clinical presentation and participation in MMRP in real-life practice settings. Moreover, the intercorrelations of most changes in outcomes also opens up the possibility of reducing the number of outcome variables and hereby reduce the burden upon patients included in the SQRP.

4.2. Strengths and Limitations

This study's strengths include a large number of patients with complex chronic pain conditions with a nation-wide representation. However, these patients were referred to specialist clinics and thus represent a selection of the most difficult cases, so our results cannot be generalised to other settings. Another strength was the use of MVDA methods such as PCA and OPLS to handle correlation patterns, repeated measures, and regressions when there were obvious risks for multicollinearity. Changes in the social context may have changed and influenced the longitudinal analyses; however, we used validated and well-known instruments. Repeated evaluations using PROM questionnaires in treatment studies may be problematic [85]. Thus, the changes that the patient undergo because of the intervention (i.e., IMMRP) may affect the interpretations of the questions when presented at follow-up. The fact that no control group or treatment-as-usual group was available, which ethically is complicated to arrange for a registry of real-life practice patients, might have influenced our interpretation of changes after IMMRP. Data for the time period 2008–2016 from the SQRP was used in the present study, and changes in the content of IMMRP may have occurred. Unfortunately, no data concerning such changes are available.

5. Conclusions

This large-scale study of IMMRPs in real life practise settings demonstrates significant outcome changes in almost all measures. Most short-term and long-term effect sizes were small, but interestingly, moderate long-term effect sizes were demonstrated for pain, pain interference in daily life, and perceived health. In addition, patients reporting higher levels of perceived disability and suffering displayed greater improvement.

Author Contributions: Conceptualization, Å.R., E.D., M.B., B.L. and B.G.; Data curation, Å.R. and B.G.; Formal analysis, B.L. and B.G.; Methodology, Å.R., M.B. and B.G.; Validation, E.D.; Writing—original draft, B.G.; Writing—review & editing, Å.R., E.D., M.B. and B.L. All authors commented on different versions of the manuscript and all authors have approved the final version of the manuscript.

Acknowledgments: The authors are very grateful for valuable comments from Marcelo Rivano Fischer, PhD.

List of Abbreviations

ACT	Acceptance Commitment Therapy
ANOVA	Analysis of Variance
BPS	biopsychosocial
CBT	Cognitive Behavioral Therapy
Change-pain	positive change in pain
Change-life situation	change in ability to handle life situations in general
CI	confidence interval
CV-ANOVA	ANOVA of the cross-validated residuals
ES	effect size
EQ-5D	European Quality of Life instrument
EQ-5D-index	index of EQ-5D based on five items
EQ-VAS	health scale of EQ-5D
FU	follow-up
GRADE	Grading of Recommendations Assessment, Development and Evaluation
HADS	Hospital Anxiety and Depression Scale
HADS-A	Hospital Anxiety and Depression Scale—anxiety subscale
HADS-D	Hospital Anxiety and Depression Scale—depression subscale
HCA	Hierarchical Clustering Analysis
HR-QoL	health-related quality of life
IASP	the International Association for the Study of Pain
IMMPACT	the Initiative on Methods, Measurement, and Pain Assessment in Clinical Trials
IMMRP	Interdisciplinary Multimodal Pain Rehabilitation Program
LR	logistic regression
MIS	Multivariate Improvement Score
MLR	multiple linear regression

MPI	Multidimensional Pain Inventory
MPI-Pain-severity	MPI subscale concerning pain severity
MPI-Pain-interfer	MPI subscale concerning pain-related interference
MPI-Distress	MPI-SocSupp affective distress
MPI-LifeCon	MPI subscale concerning life control
MPI-SocSupp	MPI subscale concerning social support
MPI-Punish	MPI subscale concerning punishing responses
MPI-Solict	MPI subscale concerning solicitous responses
MPI-Distract	MPI subscale concerning distracting responses
MPI-GAI	MPI subscale General Activity Index
MVDA	advanced multivariate analysis
NIPALS	Non-linear Iterative Partial Least Squares
NRS	Numeric Rating Scale
NRS-7days	average pain intensity the last week
OPLS	Orthogonal Partial Least Square Regression
Outside-Europe	born outside Europe
PBE	practice-based evidence
P(corr)	loading scaled as a correlation coefficient between −1.0 and
PCA	Principal Component Analysis
PLS-DA	partial least square discriminant analysis
PRI	Pain Region Index
PROM	patient reported outcome measures
RCT	Randomised Controlled Trial
SQRP	Swedish Quality Registry for Pain Rehabilitation
sf36	Short Form Health Survey
sf36-pf	sf36 subscale concerning physical functioning
sf36-rp	sf36 subscale concerning role limitations due to physical functioning
sf36-bp	sf36 subscale concerning bodily pain
sf36-gh	sf36 subscale concerning general health
sf36-vt	sf36 subscale concerning vitality
sf36-sf	sf36 subscale concerning social functioning
sf36-re	sf36 subscale concerning role limitations due to emotional problems
sf36-mh	sf36 subscale concerning mental health
SR	systematic review
University	University education
VAPAIN	Validation and Application of a patient-relevant core set of outcome domains to assess multimodal PAIN therapy
VIP	variable influence on projection

References

1. Linton, S.J.; Bergbom, S. Understanding the link between depression and pain. *Scand. J. Pain* **2011**, *2*, 47–54. [CrossRef] [PubMed]
2. Ossipov, M.H.; Dussor, G.O.; Porreca, F. Central modulation of pain. *J. Clin. Investig.* **2010**, *120*, 3779–3787. [CrossRef] [PubMed]
3. Gatchel, R.J.; Peng, Y.B.; Peters, M.L.; Fuchs, P.N.; Turk, D.C. The biopsychosocial approach to chronic pain: Scientific advances and future directions. *Psychol. Bull.* **2007**, *133*, 581–624. [CrossRef]
4. Breivik, H.; Collett, B.; Ventafridda, V.; Cohen, R.; Gallacher, D. Survey of chronic pain in Europe: Prevalence, impact on daily life, and treatment. *Eur. J. Pain* **2006**, *10*, 287. [CrossRef] [PubMed]
5. Bergman, S. *Chronic Musculoskeletal Pain: A Multifactorial Process*; Lund University: Lund, Sweden, 2001.
6. World Health Organization (WHO). *International Classification of Functioning, Disability and Health (ICF)* World Health Organization: Geneva, Switzerland, 2001.

7. Dworkin, R.H.; Turk, D.C.; Farrar, J.T.; Haythornthwaite, J.A.; Jensen, M.P.; Katz, N.P.; Kerns, R.D.; Stucki, G.; Allen, R.R.; Bellamy, N.; et al. Core outcome measures for chronic pain clinical trials: IMMPACT recommendations. *Pain* **2005**, *113*, 9–19. [CrossRef] [PubMed]
8. Fillingim, R.B. Individual Differences in Pain: Understanding the Mosaic that Makes Pain Personal. *Pain* **2017**, *158*, S11–S18. [CrossRef] [PubMed]
9. Bennett, M.; Closs, S. Methodological issues in nonpharamacological trials for chronic pain. *Pain Clin. Updates* **2010**, *18*, 1–6.
10. Swedish Council on Health Technology Assessment (SBU). *Methods for Treatment of Chronic Pain a Systematic Review of the Literature*; SBU-Rapport; Swedish Council on Health Technology Assessment: Stockholm, Sweden, 2006; Volume 177, (In Swedish: Metoder för behandling av långvarig smärta: En systematisk litteraturöversikt).
11. Swedish Council on Health Technology Assessment (SBU). *Rehabilitation of Chronic Pain*; SBU-Rapport; Swedish Council on Health Technology Assessment: Stockholm, Sweden, 2010; Volume 198, (In Swedish: Rehabilitering vid långvarig smärta. En systematisk litteraturöversikt).
12. Scascighini, L.; Toma, V.; Dober-Spielmann, S.; Sprott, H. Multidisciplinary treatment for chronic pain: A systematic review of interventions and outcomes. *Rheumatology* **2008**, *47*, 670–678. [CrossRef] [PubMed]
13. Wade, D.T. Describing rehabilitation interventions. *Clin. Rehabil.* **2005**, *19*, 811–818. [CrossRef]
14. Kaiser, U.; Kopkow, C.; Deckert, S.; Neustadt, K.; Jacobi, L.; Cameron, P.; De Angelis, V.; Apfelbacher, C.; Arnold, B.; Birch, J.; et al. Developing a core outcome-domain set to assessing effectiveness of interdisciplinary multimodal pain therapy: The VAPAIN consensus statement on core outcome-domains. *Pain* **2017**, *159*, 673–683. [CrossRef] [PubMed]
15. Campbell, M.; Fitzpatrick, R.; Haines, A.; Kinmonth, A.L.; Sandercock, P.; Spiegelhalter, D.; Tyrer, P. Framework for design and evaluation of complex interventions to improve health. *BMJ* **2000**, *321*, 694–696. [CrossRef] [PubMed]
16. Paterson, C.; Baarts, C.; Launsø, L.; Verhoef, M.J. Evaluating complex health interventions: A critical analysis of the 'outcomes' concept. *BMC Complement. Altern. Med.* **2009**, *9*, 18. [CrossRef] [PubMed]
17. Shiell, A.; Hawe, P.; Gold, L. Complex interventions or complex systems? Implications for health economic evaluation. *BMJ* **2008**, *336*, 1281–1283. [CrossRef] [PubMed]
18. Hawe, P.; Shiell, A.; Riley, T. Complex interventions: How "out of control" can a randomised controlled trial be? *BMJ* **2004**, *328*, 1561–1563. [CrossRef] [PubMed]
19. Weiner, S.S.; Nordin, M. Prevention and management of chronic back pain. *Best Pract. Res. Clin. Rheumatol.* **2010**, *24*, 267–279. [CrossRef] [PubMed]
20. Kamper, S.J.; Apeldoorn, A.T.; Chiarotto, A.; Smeets, R.J.E.M.; Ostelo, R.W.J.G.; Guzman, J.; Van Tulder, M.W.; Van Tulder, M. Multidisciplinary biopsychosocial rehabilitation for chronic low back pain: Cochrane systematic review and meta-analysis. *BMJ* **2015**, *350*, h444. [CrossRef] [PubMed]
21. Norlund, A.; Ropponen, A.; Alexanderson, K. Multidisciplinary interventions: Review of studies of return to work after rehabilitation for low back pain. *J. Rehabil. Med.* **2009**, *41*, 115–121. [CrossRef] [PubMed]
22. Busch, H.; Bodin, L.; Bergström, G.; Jensen, I.B. Patterns of sickness absence a decade after pain-related multidisciplinary rehabilitation. *Pain* **2011**, *152*, 1727–1733. [CrossRef] [PubMed]
23. Jensen, I.B.; Busch, H.; Bodin, L.; Hagberg, J.; Nygren, A.; Bergström, G. Cost effectiveness of two rehabilitation programmes for neck and back pain patients: A seven year follow-up. *Pain* **2009**, *142*, 202–208. [CrossRef] [PubMed]
24. Munder, T.; Brütsch, O.; Leonhart, R.; Gerger, H.; Barth, J. Researcher allegiance in psychotherapy outcome research: An overview of reviews. *Clin. Psychol. Rev.* **2013**, *33*, 501–511. [CrossRef]
25. Margison, F.R.; Barkham, M.; Evans, C.; McGrath, G.; Clark, J.M.; Audin, K.; Connell, J. Measurement and psychotherapy. Evidence-based practice and practice-based evidence. *Br. J. Psychiatry* **2000**, *177*, 123–130. [CrossRef] [PubMed]
26. Preis, M.A.; Vögtle, E.; Dreyer, N.; Seel, S.; Wagner, R.; Hanshans, K.; Reyersbach, R.; Pieh, C.; Mühlberger, A.; Probst, T. Long-Term Outcomes of a Multimodal Day-Clinic Treatment for Chronic Pain under the Conditions of Routine Care. *Pain Res. Manag.* **2018**. [CrossRef] [PubMed]
27. Whiteneck, G.G.; Gassaway, J. SCIRehab Uses Practice-Based Evidence Methodology to Associate Patient and Treatment Characteristics with Outcomes. *Arch. Phys. Med. Rehabil.* **2013**, *94*, S67–S74. [CrossRef] [PubMed]

28. Malmivaara, A. Assessing the effectiveness of rehabilitation and optimizing effectiveness in routine clinical work. *J. Rehabil. Med.* **2018**, *50*, 849–851. [CrossRef] [PubMed]
29. Gerdle, B.; Molander, P.; Stenberg, G.; Stålnacke, B.-M.; Enthoven, P. Weak outcome predictors of multimodal rehabilitation at one-year follow-up in patients with chronic pain—A practice based evidence study from two SQRP centres. *BMC Musculoskelet. Disord.* **2016**, *17*, 287. [CrossRef]
30. Craig, P.; Dieppe, P.; MacIntyre, S.; Michie, S.; Nazareth, I.; Petticrew, M. Medical Research Council Guidance. Developing and evaluating complex interventions: The new Medical Research Council guidance. *BMJ* **2008**, *337*, a1655. [CrossRef]
31. Bromley Milton, M.; Borsbo, B.; Rovner, G.; Lundgren-Nilsson, A.; Stibrant-Sunnerhagen, K.; Gerdle, B. Is Pain Intensity Really That Important to Assess in Chronic Pain Patients? A Study Based on the Swedish Quality Registry for Pain Rehabilitation (SQRP). *PLoS ONE* **2013**, *8*, e65483. [CrossRef]
32. Hasselström, J.; Liu-Palmgren, J.; Rasjö-Wrååk, G.; Liu-Palmgren, J.; Rasjö-Wrååk, G. Prevalence of pain in general practice. *Eur. J. Pain* **2002**, *6*, 375–385. [CrossRef]
33. Mäntyselkä, P.; Kumpusalo, E.; Ahonen, R.; Kumpusalo, A.; Kauhanen, J.; Viinamäki, H.; Halonen, P.; Takala, J. Pain as a reason to visit the doctor: A study in Finnish primary health care. *Pain* **2001**, *89*, 175–180. [CrossRef]
34. Gerdle, B.; Åkerblom, S.; Brodda Jansen, G.; Enthoven, P.; Ernberg, M.; Dong, H.-J.; Stålnacke, B.; Äng, B.; Boersma, K. Who benefit from multimodal rehabilitation—An exploration of pain, psychological distress and life impacts in over 35,000 chronic pain patients identified in the Swedish Quality Registry for Pain Rehabilitation (SQRP). *J. Pain Res.* **2019**, *12*, 891–908. [CrossRef]
35. Rovner, G.S.; Sunnerhagen, K.S.; Björkdahl, A.; Gerdle, B.; Börsbo, B.; Johansson, F.; Gillanders, D. Chronic pain and sex-differences; women accept and move, while men feel blue. *PLoS ONE* **2017**, *12*, 0175737. [CrossRef] [PubMed]
36. Bernfort, L.; Gerdle, B.; Husberg, M.; Levin, L.-A. People in states worse than dead according to the EQ-5D UK value set: Would they rather be dead? *Qual. Life Res.* **2018**, *27*, 1827–1833. [CrossRef] [PubMed]
37. Turk, D.C.; Rudy, T.E. Toward an empirically derived taxonomy of chronic pain patients: Integration of psychological assessment data. *J. Consult. Clin. Psychol.* **1988**, *56*, 233–238. [CrossRef] [PubMed]
38. Turk, D.C.; Rudy, T.E. Towards a comprehensive assessment of chronic pain patients. *Behav. Res. Ther.* **1987**, *25*, 237–249. [CrossRef]
39. Bergström, G.; Jensen, I.B.; Bodin, L.; Linton, S.J.; Nygren, A.L.; Carlsson, S.G. Reliability and factor structure of the Multidimensional Pain Inventory—Swedish Language Version (MPI-S). *Pain* **1998**, *75*, 101–110. [CrossRef]
40. Zigmond, A.S.; Snaith, R.P. The Hospital Anxiety and Depression Scale. *Acta Psychiatr. Scand.* **1983**, *67*, 361–370. [CrossRef]
41. Bjelland, I.; Dahl, A.A.; Haug, T.T.; Neckelmann, D. The validity of the Hospital Anxiety and Depression Scale. *J. Psychosom. Res.* **2002**, *52*, 69–77. [CrossRef]
42. Sullivan, M.; Karlsson, J.; Ware, J. The Swedish 36 Health survey. Evaluation of data quality, scaling assumption, reliability and construct validity across general populations in Sweden. *Soc. Sci. Med.* **1995**, *41*, 1349–1358. [CrossRef]
43. EuroQol Group. EuroQol—A new facility for the measurement of health-related quality of life. *Health Policy* **1990**, *16*, 199–208. [CrossRef]
44. Brooks, R. EuroQol: The current state of play. *Health Policy* **1996**, *37*, 53–72. [CrossRef]
45. Dolan, P.; Sutton, M.; Sutton, M. Mapping visual analogue scale health state valuations onto standard gamble and time trade-off values. *Soc. Sci. Med.* **1997**, *44*, 1519–1530. [CrossRef]
46. Bäckryd, E.; Persson, E.B.; Larsson, A.I.; Fischer, M.R.; Gerdle, B. Chronic pain patients can be classified into four groups: Clustering-based discriminant analysis of psychometric data from 4665 patients referred to a multidisciplinary pain centre (a SQRP study). *PLoS ONE* **2018**, *13*, e0192623. [CrossRef] [PubMed]
47. Jansen, J.J.; Szymanska, E.; Hoefsloot, H.C.; Jacobs, D.M.; Strassburg, K.; Smilde, A.K. Between Metabolite Relationships: An essential aspect of metabolic change. *Metabolomics* **2012**, *8*, 422–432. [CrossRef] [PubMed]
48. Pohjanen, E.; Thysell, E.; Jonsson, P.; Eklund, C.; Silfver, A.; Carlsson, I.-B.; Lundgren, K.; Moritz, T.; Svensson, M.B.; Antti, H. A Multivariate Screening Strategy for Investigating Metabolic Effects of Strenuous Physical Exercise in Human Serum. *J. Proteome Res.* **2007**, *6*, 2113–2120. [CrossRef] [PubMed]

49. Eriksson, L.; Byrne, T.; Johansson, E.; Trygg, J.; Vikström, C. *Multi—And Megavariate Data Analysis—Basic Principles and Applications*, 3rd ed.; Umetrics Academy: Umeå, Sweden, 2013.
50. Wheelock Åsa, M.; Wheelock, C.E. Trials and tribulations of 'omics data analysis: Assessing quality of SIMCA-based multivariate models using examples from pulmonary medicine. *Mol. BioSyst.* **2013**, *9*, 2589. [CrossRef] [PubMed]
51. Eriksson, L.; Johansson, E.; Kettaneh-Wold, N.; Trygg, J.; Wikström, C.; Wold, S. *Multi—And Megavariate Data Analysis: Part I and II*, 2nd ed.; Umetrics AB: Umeå, Sweden, 2006.
52. Turk, D.C.; Dworkin, R.H.; Allen, R.R.; Bellamy, N.; Brandenburg, N.; Carr, D.B.; Cleeland, C.; Dionne, R.; Farrar, J.T.; Galer, B.S.; et al. Core outcome domains for chronic pain clinical trials: IMMPACT recommendations. *Pain* **2003**, *106*, 337–345. [CrossRef] [PubMed]
53. Norrefalk, J.; Ekholm, K.; Linder, J.; Borg, K.; Ekholm, J. Evaluation of a multiprofessional rehabilitation programme for persistent musculoskeletal-related pain: Economic benefits of return to work. *Acta Derm. Venereol.* **2008**, *40*, 15–22. [CrossRef] [PubMed]
54. Matthias, M.S.; Miech, E.J.; Myers, L.J.; Sargent, C.; Bair, M.J. There's more to this pain than just pain: How patients' understanding of pain evolved during a randomized controlled trial for chronic pain. *J. Pain* **2012**, *13*, 571–578. [CrossRef] [PubMed]
55. Rivano-Fischer, M.; Persson, E.; Stålnacke, B.; Schult, M.; Löfgren, M. Return to work after interdisciplinary pain rehabilitation: One- and two-years follow-up based on the Swedish Quality Registry for pain rehabilitation. *J. Rehabil. Med.* **2019**, *51*, 281–289. [CrossRef] [PubMed]
56. Busse, J.W.; Wang, L.; Kamaleldin, M.; Craigie, S.; Riva, J.J.; Montoya, L.; Mulla, S.M.; Lopes, L.C.; Vogel, N.; Chen, E.; et al. Opioids for Chronic Noncancer Pain: A Systematic Review and Meta-analysis. *JAMA* **2018**, *320*, 2448–2460. [CrossRef] [PubMed]
57. Enthoven, W.T.; Roelofs, P.D.; Deyo, R.A.; Van Tulder, M.W.; Koes, B.W. Non-steroidal anti-inflammatory drugs for chronic low back pain. *Cochrane Database Syst. Rev.* **2016**, *2*, 012087. [CrossRef] [PubMed]
58. Saragiotto, B.T.; Machado, G.C.; Ferreira, M.L.; Pinheiro, M.B.; Abdel Shaheed, C.; Maher, C.G. Paracetamol for low back pain. *Cochrane Database Syst. Rev.* **2016**. [CrossRef] [PubMed]
59. Henry, S.G.; Bell, R.A.; Fenton, J.J.; Kravitz, R.L. Goals of Chronic Pain Management: Do Patients and Primary Care Physicians Agree and Does It Matter? *Clin. J. Pain* **2017**, *33*, 955–961. [CrossRef] [PubMed]
60. Thompson, M.; McCracken, L.M. Acceptance and Related Processes in Adjustment to Chronic Pain. *Curr. Pain Headache Rep.* **2011**, *15*, 144–151. [CrossRef] [PubMed]
61. McCracken, L.M.; Zhao-O'Brien, J.; Zhao-O'Brien, J. General psychological acceptance and chronic pain: There is more to accept than the pain itself. *Eur. J. Pain* **2010**, *14*, 170–175. [CrossRef] [PubMed]
62. Skelly, A.; Chou, R.; Dettori, J.; Turner, J.; Friedly, J.; Rundell, S.; Fu, R.; Brodt, E.; Wasson, N.; Winter, C.; et al. *Noninvasive Nonpharmacological Treatment for Chronic Pain: A Systematic Review [Internet]*; Agency for Healthcare Research and Quality (US): Rockville, MD, USA, 2018.
63. Salathé, C.R.; Melloh, M.; Crawford, R.; Scherrer, S.; Boos, N.; Elfering, A. Treatment Efficacy, Clinical Utility, and Cost-Effectiveness of Multidisciplinary Biopsychosocial Rehabilitation Treatments for Persistent Low Back Pain: A Systematic Review. *Glob. Spine J.* **2018**, *8*, 872–886. [CrossRef] [PubMed]
64. Ruscheweyh, R.; Dany, K.; Marziniak, M.; Gralow, I. Basal Pain Sensitivity does not Predict the Outcome of Multidisciplinary Chronic Pain Treatment. *Pain Med.* **2015**, *16*, 1635–1642. [CrossRef] [PubMed]
65. Borys, C.; Lutz, J.; Strauss, B.; Altmann, U. Effectiveness of a Multimodal Therapy for Patients with Chronic Low Back Pain Regarding Pre-Admission Healthcare Utilization. *PLoS ONE* **2015**, *10*, 0143139. [CrossRef] [PubMed]
66. Letzel, J.; Angst, F.; Weigl, M.B. Multidisciplinary biopsychosocial rehabilitation in chronic neck pain: A naturalistic prospective cohort study with intraindividual control of effects and 12-month follow-up. *Eur. J. Phys. Rehabil. Med.* **2018**, in press. [CrossRef]
67. Moradi, B.; Hagmann, S.; Zahlten-Hinguranage, A.; Caldeira, F.; Putz, C.; Rosshirt, N.; Schonit, E.; Mesrian, A.; Schiltenwolf, M.; Neubauer, E. Efficacy of multidisciplinary treatment for patients with chronic low back pain: A prospective clinical study in 395 patients. *J. Clin. Rheumatol.* **2012**, *18*, 76–82. [CrossRef]
68. Boersma, K.; Södermark, M.; Hesser, H.; Flink, I.; Gerdle, B.; Linton, S. The efficacy of a transdiagnostic emotion-focused exposure treatment for chronic pain patients with comorbid anxiety and depression: A randomized controlled trial. *Pain* **2019**, in press. [CrossRef] [PubMed]

69. Craig, P.; Dieppe, P.; Macintyre, S.; Michie, S.; Nazareth, I.; Petticrew, M. Developing and Evaluating Complex Interventions: New Guidance. 2008. Available online: https://www.researchgate.net/publication/32899190_Developing_and_Evaluating_Complex_Interventions_New_Guidance_Online (accessed on 4 June 2019).
70. Kamper, S.J.; Apeldoorn, A.T.; Chiarotto, A.; Smeets, R.J.; Ostelo, R.W.J.G.; Guzman, J.; Van Tulder, M.W. Multidisciplinary biopsychosocial rehabilitation for chronic low back pain. *Cochrane Database Syst. Rev.* **2014**, *350*. [CrossRef] [PubMed]
71. Movsisyan, A.; Melendez-Torres, G.; Montgomery, P. Outcomes in systematic reviews of complex interventions never reached "high" GRADE ratings when compared with those of simple interventions. *J. Clin. Epidemiol.* **2016**, *78*, 22–33. [CrossRef] [PubMed]
72. Feise, R.J. Do multiple outcome measures require p-value adjustment? *BMC Med. Res. Methodol.* **2002**, *2*, 8. [CrossRef]
73. Turk, D.C.; Dworkin, R.H.; McDermott, M.P.; Bellamy, N.; Burke, L.B.; Chandler, J.M.; Cleeland, C.S.; Cowan, P.; Dimitrova, R.; Farrar, J.T.; et al. Analyzing multiple endpoints in clinical trials of pain treatments: IMMPACT recommendations. *Pain* **2008**, *139*, 485–493. [CrossRef] [PubMed]
74. Bagiella, E. Clinical Trials in Rehabilitation: Single or Multiple Outcomes? *Arch. Phys. Med. Rehabil.* **2009**, *90*, S17–S21. [CrossRef] [PubMed]
75. Tyler, K.M.; Normand, S.L.; Horton, N.J. The use and abuse of multiple outcomes in randomized controlled depression trials. *Contemp. Clin. Trials* **2011**, *32*, 299–304. [CrossRef] [PubMed]
76. Teixeira-Pinto, A.; Mauri, L. Msc Statistical Analysis of Noncommensurate Multiple Outcomes. *Circ. Cardiovasc. Qual. Outcomes* **2011**, *4*, 650–656. [CrossRef]
77. Boonstra, A.M.; Reneman, M.F.; Waaksma, B.R.; Schiphorst Preuper, H.R.; Stewart, R.E. Predictors of multidisciplinary treatment outcome in patients with chronic musculoskeletal pain. *Disabil. Rehabil.* **2015**, *37*, 1242–1250. [CrossRef]
78. Morley, S.; Williams, A.; Hussain, S. Estimating the clinical effectiveness of cognitive behavioural therapy in the clinic: Evaluation of a CBT informed pain management programme. *Pain* **2008**, *137*, 670–680. [CrossRef]
79. Pina-Sánchez, J.; Koskinen, J.; Plewis, I. *Measurement Error in Retrospective Reports of Unemployment*; CCSR Working Paper; The Cathie Marsh Centre for Census and Survey Research, University of Manchester: Manchester, UK, 2012; pp. 1–56.
80. Bernard, H.R.; Killworth, P.; Kronenfeld, D.; Sailer, L. The Problem of Informant Accuracy: The Validity of Retrospective Data. *Annu. Rev. Anthropol.* **1984**, *13*, 495–517. [CrossRef]
81. Van Der Vaart, W.; Van Der Zouwen, J.; Dijkstra, W. Retrospective questions: Data quality, task difficulty, and the use of a checklist. *Qual. Quant.* **1995**, *29*, 299–315. [CrossRef]
82. Schwartz, N. Retrospective and concurrent self-reports: The rationale for real-time data capture. In *The Science of Real-Time Data CAPTURE: Self-Reports in Health Research*; Oxford University Press: New York, NY, USA, 2007; pp. 11–26.
83. Schatman, M. Interdisciplinary Chronic Pain Management: International Perspectives. *Pain Clin. Updates* **2012**, *20*, 1–6.
84. Tseli, E.; Stalnacke, B.M.; Boersma, K.; Enthoven, P.; Gerdle, B.; Ang, B.O.; Grooten, W.J.A. Prognostic Factors for Physical Functioning After Multidisciplinary Rehabilitation in Patients with Chronic Musculoskeletal Pain: A Systematic Review and Meta-analysis. *Clin. J. Pain* **2018**, *35*, 148. [CrossRef] [PubMed]
85. Westlander, G. Refined use of standardized self-reporting in intervention studies (In Swedish: Förfinad användning av standardiserad självrapportering i interventionstudier). *Soc. Tidskr.* **2004**, *2*, 168–181.

8

The Relationship between Pain Beliefs and Physical and Mental Health Outcome Measures in Chronic Low Back Pain: Direct and Indirect Effects

Andrew Baird * and David Sheffield

Centre for Psychological Research, Kedleston Road Campus, University of Derby, Derby DE22 1GB, UK; d.sheffield@derby.ac.uk
* Correspondence: A.Baird@derby.ac.uk

Academic Editor: Robert J. Gatchel

Abstract: Low back pain remains a major health problem with huge societal cost. Biomedical models fail to explain the disability seen in response to reported back pain and therefore patients' beliefs, cognitions and related behaviours have become a focus for both research and practice. This study used the Pain Beliefs Questionnaire and had two aims: To examine the extent to which pain beliefs are related to disability, anxiety and depression; and to assess whether those relationships are mediated by pain self-efficacy and locus of control. In a sample of 341 chronic low back pain patients, organic and psychological pain beliefs were related to disability, anxiety and depression. However, organic pain beliefs were more strongly related to disability and depression than psychological pain beliefs. Regression analyses revealed that these relationships were in part independent of pain self-efficacy and locus of control. Further, mediation analyses revealed indirect pathways involving self-efficacy and, to a lesser extent chance locus of control, between organic pain beliefs, on the one hand, and disability, anxiety and depression, on the other. In contrast, psychological pain beliefs were only directly related to disability, anxiety and depression. Although longitudinal data are needed to corroborate our findings, this study illustrates the importance of beliefs about the nature of pain and beliefs in one's ability to cope with pain in determining both physical and mental health outcomes in chronic low back pain patients.

Keywords: low back pain; pain beliefs; disability; pain self-efficacy; anxiety; depression; locus of control

1. Introduction

Despite considerable attention, low back pain remains one of medicine's most enigmatic problems, particularly in its chronic form. The majority of people will experience back pain at some point in their lives [1], but only a minority will receive a definitive diagnosis [2,3]. Most low back pain is largely non-specific in nature, but nevertheless has a societal cost greater than that for cancer, coronary artery disease and AIDS combined [4]. A systematic review by Dagenais, Caro and Haldeman [5] showed inconsistencies in the calculation of costs but found all studies to indicate back pain to be a substantial burden on society. In terms of healthcare costs, a recent study from the UK indicates that costs associated with chronic low back pain sufferers were twice that of matched controls [6]. The situation has been described in terms of an "epidemic" [7] and as a "20th Century medical disaster" [8] and is still perhaps one of the greatest examples of the failure of biomedical approaches. Biopsychosocial perspectives now dominate the literature, with psychosocial factors recognized as being fundamental in both assessment [9,10] and treatment/management [11,12]. Key to understanding the psychosocial influence is the consideration of individuals' beliefs, cognitions and behaviours.

Therefore, addressing patients' pain beliefs, cognitions and associated behaviours has become a major issue in pain management, particularly in chronic pain. Beliefs and associated behaviours have been associated with: The level of activity interference [13]; the frequency of pain behaviour [14]; the severity of pain experienced [15]; and levels of associated depression [16]. Two of the most important constructs in this area, which are driven by beliefs and which influence subsequent cognition and behaviour, are fear and catastrophising. These overlapping constructs impact upon vigilance to pain which can in turn also lead to increases in perceived pain severity [17]. A recent meta-analysis showed the relationship between fear and disability to be moderate to large in magnitude [18].

Ultimately, pain-related fear is more disabling than pain itself [19] as fear motivates avoidance behaviours [20,21]. In turn, avoidance behaviour affects activities of daily living and has a role in the transition from acute to chronic pain [22]. One of the key elements of fear is that of fear of further injury and re-injury [23], which can be a major barrier to recovery. In addition, expectancy beliefs are also a key factor in chronic pain. Ashari and Nicholas [24] showed pain self-efficacy beliefs to be an important determinant of pain behaviours and the disability associated with pain. More recently, Denison et al.'s [25] findings suggest that self-efficacy beliefs are even more important determinants of disability than fear avoidance beliefs in primary health care patients with musculoskeletal pain. Pain self-efficacy can mediate the relationship between clinical predictors and outcome measures. Pain self-efficacy mediates the relationship between pain severity and associated disability [26,27] and between pain related fear and disability [28]. It also mediates the relationship between fear and pain intensity [28] and between pain intensity and related depression [26]. Internal pain control can mediate reduction in levels of depression and pain behaviour following treatment [29].

Addressing problematic beliefs and related cognitions and behaviours can however, bring improvement in function [30]. Modern back pain management programmes are frequently grounded in the proven effectiveness of cognitive behavioural approaches [31–33] and exercise [34,35].

In the current study, participants were from a programme that explicitly addresses pain beliefs with participants [36], particularly the erroneous notion that "hurt = harm" and "more hurt = more harm". Addressing these "organic" pain beliefs has been shown to be associated with improvements in function following a rehabilitation programme [37] and the strength of these beliefs has been shown to clearly differentiate patients with chronic low back pain from the general population [38]. This study aims to assess the extent to which pain related physical and mental outcome measures can be explained by individuals' pain beliefs as measured with the Pain Beliefs Questionnaire (PBQ) [39]. Furthermore, it aims to assess the extent to which the relationship between pain beliefs and physical and mental outcome measures is mediated by pain self-efficacy and locus of control.

2. Materials and Methods

2.1. Sample

The sample comprised 341 individuals who had been referred to the Nottingham Back Team programme located in Nottinghamshire, England. It is multi-disciplinary back pain management programme for individuals with chronic low back pain, delivered using 7 half day sessions on consecutive weeks. It is undertaken in community settings, i.e., utilising facilities at leisure centres as an alternative to requiring participants to visit a hospital site. The programme takes a cognitive behavioural approach and patients were informed that each session would incorporate, education, exercise, relaxation and discussions with a key worker (including goal setting). The sessions are delivered by a combination of physiotherapists, occupational therapists and nurses, with additional input from a clinical psychologist. The authors are independent of the programme and have no clinical role within it. Participants completed the standard battery of tests used within the programme together with the Pain Beliefs Questionnaire. Every patient that attended for assessment during the research period consented for their data to be used in the research, but not all responses were complete (n = 290). All data was gathered at assessment, before commencement of the programme.

2.2. Measures

The PBQ consists of 12 items representing two scales, which the authors described as "organic" (8 items) and "psychological" (4 items) [37]. One advantage of this questionnaire is that it is designed such that it is not necessary for the completer to be in pain or suffering from a specific condition (i.e., it is condition independent). The PBQ has previously been used successfully in research investigating chronic back pain [37–40] and with a UK general population [38]. On this occasion, the original 6 point ("always" to "never") scale response was modified to a 5 point scale fit better with other questionnaires it was being used with, as part of the broader research [38]. The five items were "All of the time", "Most of the time", "Some of the time", "A little of the time", "None of the time". In their study with patients experiencing chronic low back pain, Walsh and Radcliffe also describe using a 5-point scale [37]. The PBQ organic and psychological sub-scales are scored using the sum of the items for each scale respectively.

The Roland-Morris Disability Questionnaire (RDQ) [41] is one of the most widely used measures of back pain related disability and was originally derived from the Sickness Impact Profile (SIP). Twenty-four items that related to physical functions potentially affected by back pain were selected from the SIP. Each item was then qualified with the phrase "because of my back pain" to differentiate back pain disability from disability due to other causes [42]. Patients are asked to indicate which of the series of statements applies to them on the day of completing the questionnaire. The RDQ provides a single score which is calculated by summing the number of items selected. The items are not weighted in any way. The scores therefore range from 0 (no disability) to 24 (maximum disability). The RDQ is short, easy to understand and simple to complete [42].

The Pain Self-efficacy Questionnaire [43] is a ten item questionnaire, with each item assessed on a scale from 0 to 6 where 0 indicates no confidence and 6 indicates complete confidence. The 10 items are designed to cover a range of factors relating to activities of daily living. The items are not weighted and the questionnaire provides a single scale. The scores therefore range from 0, indicating no confidence in carrying out activities of daily living, to 60, indicating complete confidence in carrying out normal activities of daily living.

The Hospital Anxiety and Depression Scale (HADS) [44] is a 14 item screening tool comprising two seven item scales—anxiety and depression. To ensure a focus on anxiety and depression, symptoms which could also be associated with somatic disorders were excluded as were those indicative of more complex/serious psychiatric conditions. It is a widely used instrument in both clinical practice and research. A review by Bjellanda et al. [45] identified over seven hundred papers reporting use of HADS. It has been found to have good psychometric properties and performed well in assessing the general severity and 'caseness' of both anxiety disorders and depression. It has been widely used in trials relating to back pain including the large STarT Back trial [46].

The Multi-Dimensional Health Locus of Control Questionnaire [47] is an 18 item questionnaire comprising 3 scales—internal, chance and powerful others. The measure has been used for several decades and the scales are considered reliable and valid [48]. It is a general measure; not specific to particular symptoms or conditions. The measure has been used in back pain research in the past [49] and it was used during the development of the Pain Beliefs Questionnaire [39].

2.3. Analytic Strategy and Scoring

Initial analyses focused on examining differences in age and gender between those who completed the questionnaires and those that did not. Gender data was not available from one completer and one non-completer of all questionnaires. Then attention focused on correlations between beliefs, self-efficacy, locus of control, and depression, anxiety and disability. Next, regression analysis was used to examine the independent contributions that beliefs, self-efficacy, and locus of control variables make to the prediction of depression, anxiety and disability. Finally, a bootstrapped mediation model tested the conceptual model outlined in Figure 1. For each belief-mental or physical outcome relationship hypotheses were tested simultaneously using the "Process" macro for SPSS [50], with

5,000 bootstrapping re-samples and bias-corrected 95% confidence intervals (CIs) for each indirect effect. In bootstrapping analyses, bias corrected CIs that do not contain 0 signify a significant indirect effect [51,52]. Direct effects estimate how much two cases differing on the independent variable (organic or psychological belief) also differ on the dependent variable (disability, anxiety, or depression) independent of the effect of the mediator variables (self-efficacy and locus of control variables) on the dependent variable. Total effects are the sum of the indirect and direct effects of the independent variables on the dependent variable [50]. Alternate models were tested and these are presented in the Appendix. Analysis was conducted using IBM SPSS 22 for Windows with an alpha = 0.05. No participants were excluded from the analysis.

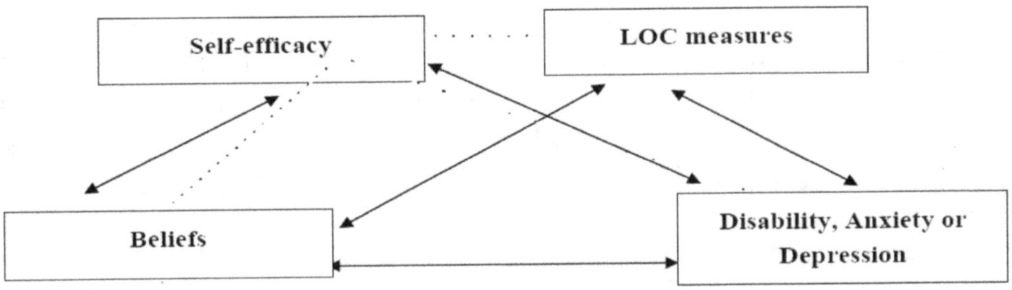

Figure 1. Conceptual Model of Bootstrapped Mediation Model.

2.4. Ethics

Ethical approval for the study was provided through the Nottingham Back Team via National Health Service processes. Participants received both written and verbal explanation during their assessment before informed consent was sought for their data to be used for the purposes of this research.

3. Results

3.1. Gender and Age Differences

Individuals who completed all questionnaires were significantly older (mean ± S.D. = 45.35 ± 13.14 vs. 48.02 ± 13.61 years) and more likely to be men (43.8% vs. 31.8%) than those who did not, $p < 0.05$.

3.2. Demographics

Examination of the mean and standard deviations suggested that participants were similar to previous low back pain samples [46]; see Table 1.

Table 1. Bivariate correlations and Means (SDs).

Variables	2	3	4	5	6	7	8	9	Mean (SD)
1. Disability	0.41 ***	0.57 ***	0.56 ***	0.21 ***	−0.70 ***	−0.19 ***	0.14 *	0.12 *	9.58 (5.34)
2. Anxiety	–	0.58 ***	0.34 ***	0.26 ***	−0.45 ***	−0.03	0.35 ***	0.21 ***	8.22 (3.97)
3. Depression	0.58 ***	- -	0.50 ***	0.15 **	−0.70 ***	−0.13 **	0.26 ***	0.17 **	5.96 (3.54)
4. Organic Beliefs	0.34 ***	0.50 ***	- -	0.13 **	−0.59 ***	−0.22 ***	0.27 ***	0.18 **	25.91 (4.90)
5. Psychological Beliefs	0.26 ***	0.15 **	0.13 **	- -	−0.08	0.17 **	0.00	0.02	11.28 (3.50)
6. Self-efficacy	0.45 ***	−0.70 ***	−0.59 ***	−0.08	- -	0.22 ***	−0.19 ***	−0.19 ***	34.09 (13.39)
7. LOC—Internal	−0.03	−0.13 **	−0.22 ***	0.17 **	0.22 ***	- -	−0.01	0.06	26.58 (4.75)
8. LOC—Chance	0.35 ***	0.26 ***	0.27 ***	0.00	−0.19 ***	−0.01	- -	0.39 ***	19.02 (5.27)
9. LOC—Other	0.21 ***	0.17 **	0.18 **	0.02	−0.19 ***	0.06	0.39 ***	- -	20.07 (6.23)

LOC: locus of control; * $p < 0.05$; ** $p < 0.01$; *** $p < 0.001$; - - There is perfect correlation between the same variable/s.

3.3. Bivariate Correlations

There were no gender differences in any predictor or outcome measures, $p > 0.1$. Age was negatively related to anxiety, $r = -0.15$, $p < 0.01$, and internal locus of control, $r = -0.13$, $p < 0.05$.

Accordingly, age was entered in subsequent regression analyses. Pearson's correlations revealed that disability, anxiety and depression were strongly inter-related but as the proportion of shared variance was less than 50% regression models with each as an outcome variable were calculated. Disability was strongly related to organic pain beliefs and self-efficacy, and more weakly, but significantly, related to psychological pain beliefs and locus of control measures. Anxiety was related to organic and psychological pain beliefs and self-efficacy, and more weakly, but significantly, related to internal and other locus of control measures; it was unrelated to chance locus of control. Depression was strongly related to organic pain beliefs and self-efficacy and more weakly related to psychological pain beliefs and locus of control measures. Fisher transformations revealed that organic pain beliefs were more strongly related to disability and depression than psychological pain beliefs ($p < 0.05$); correlations between organic and psychological pain beliefs and anxiety were not different. Organic pain beliefs were strongly related to self-efficacy and more weakly related to locus of control measures. Psychological pain beliefs were related to internal locus of control, but were not related to self-efficacy or chance and other locus of control (see Table 1).

3.4. Regression Analyses: Disability

After testing for multi-collinearity (all VIF < 2; all tolerances > 0.5), analysis revealed that the regression model was significant ($F(7, 333) = 56.82$, $p < 0.001$), with 54% of the variance in the outcome being explained by the predictors ($R^2 = 0.544$, adjusted $R^2 = 0.535$). There were significant positive relationships between organic pain beliefs and disability and between psychological pain beliefs and disability, and a significant negative relationship between pain self-efficacy and disability; there were no other significant relationships (see Table 2).

Table 2. Beta (standard deviation) and *t*-values for Regression Models.

Variables	Disability Beta (SD)	*T*	Anxiety	*t*	Depression	*t*
Age	0.011 (0.016)	0.71	−0.046 (0.014)	−3.24 **	−0.014 (0.011)	−1.33
Organic Beliefs	0.222 (0.052)	4.26 ***	0.035 (0.046)	0.76	0.071 (0.035)	2.01 *
Psychological Beliefs	0.229 (0.058)	3.94 ***	0.259 (0.052)	5.02 ***	0.086 (0.039)	2.19 *
Self-efficacy	−0.225 (0.019)	−12.31 ***	−0.103 (0.017)	−6.24 ***	−0.163 (0.013)	−12.93 ***
LOC—Internal	−0.041 (0.044)	−0.93	−0.003 (0.040)	−0.07	0.002 (0.030)	0.07
LOC—Chance	−0.015 (0.043)	−0.34	0.170 (0.038)	4.47 ***	0.074 (0.029)	2.55 *
LOC—Other	−0.021 (0.036)	−0.57	0.048 (0.032)	1.49	−0.001 (0.024)	−0.06

* $p < 0.05$; ** $p < 0.01$; *** $p < 0.001$.

Results of the mediation analyses indicated that there was a significant indirect effect of organic pain beliefs on disability through self-efficacy, $b = -0.23$, $p < 0.01$, BCa CI (-0.27, -0.19), which explained 36% of the total effect. In contrast, there were no significant indirect effects of organic pain beliefs on disability through LOC measures. The direct effect of organic pain beliefs on disability was also significant, $b = 0.25$, $t = 4.79$, $p < 0.0001$. In contrast, there was no significant indirect effect of organic pain beliefs on disability through LOC measures. For psychological pain beliefs on disability, there were no significant indirect effects through self-efficacy or LOC measures. The direct effect of psychological pain beliefs on disability was significant, $b = 0.26$, $t = 4.35$, $p < 0.0001$. Analyses with belief and locus of control measures as mediators of the self-efficacy-disability relationship were also examined. These suggest that the model is less parsimonious than the one proposed; these are presented in the Appendix.

3.5. Regression Analyses: Anxiety

The regression model was significant ($F(7, 333) = 25.39$, $p < 0.001$), with 35% of the variance in the outcome being explained by the predictors ($R^2 = 0.348$, adjusted $R^2 = 0.334$). There were significant positive relationships between psychological pain beliefs and anxiety and between chance locus of control and anxiety, and significant negative relationships between age and anxiety and pain self-efficacy and anxiety; there were no other significant relationships (see Table 2).

Results of the mediation analyses indicated that there was a significant indirect effect of organic pain beliefs on anxiety through self-efficacy, $b = -0.11$, $p < 0.0001$, BCa CI (−0.15, −0.07), which explained 18% of the total effect, and through chance locus of control, $b = 0.19$, $p < 0.0001$, BCa CI (0.11, 0.27), which explained 5% of the total effect. There were no significant indirect effects of organic pain beliefs on anxiety through other LOC measures and there was no direct effect of organic pain beliefs on anxiety, $b = 0.05$, $t = 1.06$, $p = 0.29$. For psychological pain beliefs on anxiety, there were no significant indirect effects through self-efficacy or LOC measures. The direct effect of psychological pain beliefs on anxiety was significant, $b = 0.26$, $t = 4.70$, $p < 0.0001$.

3.6. Regression Analyses: Depression

The regression model was significant ($F(7, 333) = 52.23$, $p < 0.001$), with 52% of the variance in the outcome being explained by the predictors ($R^2 = 0.523$, adjusted $R^2 = 0.513$). There were significant positive relationships between organic pain beliefs and depression, psychological pain beliefs and depression, and between chance locus of control and depression, and a significant negative relationship between pain self-efficacy and depression; there were no other significant relationships (see Table 2).

Results of the mediation analyses indicated that there was a significant indirect effect of organic pain beliefs on depression through self-efficacy, $b = -0.17$, $p < 0.0001$, BCa CI (−0.19, −0.14), which explained 27% of the total effect, and through chance locus of control, $b = 0.08$, $p < 0.005$, BCa CI (−0.02, 0.13), which explained 2% of the total effect. There were no significant indirect effects of organic pain beliefs on depression through other LOC measures. There was a direct effect of organic pain beliefs on depression, $b = 0.07$, $t = 2.20$, $p = 0.03$. For psychological pain beliefs on depression, there were no significant indirect effects through self-efficacy or LOC measures. The direct effect of psychological pain beliefs on depression was significant, $b = 0.10$, $t = 2.42$, $p = 0.01$.

4. Discussion

This study had two aims: To examine the extent to which pain beliefs are related to disability, anxiety and depression; and to assess whether those relationships are mediated by pain self-efficacy and locus of control. In a sample of 341 low back pain patients, organic and psychological pain beliefs were related to disability, anxiety and depression. However, organic pain beliefs were more strongly related to disability and depression than psychological pain beliefs. Regression analyses revealed that these relationships were in part independent of pain self-efficacy and locus of control. Further, mediation analyses revealed indirect pathways involving self-efficacy and, to a lesser extent chance locus of control, between organic pain beliefs, on the one hand, and disability, anxiety and depression, on the other. In contrast, psychological pain beliefs were only directly related to disability, anxiety and depression.

The gender split of the 341 participants included in the study was comparable with other studies of chronic low back pain [46,53]. Consideration of the descriptive statistics for the commonly taken measures—RMDQ, PSEQ and HADS—shows a pattern fairly typical of chronic low back pain patients. A mean disability of 9.6 is similar to that found by Hill et al. within the STarT Back trial [46] (9.8), though slightly higher than in the large study by Foster et al. [53] (8.6). The PSEQ mean of 34.1 was similar to that found by Foster et al. [53] (37.8). This is higher than reported by Nicholas [54] (25.8), but lower than reported by Costa et al. [55] (44.4) in chronic low back pain patients, so it appears to be in the range reported for chronic low back pain patients. A mean anxiety score of 8.2 was again similar to that reported by Foster et al. [53] (8.3) albeit slightly higher than that reported by Hill et al. [46] (7.5). Depression scores were lower than anxiety scores as is consistent within the literature and the mean of 6.0 is in line with that reported by Foster et al. [53] (6.5) and Hill et al. [46] (5.9). Overall, therefore this could be said to be an 'unremarkable' sample of chronic low back pain patients.

Organic pain beliefs deal with both the perceived cause of an individual's pain ("hurt = harm") and its management (issues of control and exercise/activity). As such, they could be considered a measure of 'biomedical thinking' [38]. These organic beliefs are associated with the outcome measures of disability, anxiety and depression. Higher organic pain beliefs are associated with higher levels of disability, depression and anxiety. On its own it could interpreted to be a good predictor of these outcomes, but mediation analyses show that much of the effect (all in the case of anxiety) is indirect through self-efficacy and to a lesser extent chance locus of control. The cross-sectional nature of the data is such that different mediation models could be described, but the defined model is in keeping with the literature on pain self-efficacy [26–28] and was the most parsimonious one (see Appendix).

Psychological pain beliefs are concerned with the impact of anxiety, depression, attention to pain and the issue of relaxation. These beliefs are also associated with the outcome measures, but the strength of the belief was much lower than for the organic beliefs. Higher levels of psychological pain beliefs are associated with higher levels of disability, depression and anxiety, but the relationship is relatively weak. Moreover, the mediation analyses showed that none of the effects were indirect through self-efficacy or locus of control measures. Thus, psychological pain beliefs are directly related to disability, depression and anxiety. Moreover, they appear to relate to markedly different constructs than other commonly used belief measures, such as fear avoidance beliefs, which like organic beliefs are mediated by self-efficacy [28]. Baird and Haslam [38] found that psychological beliefs differentiated between chronic low back pain patients and a non-clinical sample, but unlike with organic beliefs, there was no difference within the non-clinical sample between those who experienced frequent pain and those who did not. It was suggested that this may indicate that psychological pain beliefs are uniquely influenced by chronicity and not simply the presence of pain.

The PBQ has been used successfully with chronic low back pain samples [37,38,40] and this study supports the value of the measure. The scales illustrate both direct and mediated effects on key physical and mental health outcome measures. The measure has utility in both research and practice as it taps into clinically relevant beliefs that are amenable to change and are the focus of many rehabilitation programmes. Indeed, efforts to reduce the strength of these beliefs about the origins, nature and treatment of pain, particularly the 'biomedical' beliefs, should yield positive results in chronic low back pain rehabilitation [37,40].

This study supports the view that self-efficacy is an important predictor of disability [24,25,53]. It has a strong relationship with disability in bivariate analysis and its importance as an independent predictor of disability is confirmed in the regression models. Self-efficacy also has a strong association with mental health outcome measures, particularly depression. Further, the findings support previous studies indicating a role for self-efficacy as mediator between beliefs and outcomes [26–28]. Although Schiphorst Preuper et al. [56] questioned the impact of psychological variables, including self-efficacy, in a study in which psychological variables explained only 19% of the variance in self-reported disability, it was noticeable that the research used a general measure of self-efficacy and not a pain-specific measure as used in the current study and in previous studies mentioned above [24,28,53]. Pain self-efficacy may represent one of the most influential and most valuable psychological constructs in chronic low back pain [53] and it may be wise to measure this construct in both practice and research. These beliefs may be the target of clinical intervention via cognitive-behavioural, exercise-based programmes using both education and graded exposure.

The Multidimensional Health Locus of Control (MHLC) measure is a generic measure rather than a pain-specific questionnaire like the other scales used within the study. As such it may lack a degree of sensitivity with this patient population. The MHLC was used in the development of the Pain Beliefs Questionnaire [39] but it is noticeable that the correlations found in this study are weaker than those found by Edwards et al. [39]. The PBQ developers found no relationship between internal locus of control and organic pain beliefs, but this study indicated a negative relationship, albeit a relatively weak one. The regression analyses in this study illustrate that internal and powerful other locus of control are not predictors of any of the outcomes. Chance locus of control does however predict anxiety and, to a lesser extent, depression. Mediation analyses showed that there was some effect of organic pain beliefs on anxiety and depression which was indirect, through chance locus of control. Overall MHLC appears to have limited utility in relation to chronic low back pain.

This study utilises a suitably large sample whose characteristics indicate it to be a fairly typical chronic low back pain population. However, there were differences between questionnaire battery completers and non-completers. Failure to fully complete the questionnaire battery was perceived to be a consequence of time pressures during the assessment process. The difference in age (mean of 45 v 48 years) was not large however, given the nature of the sample. It was surprising that a higher proportion of men completed the battery than did not. Given the time pressure at initial assessment, men, who tend to be less conscientious than women [57], may have attempted the battery more quickly and so completed it.

Finally, the study is cross-sectional so causal inferences cannot be made from this data. The mediation models tested do reflect the literature, but it must be recognized that alternative models could be produced which could also fit with the available data, for example beliefs may mediate the relationships observed between self-efficacy and outcomes however this was a less good fit. Alternatively, unmeasured variables such as pain catastrophizing, may play a role in these relationships. Future longitudinal studies using the Pain Beliefs Questionnaire could further assess the usefulness of the measure in predicting and explaining variations in disability, anxiety and depression following low back pain rehabilitation programmes. In addition, controlled trials would help provide causal information about the role of beliefs in pain rehabilitation.

5. Conclusions

Overall, this study illustrates the importance of beliefs about the nature of pain and beliefs in one's ability to cope with pain in determining both physical and mental health outcomes amongst chronic low back pain patients. The pain beliefs questionnaire is a simple measure that is independent of condition or the presence of pain, but nevertheless provides two scales that are useful in predicting disability and mental health outcomes. Pain self-efficacy is an excellent predictor of physical and mental pain-related outcomes and can act indirectly in the relationship between organic ('biomedical') beliefs about pain and disability, anxiety and depression.

Acknowledgments: The authors would like to acknowledge the generous support offered by all staff at the Nottingham Back Team.

Author Contributions: Andrew Baird conceived, designed and undertook the study. Andrew Baird and David Sheffield analyzed the results and wrote the paper.

Appendix

The main body of the paper describes the most parsimonious model, but further analyses were undertaken to consider alternatives in relation to disability, anxiety and depression as described below:

Disability: In order to test the possibility that a third unmeasured variable may account for these relationships, further mediation analysis was conducted, with belief and LOC measures as mediators of the self-efficacy-disability relationship. There was a significant indirect effect of self-efficacy on disability through organic pain beliefs, $b = -0.23$, $p < 0.0001$, BCa CI (-0.07, -0.03), which explained 5% of the total effect. The direct effect of self-efficacy on disability was also significant, $b = -0.22$, $t = -12.13$, $p < 0.0001$.

Anxiety: In order to test the possibility that a third unmeasured variable may account for these relationships, further mediation analysis was again conducted, with belief and LOC measures as mediators of the self-efficacy-anxiety relationship. There was a significant indirect effect of self-efficacy on anxiety through chance LOC, $b = -0.20$, $p < 0.0001$, BCa CI (-0.03, -0.01), which explained 1% of the total effect. The direct effect of self-efficacy on anxiety was also significant, $b = -0.11$, $t = -6.50$, $p < 0.0001$.

Depression: Again, to test the possibility that a third unmeasured variable may account for these relationships, further mediation analysis was conducted, with belief and LOC measures as mediators of the self-efficacy-depression relationship. There was a significant indirect effect of self-efficacy on depression through chance LOC, $b = -0.08$, $p < 0.005$, BCa CI (-0.01, 0.00), which explained 1% of the total effect. The direct effect of self-efficacy on depression was also significant, $b = -0.16$, $t = -13.11$, $p < 0.0001$.

References

1. Balague, F.; Manion, A.F.; Pellise, F.; Cedraschi, C. Non-specific low back pain. *Lancet* **2012**, *379*, 482–491. [PubMed]
2. Snook, S. Work-related low back pain: Secondary intervention. *J. Electromyogr. Kinesiol.* **2004**, *14*, 153–160. [CrossRef] [PubMed]
3. Deyo, R.; Weinstein, J. Low back pain. *N. Engl. J. Med.* **2001**, *344*, 363–370. [CrossRef] [PubMed]
4. Thomsen, A.; Sorenson, J.; Sjorgen, P.; Eriksen, J. Chronic non-malignant pain patients and health economic consequences. *Eur. J. Pain* **2002**, *6*, 341–352. [PubMed]
5. Dagenais, G.; Caro, J.; Haldeman, S. A systematic review of low back pain cost of illness studies in the United States and internationally. *Spine J.* **2008**, *8*, 8–20. [CrossRef] [PubMed]
6. Hong, J.; Reed, C.; Novick, D.; Happich, M. Costs associated with treatment of chronic low back pain: An analysis of the UK General Practice Research Database. *Spine* **2013**, *38*, 75–82. [CrossRef] [PubMed]
7. Lidgren, L. The Bone and Joint Decade and the global economic and healthcare burden of musculoskeletal disease. *J. Rheumatol.* **2003**, *67*, 4–5.
8. Waddell, G. *The Back Pain Revolution*, 2nd ed.; Churchill Livingstone: Edinburgh, UK, 2004.
9. Waddell, G.; Burton, A.K. Occupational health guidelines for the management of low back pain at work: Evidence review. *Occup. Med. (Lond.)* **2001**, *51*, 124–135. [CrossRef] [PubMed]
10. Main, C.J.; George, S.Z. Psychologically informed practice for management of low back pain: Future directions in practice and research. *Phys. Ther.* **2011**, *91*, 820–824. [CrossRef] [PubMed]
11. Burton, A.K.; Balague, F.; Cardon, G.; Eriksen, H.R.; Henrotin, Y.; Lahad, A.; Leclerc, A.; Müller, G.; van der Beek, A.J. Chapter 2. European guidelines for prevention in low back pain. *Eur. Spine J.* **2006**, *15*, S136–S168. [CrossRef] [PubMed]
12. Chou, R.; Qaseem, A.; Snow, V.; Casey, D.; Cross, J.T.; Shekelle, P.; Owens, D. Diagnosis and treatment of low back pain: A joint clinical practice guideline from the American College of Physicians and the American Pain Society. *Ann. Intern. Med.* **2007**, *147*, 478–491. [CrossRef] [PubMed]
13. Turner, J.; Dworkin, S.; Mancl, L.; Huggins, K.; Truelove, E. The roles of beliefs, catastrophizing, and coping in the functioning of patients with temporomandibular disorders. *Pain* **2001**, *92*, 41–51. [CrossRef]
14. Jensen, M.; Romano, J.; Turner, J.; Good, A.; Wald, L. Patient beliefs predict patient functioning: Further support for a cognitive-behavioural model of chronic pain. *Pain* **1999**, *81*, 95–104. [CrossRef]
15. Vowle, K.E.; Gross, R.T. Work-related beliefs about injury and physical capability for work in individuals with chronic pain. *Pain* **2003**, *101*, 291–298. [CrossRef]
16. Turner, J.; Jensen, M.; Romano, J. Do beliefs, coping, and catastrophizing independently predict functioning in patients with chronic pain? *Pain* **2000**, *85*, 115–125. [CrossRef]
17. Goubert, L.; Crombez, G.; Van Damme, S. The role of neuroticism, pain catastrophizing and pain-related fear in vigilance to pain: A structural equations approach. *Pain* **2004**, *107*, 234–241. [CrossRef] [PubMed]
18. Zale, E.L.; Lange, K.L.; Fields, S.A.; Ditre, J.W. The relation between pain-related fear and disability: A meta-analysis. *J. Pain* **2013**, *14*, 1019–1030. [CrossRef] [PubMed]
19. Crombez, G.; Vlaeyen, J.W.; Heuts, P.; Lysens, R. Pain-related fear is more disabling than pain itself: Evidence on the role of pain-related fear in chronic back pain disability. *Pain* **1999**, *80*, 329–339. [CrossRef]
20. Vlaeyen, J.W.; Linton, S.J. Fear-avoidance and its consequences in chronic musculoskeletal pain: A state of the art. *Pain* **2000**, *85*, 317–332. [CrossRef]

21. Pfingsten, M.; Leibing, E.; Harter, W.; Kroner-Herwig, B.; Hempel, D.; Kronshage, U.; Hildebrandt, J. Fear-avoidance behavior and anticipation of pain in patients with chronic low back pain: A randomized controlled study. *Pain Med.* **2001**, *2*, 259–266. [CrossRef] [PubMed]
22. Buer, N.; Linton, S.J. Fear-avoidance beliefs and catastrophizing: Occurrence and risk factor in back pain and ADL in the general population. *Pain* **2002**, *99*, 485–491. [CrossRef]
23. Shaw, W.S.; Main, C.J.; Johnston, V. Addressing occupational factors in the management of low back pain: Implications for physical therapist practice. *Phys. Ther.* **2011**, *91*, 777–789. [CrossRef] [PubMed]
24. Ashari, A.; Nicholas, M.K. Pain self-efficacy beliefs and pain behaviour. A prospective study. *Pain* **2001**, *94*, 85–100. [CrossRef]
25. Denison, E.; Asenlof, P.; Lindberg, P. Self-efficacy, fear avoidance, and pain intensity as predictors of disability in subacute and chronic musculoskeletal pain patients in primary health care. *Pain* **2004**, *111*, 245–252. [CrossRef] [PubMed]
26. Amstein, P.; Caudill, M.; Mandler, C.; Norris, A.; Beasley, R. Self-efficacy as a mediator of the relationship between pain intensity, disability and depression in chronic pain patients. *Pain* **1999**, *80*, 483–491.
27. Arnstein, P. The mediation of disability by self-efficacy in different samples of chronic pain patients. *Disabil. Rehabil.* **2000**, *22*, 794–801. [CrossRef] [PubMed]
28. Woby, S.; Urmston, M.; Watson, P. Self-efficacy mediates the relation between pain-related fear and outcome in chronic low back pain patients. *Eur. J. Pain* **2007**, *11*, 711–718. [CrossRef] [PubMed]
29. Spinhoven, P.; ter Kuile, A.; Mansfeld, M.H.; den Ouden, D.J.; Vlaeyen, J.W.S. Catastrophizing and internal pain control as mediators of outcome in the multidisciplinary treatment of chronic low back pain. *Eur. J. Pain* **2004**, *8*, 211–219. [CrossRef] [PubMed]
30. Woby, S.; Watson, P.; Roach, N.; Urmston, M. Are changes in fear-avoidance beliefs, catastrophizing, and appraisals of control, predictive of changes in chronic low back pain and disability? *Eur. J. Pain* **2004**, *8*, 201–210. [CrossRef] [PubMed]
31. Morley, S.; Eccleston, C.; Williams, A. Systematic review and meta-analysis of randomized controlled trials of cognitive behaviour therapy and behaviour therapy for chronic pain in adults, excluding headache. *Pain* **1999**, *80*, 1–13. [CrossRef]
32. van Tulder, M.; Ostelo, R.; Vlaeyen, J.; Linton, S.; Morley, S.; Assendelft, W. Behavioral treatment for chronic low back pain: A systematic review within the framework of the Cochrane Back Review Group. *Spine* **2000**, *25*, 2688–2699. [CrossRef] [PubMed]
33. Linton, S.J.; Ryberg, M. A cognitive-behavioral group intervention as prevention for persistent neck and back pain in a non-patient population: A randomized controlled trial. *Pain* **2001**, *90*, 83–90. [CrossRef]
34. Abenhaim, L.; Rossignol, M.; Valat, J.P.; Nordin, M.; Avouac, B.; Blotman, F.; Charlot, J.; Dreiser, R.; Legrand, E.; Rozenberg, S.; et al. The role of activity in the therapeutic management of back pain. Report of the International Paris Task Force on Back Pain. *Spine* **2000**, *25*, 1S–33S. [CrossRef] [PubMed]
35. Liddle, S.; Baxter, G.; Gracey, J. Exercise and chronic low back pain: What works? *Pain* **2004**, *107*, 176–190. [CrossRef] [PubMed]
36. Baird, A.; Worral, L.; Haslam, C.; Haslam, R. Evaluation of a multi-disciplinary back pain rehabilitation programme—Individual and group perspectives. *Qual. Life Res.* **2008**, *17*, 357–366. [CrossRef] [PubMed]
37. Walsh, D.A.; Radcliffe, J.C. Pain beliefs and perceived physical disability of patients with chronic low back pain. *Pain* **2002**, *97*, 23–31. [CrossRef]
38. Baird, A.J.; Haslam, R.A. Exploring differences in pain beliefs within and between a large nonclinical (workplace) population and a clinical (chronic low back pain) population using the pain beliefs questionnaire. *Phys. Ther.* **2013**, *12*, 1615–1624. [CrossRef] [PubMed]
39. Edwards, L.; Pearce, S.; Turner-Stokes, L.; Jones, A. The Pain Beliefs Questionnaire: An investigation of beliefs in the causes and consequences of pain. *Pain* **1992**, *51*, 267–272. [CrossRef]
40. Sloan, T.; Gupta, R.; Zhang, W.; Walsh, D. Beliefs about the causes and consequences of pain in patients with chronic inflammatory or non-inflammatory low back pain and in pain-free individuals. *Spine* **2008**, *33*, 966–972. [CrossRef] [PubMed]
41. Roland, M.; Morris, R. A study of the natural history of low back pain. Part 1: Development of a reliable and sensitive measure of disability in low-back pain. *Spine* **1983**, *8*, 141–144. [CrossRef] [PubMed]
42. Roland, M.; Fairbank, J. The Roland–Morris Disability questionnaire and the oswestry disability questionnaire. *Spine* **2000**, *25*, 3115–3124. [CrossRef] [PubMed]

43. Nicholas, M.K. Self-efficacy and Chronic Pain. In Proceedings of the Annual Conference of the British Psychological Society, St. Andrews, Scotland, 1 April 1989.
44. Zigmond, A.S.; Snaith, R.P. The Hospital Anxiety and Depression Scale. *Acta. Psychiatr. Scand.* **1983**, *67*, 361–370. [CrossRef] [PubMed]
45. Bjellanda, I.; Dahlb, A.A.; Tangen Haugc, T.; Neckelmann, D. The validity of the Hospital Anxiety and Depression Scale: An updated literature review. *J. Psychosom. Res.* **2002**, *52*, 69–77. [CrossRef]
46. Hill, J.C.; Whitehurst, D.G.T.; Lewis, M.; Dunn, K.M.; Foster, N.E.; Konstantinou, K.; Main, C.J.; Mason, E.; Somerville, S.; Sowden, G.; Vohora, K.; Hay, E.M. Comparison of stratified primary care management for low back pain with current best practice (STarT Back): A randomised controlled trial. *Lancet* **2011**, *378*, 1560–1571. [CrossRef]
47. Wallston, K.A.; Wallston, B.S.; DeVellis, R. Development of the multidimensional health locus of control (MHLC) scales. *Health Educ. Monogr.* **1978**, *6*, 160–170. [CrossRef] [PubMed]
48. Wallston, K.A. The Validity of the Multidimensional Health Locus of Control Scales. *J. Health Psychol.* **2005**, *10*, 623–631. [CrossRef] [PubMed]
49. Harkapaa, K.; Jarvikovski, A.; Mellin, G.; Hurri, H.; Luoma, J. Health locus of control beliefs and psychological distress as predictors for treatmeant outcome in low-back pain patients: Results of a 3-month follow-up of a controlled intervention study. *Pain* **1991**, *46*, 35–41. [CrossRef]
50. Hayes, A.F. PROCESS: A versatile computational tool for observed variable mediation, moderation, and conditional process modelling. Available online: http://afhayes.com/public/process2012.png (accessed on 10 April 2015).
51. Preacher, K.J.; Hayes, A.F. SPSS and SAS procedures for estimating indirect effects in simple mediation models. *Behav. Res. Methods Instrum. Comput.* **2004**, *36*, 717–731. [CrossRef] [PubMed]
52. Preacher, K.J.; Hayes, A.F. Asymptotic and resampling strategies for assessing and comparing indirect effects in multiple mediator models. *Behav. Res. Methods* **2008**, *40*, 879–891. [CrossRef] [PubMed]
53. Foster, N.E.; Thomas, E.; Bishop, A.; Dunn, K.M.; Main, C.J. Distinctiveness of psychological barriers to recovery in low back pain patients in primary care. *Pain* **2010**, *148*, 398–406. [CrossRef] [PubMed]
54. Nicholas, M.K. The pain self-efficacy questionnaire: Taking pain into account. *Eur. J. Pain* **2007**, *11*, 153–163. [CrossRef] [PubMed]
55. Costa, L.D.C.M.; Maher, C.G.; McAuley, J.H.; Hancock, M.J. Self-efficacy is more important than fear of movement in mediating the relationship between pain and disability in chronic low back pain. *Eur. J. Pain* **2011**, *15*, 213–219. [CrossRef] [PubMed]
56. Schiphorst Preuper, H.R.; Reneman, M.F.; Boonstra, A.M.; Dijkstra, P.U.; Versteegen, G.J.; Geertzen, J.H.B.; Brouwer, S. Relationship between psychological factors and performance-based and self-reported disability in chronic low back pain. *Eur. Spine J.* **2008**, *17*, 1448–1456. [CrossRef] [PubMed]
57. Vianello, M.; Schnabel, C.; Sriram, N.; Nosek, B. Gender differences in implicit and explicit personality traits. *Pers. Individid. Dif.* **2013**, *55*, 994–999. [CrossRef]

9

Differences in the Association between Depression and Opioid Misuse in Chronic Low Back Pain *versus* Chronic Pain at Other Locations

Arpana Jaiswal [1], Jeffrey F. Scherrer [1,*], Joanne Salas [1], Carissa van den Berk-Clark [1], Sheran Fernando [1] and Christopher M. Herndon [1,2]

1 Department of Family and Community Medicine, Saint Louis University School of Medicine, St. Louis, MO 63104, USA; jaiswala@slu.edu (A.J.); salasj@slu.edu (J.S.); cvanden1@slu.edu (C.B.-C.); fernandos@slu.edu (S.F.); cherndo@siue.edu (C.M.H.)

2 Department of Pharmacy Practice, School of Pharmacy, Southern Illinois University Edwardsville, Edwardsville, IL 62026, USA

* Correspondence: scherrjf@slu.edu

Academic Editor: Robert J. Gatchel

Abstract: Patients with chronic pain and depression are more likely to develop opioid abuse compared to patients without depression. It is not known if this association differs by pain location. We compared the strength of association between depression and opioid misuse in patients with chronic low back pain (CLBP) *vs.* chronic pain of other location (CPOL). Chart abstracted data was obtained from 166 patients seeking care in a family medicine clinic. Depression was measured by the PHQ-9 and opioid misuse was measured using the Current Opioid Misuse Measure. Pain severity and interference questions came from the Brief Pain Inventory. Cross-tabulations were computed to measure the association between depression and opioid misuse stratified on pain location. Exploratory logistic regression modeled the association between depression and opioid misuse after adjusting for pain location and pain severity and interference. Depression was significantly associated with opioid misuse in CPOL but not in CLBP. Regression results indicate pain interference partly accounts for the depression–opioid misuse association. These preliminary results from a small patient sample suggest depression may co-occur with opioid misuse more often in CPOL than in CLBP. Further research is needed to compare this comorbidity in specific pain diagnoses such as arthritis, fibromyalgia and CLBP.

Keywords: chronic pain; pain location; depression; opioid misuse

1. Introduction

Patients with comorbid chronic pain and depression are more likely to receive a longer duration of opioid treatment at higher doses and are more likely to develop opioid abuse compared to non-depressed patients [1,2]. To our knowledge, it is not known if the link between depression and opioid abuse is similarly present in all types of chronic pain or is more common in chronic low back pain (CLPB). We are aware of one study of pain location and opioid misuse which found prevalence of opioid misuse was 82.8% in CLBP, 76.8% in those with arthritis, and 87.9% in neck/joint pain diagnosis suggesting some variation in opioid misuse by pain location [3]. The association between opioid misuse and depression could be stronger in CLBP given some evidence from patient populations that this pain location is associated with more depression than other pain types such as migraine and nerve root pain [4]. Comparison of fibromyalgia to other pain diagnostic groups found prevalence of the personality profile for neuroticism was greatest in fibromyalgia (46.2%) followed by 29.2% for lumbar, 20.5% for lower extremity and 15.4% for thoracic [5]. These results indicate that back pain patients have higher neuroticism compared to patients with other pain diagnoses with the exception of fibromyalgia. Significantly greater psychological distress and higher geriatric depression measures were reported for geriatric patients with CLBP compared to those with joint pain [6]. Data from survey studies indicate the prevalence and incidence of depression varies by pain location [7–9].

Thus, this limited literature provides some evidence that CLBP is associated with more depression and psychological distress than other pain types with the exception of fibromyalgia when data are obtained from patient populations. Given the strong association between opioid misuse and depression, we hypothesized that patients with CLBP would have a higher prevalence of depression and opioid misuse and this association would be stronger in CLBP than in patients with Chronic Pain of Other Location (CPOL).

We computed exploratory analysis to determine if: (1) the prevalence of depression and risk of opioid misuse differed among patients with CLBP *vs.* those with CPOL; and (2) the association between depression and risk of opioid misuse differed in patients with CLBP *vs.* those with CPOL.

2. Materials and Methods

2.1. Study Design and Population

Data for this cross-sectional study were obtained from a retrospective chart review of 166 chronic pain patients receiving pain management services at an academic family medicine clinic between January 2013 and December 2014. As part of routine care, patients presenting to the service completed the Brief Pain Inventory (BPI), Patient Health Questionnaire-9 (PHQ-9) and the Current Opioid Misuse Measure (COMM) at each visit. Data from initial clinical encounters were abstracted into an anonymized data set for the present study. After removing patients with missing data on any variable, the analytic data file contained 122 patients.

Pain conditions: From 22 primary pain diagnoses, we created a binary variable indicating the patient had CLBP, (n = 61) or CPOL (n = 61). Conditions among the CPOL group were osteoarthritis (n = 18), cervicalgia (n = 10), fibromyalgia (n = 7), migraine (n = 6), rheumatoid arthritis (n = 4), neuropathic pain (n = 4), HIV neuropathy (n = 2), avascular necrosis of the hip (n = 2), temporomandibular joint pain (n = 1), osteogenesis imperfecta (n = 1), lymphedema (n = 1), lower extremity trauma (n = 1), diffuse idiopathic skeletal hyperostosis (n = 1), complex regional pain syndrome (n = 1), chronic post stroke pain (n = 1) and abdominal pain (n = 1).

2.2. Measures

The three main measures assessed in this study were depression, risk of opioid misuse and pain interference.

2.2.1. Depression

The PHQ-9 questionnaire was utilized to assess depression. PHQ-9 is a self-report tool used in screening, diagnosing, monitoring and measuring severity of depression. The tool measures Diagnostic and Statistical Manual of Mental Disorders—4th Edition (DSM-IV) depression symptoms with nine items. Scores range from 0–27 and suggested thresholds are 5 (mild), 10 (moderate), 15 (moderately severe) and 20 (severe depression) [10]. Due to sample size, we used a binary indicator of depression with a threshold of at least 15 for depression. We used this threshold to ensure patients had clinically relevant depression associated with seeking care and receiving treatment.

2.2.2. Opioid Misuse

The Current Opioid Misuse Measure (COMM) questionnaire was used to measure risk of opioid misuse [11]. This questionnaire reflects patient's risk of medication-related aberrant behavior among chronic pain patients using prescription opioids. The COMM includes 17-items ranging from 0–4.

A summative score more than 9 is considered an elevated risk for opioid misuse. For ease of presentation, we refer to patients with this score as positive for risk of opioid misuse.

2.2.3. Pain Severity and Interference

We used the Brief Pain Inventory (BPI) short form [12] as a tool for measuring pain severity and pain interference. Pain severity had four questions measuring least pain, worst pain, average pain and current pain score, with each item measured on a 0–10 Likert scale (10 being the worst). Pain interference contained seven questions measuring interference with: activity, mood, walking, work, relationships, sleep, and joy using the same 0–10 Likert scale. Following BPI scoring instructions, we created the average pain severity score by averaging all four pain scores (least pain, worst pain, average pain and current pain score) and similarly created an average pain interference score by averaging the seven interference components.

2.2.4. Demographic Variables

Demographic data available from chart abstraction included age, gender and race. Due to small numbers of minority groups other than African-Americans (AA) we created a binary white/non-white race variable.

This study was approved by the IRBs of participating institutions.

2.3. Statistical Analysis

Frequencies, means and associations were computed using SPSS 23 [13]. Differences between CPOL and CLBP in demographics, pain indicators, depression, and opioid misuse risk were assessed using chi-square tests for categorical variables and independent samples t-tests for continuous variables. Also, chi-square and independent samples t-tests were conducted and stratified on pain location, to determine if there were differences in the association between depression and no depression with opioid misuse risk and pain. Similarly, the associations between pain characteristics and depression with opioid misuse risk were computed after stratifying by pain location. To assess whether there were any differential effects of depression or opioid misuse on other variables based on pain location strata, the interaction term in an ANOVA (for continuous variables) and the Breslow-Day test (categorical variables) were conducted. Last, a hierarchical logistic regression was conducted to calculate odds ratios and 95% confidence intervals by first adding pain characteristics and then adding depression, pain location, and the interaction of pain location and depression in successive blocks. All tests were conducted at $p < 0.05$.

3. Results

Table 1 displays the characteristics of the 122 pain patients included in our study sample. On average, patients were 49.6 ($\pm$ 12.6) years of age, 56.6% female and nearly 80% white. One-fourth were positive for opioid misuse risk and 35.2% met the criteria for depression. The average total pain score was 6.3 ($\pm$ 1.7) and average pain interference was 6.7 ($\pm$ 2.4). Comparisons between CPOL and CLBP indicated that those with CLBP had lower average pain severity, lower average least pain and lower average pain than those with CPOL.

Table 2 shows the association between opioid misuse and pain characteristics by depression, stratified by pain location. Among CPOL patients, 66.7% of depressed patients were positive for opioid misuse compared to 7.5% of non-depressed CPOL patients ($p < 0.001$). Among CLBP patients, depression was not related to positive opioid misuse ($p = 0.19$). A Breslow-Day test showed that depression and opioid misuse were more strongly associated among CPOL than among CLBP patients ($p = 0.019$). Average COMM score was significantly greater among depressed compared to non-depressed CPOL ($p < 0.0001$) and CLBP ($p < 0.01$) patients; however the difference between depressed and non-depressed was larger (interaction p-value = 0.016) among CPOL (difference = 13.0) patients than CLBP patients (difference = 5.8). Among CPOL, but not among CLBP patients, average pain severity was significantly higher among depressed *vs.* non-depressed patients. Pain interference was significantly greater among depressed *vs.* non-depressed patients in both CPOL and CLBP patients. The relationship of BPI measures and depression were similar across pain location strata.

Table 1. Characteristics of family medicine pain clinic patients, n = 122.

Variables, Mean (sd)	Total (n = 122)	CPOL (n = 61) [1]	CLBP (n = 61) [1]	*p*-value
Age	49.6 (± 2.6)	50.4 (± 11.5)	48.8 (± 13.0)	0.485
Gender, n(%)				0.100
Female	69 (56.6%)	39 (63.9%)	30 (49.2%)	
Male	53 (43.4%)	22 (36.1%)	31 (50.8%)	
Race, n(%)				0.501
White	97 (79.5%)	47 (77.0%)	50 (82.0%)	
Non-white	25 (20.5%)	14 (23.0%)	11 (18.0%)	
Positive opioid misuse (COMM [2] > 9), n(%)	30 (24.6%)	17 (27.9%)	13 (21.3%)	0.400
COMM score [2]	9.2 (± 9.1)	9.5 (± 9.8)	8.9 (± 8.5)	0.639
Depression (PHQ-9 [3] > 14), n(%)	43 (35.2%)	21 (34.4%)	22 (36.1%)	0.850
PHQ-9 [3] score	11.0 (± 6.7)	11.0 (± 6.8)	11.0 (± 6.7)	0.989
BPI [4] mean, (sd)				
Total Average pain index	6.3 (± 1.7)	6.6 (± 1.8)	5.9 (± 1.7)	0.035
Worst pain level	7.7 (± 1.7)	7.9 (± 1.7)	7.4 (± 1.6)	0.112
Least pain level	5.0 (± 2.2)	5.4 (± 2.2)	4.5 (± 2.1)	0.029
Pain level on average	6.3 (± 1.8)	6.7 (± 1.8)	6.0 (± 1.7)	0.039
Pain level right now	6.2 (± 2.3)	6.5 (± 2.3)	5.9 (± 2.2)	0.115
Total Average pain interference	6.7 (± 2.4)	6.7 (± 2.6)	6.7 (± 2.2)	0.900
General activity	7.2 (± 2.3)	7.2 (± 2.5)	7.2 (± 2.2)	0.957
Mood	6.5 (± 2.8)	6.4 (± 2.9)	6.6 (± 2.7)	0.713
Walking ability	6.7 (± 2.8)	6.7 (± 2.9)	6.7 (± 2.6)	0.987
Normal work	7.5 (± 2.6)	7.4 (± 2.7)	7.5 (± 2.5)	0.755
Relations with others	5.2 (± 3.4)	5.3 (± 3.6)	5.1 (± 3.3)	0.762
Sleep	6.8 (± 2.8)	6.8 (± 2.8)	6.8 (± 2.8)	0.987
Enjoyment of life	7.0 (± 2.9)	6.9 (± 3.2)	7.1 (± 2.7)	0.658

Note: *p*-value is for chi-square tests for categorical variables and independent samples *t*-tests for continuous variables. [1] CPOL: Chronic pain of other location, CLBP: Chronic low back pain; [2] COMM= Chronic Opioid Misuse Measure (0–68); [3] PHQ-9 = Depression scale (0–27); [4] BPI = Brief Pain Inventory (Average Severity and interference: 0–10, Individual BPI items: 0–10).

Table 2. Distribution of patient opioid misuse risk and pain characteristics by depression, stratified by pain location (n = 122).

Variables, Mean(sd)	CPOL [1] (n = 61)			CLBP [1] (n = 61)			Interaction *p*-value [4]
	Not depressed (n = 40)	Depressed (n = 21)	*p*-value	Not depressed (n = 39)	Depressed (n = 22)	*p*-value	
Positive opioid misuse (COMM [2] > 9), n(%)	3 (7.5%)	14 (66.7%)	<0.001	6 (15.4%)	7 (31.8%)	0.19	0.019
COMM [2]	5.1 (± 5.1)	18.1 (± 10.9)	<0.001	6.8 (± 7.5)	12.6 (± 9.1)	0.01	0.016
BPI [3]							
Total average pain index	6.1 (± 1.8)	7.6 (± 1.2)	<0.001	5.8 (± 1.7)	6.3 (± 1.6)	0.25	0.143
Total average pain interference	5.7 (± 2.6)	8.5 (± 0.9)	<0.001	6.1 (± 2.1)	7.8 (± 1.9)	0.004	0.151

Note: *p*-value is for chi-square tests for categorical variables and independent samples *t*-tests for continuous variables. [1] CPOL: Chronic Pain of Other Location, CLBP: Chronic Low Back Pain; [2] COMM = Current Opioid Misuse Measure (0–68); [3] BPI = Brief Pain Inventory (Average Severity and interference: 0–10); [4] *p*-value for interaction term of pain location x depression, ANOVA for continuous variables and Breslow-Day test for dichotomous variables.

Table 3 shows the association between PHQ-9 score and pain characteristics by opioid misuse, stratified by pain location. The average PHQ-9 scores were significantly higher among COMM positive CPOL patients compared to COMM negative CPOL patients. The association between COMM status and PHQ-9 score was not significant in the CLBP group. There were marginally significant between strata differences in the relationship of opioid misuse and PHQ-9 score (interaction p-value = 0.050). Both pain severity and pain interference were positively related to COMM positive status among CPOL patients. Conversely, only pain interference was higher among COMM positive CLBP patients compared to COMM negative CLBP patients. There were no between strata differences in the relationship of opioid misuse and pain characteristics.

Table 3. Distribution of depression score and pain characteristics by opioid misuse, stratified by pain location (n = 122).

Variables, mean (sd)	CPOL [1] (n = 61)			CLBP [1] (n = 61)			Interaction p-value [5]
	COMM [2] negative (n = 44)	COMM [2] positive (n = 17)	p-value *	COMM [2] negative (n = 48)	COMM [2] positive (n = 13)	p-value *	
PHQ-9 [3]	8.6 (± 5.6)	17.4 (± 5.2)	<0.001	10.3 (± 6.8)	13.9 (± 5.7)	0.08	0.050
BPI [4]							
Total Average pain index	6.3 (± 1.8)	7.5 (± 1.3)	0.017	5.8 (± 1.7)	6.6 (± 1.6)	0.101	0.638
Total Average pain interference	5.9 (± 2.6)	8.6 (± 1.0)	<0.001	6.3 (± 2.2)	8.2 (± 1.2)	0.005	0.384

Note: p-value is for chi-square tests for categorical variables and independent samples t-tests for continuous variables. [1] CPOL: Chronic Pain of Other Location, CLBP: Chronic Low Back Pain; [2] COMM = Current Opioid Misuse Measure (0–68); [3] PHQ-9 = Depression scale (0–27); [4] BPI = Brief Pain Inventory (Average Severity and interference: 0–10); [5] p-value for interaction term of pain location * COMM Opioid Misuse, ANOVA for continuous variables and Breslow-Day test for dichotomous variables.

Table 4 shows results of a hierarchical logistic regression. In model 1, pain severity and interference explain 32.0% of the variance in the likelihood of opioid misuse risk, with each unit increase in pain interference having over twice the likelihood of opioid misuse risk (OR = 2.25; 95% CI: 1.45–3.48); however, pain severity was unrelated to opioid misuse risk. Adding depression explained an additional 5.2% (p = 0.019) of the variance in opioid misuse risk and increased the odds of opioid misuse risk by over 3-fold (OR = 3.32; 95% CI: 1.20–9.16). Pain location did not significantly explain any additional variance in opioid misuse risk; however, adding an interaction term of pain location and depression in a final model explained an additional 4.5% of the variance (p = 0.025). The significant interaction term showed that the odds ratio for the relationship of depression and opioid misuse risk increased by over a factor of 10 comparing CPOL to CLBP (depression OR: 10.57 *vs.* 1.04, respectively).

Table 4. Logistic regression models for opioid misuse risk (COMM [1]) (n = 122).

Predictor Variables	Model 1. Pain severity and interference	Model 2. Add depression	Model 3. Add pain location	Model 4.Add depression * pain location
Variables	OR (95% CI)	OR (95% CI)	OR (95% CI)	OR (95% CI)
Total average pain severity [2]	0.88 (0.60–1.29)	0.92 (0.61–1.37)	0.87 (0.58–1.31)	0.81 (0.52–1.26)
Total average pain interference [2]	2.25 (1.45–3.48)	1.91 (1.21–3.01)	1.95 (1.23–3.09)	2.09 (1.26–3.47)
Depression (Yes *vs.* No)		3.32 (1.20–9.16)	3.32 (1.19–9.23)	
Pain Location [3]				
CPOL			1.00	-
CLBP			0.64 (0.23–1.77)	-
Depression * Pain Location [4]				
CPOL: Depression (Yes *vs.* No)				10.57 (2.21–50.49)
CLBP: Depression (Yes *vs.* No)				1.04 (0.25–4.41)
Chi-square change (df, *p*-value)	29.58 (2, <0.0001)	5.48 (1, 0.019)	0.74 (1, 0.390)	5.00 (1, 0.025)
Nagelkerke R-square	0.320	0.372	0.378	0.423

Note: OR = odds ratio; CI = confidence interval; [1] COMM = Chronic opioid Misuse Measure; [2] Brief Pain Inventory (Average Severity and interference: 0–10), odds ratio represents the change in odds of opioid misuse risk given one unit increase in average pain severity or interference; [3] CPOL: Chronic pain other location, CLBP: Chronic low back pain; [4] Wald Chi-square $p = 0.031$.

4. Discussion

In patients seeking treatment at a family medicine pain clinic, we observed evidence that the association between depression and opioid misuse differed in patients with CLBP compared to CPOL. Results of bivariate analysis stratified on pain location revealed that depression was more strongly associated with opioid misuse among CPOL patients than in patients with CLBP. This observation is not explained by pain interference which showed similar significant associations with depression in both CPOL and CLBP. Exploratory hierarchical logistic regression found that depression increases the odds of opioid misuse after adjusting for pain location and pain characteristics (severity and interference) and that this relationship is over 10 times stronger in CPOL than in CLBP. While pain severity was not significantly associated with opioid misuse risk in adjusted analysis, results suggest that pain interference independently contributes to opioid misuse risk after accounting for depression.

Our data expand on the existing literature on the prevalence of depression among different pain types [4–9] and the prevalence of opioid misuse across different pain types [3] by showing prevalence estimates of both opioid misuse and depression in groups stratified by pain location. Additional studies are warranted to determine if the frequent depression—opioid misuse comorbidity varies in CLBP compared to other specific types of pain such as arthritis, migraine, fibromyalgia, *etc.*

Because neuroticism is thought to be more common in CLBP [5] we expected CLBP patients to have more depression and subsequently more opioid misuse. However our results indicate the prevalence of depression does not differ by pain location. We did not expect to find a stronger association of depression and opioid misuse among CPOL patients. Though speculative, these results may be due to evidence from Morasco *et al.* [3] that neck and joint pain patients are more likely to have a history of substance use disorder compared to CLBP patients (94.4% *vs.* 83.3%).

One potential explanation for the stronger association between depression and opioid misuse in CPOL patients could be the significantly higher BPI score, higher average least pain and higher average pain level among CPOL *vs.* CLBP. In addition BPI scores were significantly greater in the depressed CPOL compared to non-depressed CPOL patients but did not differ by depression status in the CLBP patients. BPI scores were also higher in COMM positive *vs.* COMM negative patients in the CPOL patients but not CLBP patients. Greater pain severity in CPOL may lead to both depression and opioid misuse in patients with CLBP. Although pain severity was not significant when modeled with pain interference in regression analysis, this does not preclude the possibility that pain severity leads to greater pain interference which then increases depression and opioid misuse. Longitudinal data collection is needed to confirm this possibility.

There are several biological mechanisms proposed for the association between pain and depression. Common vulnerability due to past psychopathology or trauma leads to chronic pain via changes in catecholamines, substance P and cytokine activity and less responsive opioid receptors that may perpetuate or worsen depression [14]. Another biological underpinning for the pain-depression relationship is inflammatory processes and oxidative stress [15]. Studies of memantine, an NMDA receptor antagonist improves both pain and depression via reduction in glutamate activity and thereby reducing inflammatory factors related to pain and depression [16].

Limitations include small sample size which limits the precision of our conclusions. We did not have enough subjects to compare CLBP to specific types of CPOL such as arthritis or fibromyalgia; however, sensitivity analysis removing fibromyalgia which is often comorbid with depression, did not change our conclusions. We also lacked sample size to conduct stratified multivariable logistic regression models. The data did not contain type of opioid or co-medication which may bias results if CLBP or CPOL systematically differed in morphine equivalent dose because higher daily opioid morphine equivalent dose is associated with depression [17,18] and opioid misuse [19]. Comorbid conditions such as specific co-occurring pain conditions and anxiety disorders, were not available to improve control of confounding. The results may not apply to other geographic locations or to pain patients seeking care in other settings.

5. Conclusions

We found depression was more strongly associated with opioid misuse in patients with CPOL compared to patients with CLBP. The well-established association between depression and opioid misuse may be less prominent in CLBP than in other pain types. Further research with larger samples should compare this association in CLBP, arthritis, fibromyalgia and neuralgia. Refining which pain patients are most likely to develop comorbid depression and opioid misuse can inform clinical care and target limited resources to patients at greatest risk for this comorbidity.

Acknowledgments: Arpana Jaiswal and Sheran Fernando were supported by a training fellowship. No funds were received to cover the costs to publish in open access.

Author Contributions: Arpana Jaiswal and Jeffrey F. Scherrer conceived and designed the experiments; Arpana Jaiswal and Jeffrey F. Scherrer and Joanne Salas analyzed the data; Christopher M. Herndon contributed data. Jeffrey F. Scherrer, Arpana Jaiswal, Carissa van den Berk-Clarkand Joanne Salas wrote the paper. All authors contributed to revisions and approval of the final manuscript.

Abbreviations

The following abbreviations are used in this manuscript:

CLBP	Chronic low back pain
CPOL	Chronic pain of other location
COMM	Current Opioid Misuse Measure
PHQ-9	Patient Health Questionnaire-9
BPI	Brief Pain Inventory

References

1. Edlund, M.J.; Martin, B.C.; Fan, M.Y.; Devries, A.; Braden, J.B.; Sullivan, M.D. Risks for opioid abuse and dependence among recipients of chronic opioid therapy: Results from the Troup study. *Drug Alcohol Depend.* **2010**, *112*, 90–98. [CrossRef] [PubMed]

2. Sullivan, M.D.; Edlund, M.J.; Zhang, L.; Unützer, J.; Wells, K.B. Association between mental health disorders, problem drug use, and regular prescription opioid use. *Arch. Intern. Med.* **2006**, *166*, 2087–2093. [CrossRef] [PubMed]
3. Morasco, B.J.; Dobscha, S.K. Prescription medication misuse and substance use disorder in VA primary care patients with chronic pain. *Gen. Hosp. Psychiatry* **2008**, *30*, 93–99. [CrossRef] [PubMed]
4. Makovec, M.; Vintar, N.; Makovec, S. Self-reported depression, anxiety and evaluation of own pain in clinical sample of patients with different location of chronic pain. *Zdrav Var.* **2015**, *54*, 1–10.
5. Porter-Moffit, S.; Gatchel, R.J.; Robinson, R.C.; Deschner, M.; Posamentier, M.; Polatin, P.; Lou, L. Biophysical profile of different pain diagnostic groups. *J. Pain* **2006**, *7*, 308–318. [CrossRef] [PubMed]
6. Morone, N.E.; Karp, J.F.; Lynch, C.; Bost, J.E.; El Khoudhry, S.R.; Weiner, D.K. Impact of chronic musculoskeletal pathology on older adults: A study of differences between knee OA and low back pain. *Pain Med.* **2009**, *4*, 693–701. [CrossRef] [PubMed]
7. de Heer, E.W.; Gerrits, M.M.; Beekman, A.T.; Dekker, J.; van Marwijk, H.W.; de Waal, M.W.; Spinhoven, P.; Penninx, B.W.; van der Feltz-Cornelis, C.M. The association of depression and anxiety with pain: A study from NESDA. *PloS ONE* **2014**, *9*, e106907.
8. Gerritis, M.M.; van Oppen, P.; van Marwijk, H.W.; Penninx, B.W.; van der Horst, E.H. Pain and the onset of depressive and anxiety disorders. *Pain* **2014**, *155*, 53–59. [CrossRef] [PubMed]
9. Baune, B.T.; Caniato, R.N.; Garcia-Alcaraz, M.A.; Berger, K. Combined effects of major depression, pain and somatic disorders on general functioning in the general adult population. *Pain* **2008**, *138*, 310–317. [CrossRef] [PubMed]
10. Kroencke, K.; Spitzer, R.; Williams, J. The PHQ-9: Validity of a brief depression severity measure. *J. Gen. Intern. Med.* **2001**, *16*, 606–613. [CrossRef]
11. Butler, S.F.; Budman, S.H.; Fernandez, K.C.; Houle, B.; Benoit, C.; Katz, N.; Jamison, R.N. Development and validation of the current opioid misuse measure. *Pain* **2007**, *130*, 144–156. [CrossRef] [PubMed]
12. Cleeland, C.S. The Brief Pain Inventory. Available online: https://www.mdanderson.org/education-and-research/departments-programs-and-labs/departments-and-divisions/symptom-research/symptom-assessment-tools/BPI_UserGuide.pdf (accessed on 1 March 2016).
13. Statistical package for the social sciences. Available online: http://www.ibm.com/analytics/us/en/technology/spss/ (accessed on 1 March 2015).
14. Leo, R.J. Chronic pain and comorbid depression. *Curr. Treat. Options Neurol.* **2005**, *7*, 403–412. [CrossRef] [PubMed]
15. Moura, F.A.; Queiroz de Andrade, K.; dos Santos, J.C.; Araujo, O.R.; Goulart, M.O. Antioxidant therapy for treatment of inflammatory bowel disease: Does it work? *Redox Biol.* **2015**, *6*, 617–639. [CrossRef] [PubMed]
16. Olivan-Blazquez, B.; Herrera-Mercadal, P.; Puebla-Guedea, M.; Perez-Yus, M.C.; Andres, E.; Fayed, N.; Lopez-Del-Hoyo, Y.; Magallon, R.; Roca, M.; Carcia-Campayo, J. Efficacy of memantine in the treatment of fibromyalgia: A double-blind, randomised, controlled trial with 6-month follow-up. *Pain* **2014**, *155*, 2517–2525. [CrossRef] [PubMed]
17. Merrill, J.O.; Von Korff, M.; Banta-Green, C.J.; Sullivan, M.D.; Saunders, K.W.; Campbell, C.I.; Weisner, C. Prescribed Opioid difficulties, depression and opioid dose among chronic opioid therapy patients. *Gen. Hosp. Psychiatry* **2012**, *24*, 581–587. [CrossRef] [PubMed]
18. Scherrer, J.F.; Salas, J.; Lustman, P.J.; Burge, S.; Schneider, F.D. Residency Research network of Texas (RRNeT) Investigators. *Pain* **2015**, *156*, 348–355. [CrossRef] [PubMed]
19. White, A.G.; Birnbaum, H.G.; Schiller, M.; Tang, J.; Katz, N.P. Analytic models to identify patients at risk for prescription opioid abuse. *Am. J. Manag. Care* **2009**, *15*, 897–906. [PubMed]

10

Chronic Pain in Children and Adolescents: Diagnosis and Treatment of Primary Pain Disorders in Head, Abdomen, Muscles and Joints

Stefan J. Friedrichsdorf [1,2,*], James Giordano [3], Kavita Desai Dakoji [1], Andrew Warmuth [1], Cyndee Daughtry [1] and Craig A. Schulz [1,4]

1 Children's Hospitals and Clinics of Minnesota, Minneapolis, MN 55404, USA; Kavita.DesaiDakoji@childrensMN.org (K.D.D.); Andrew.Warmuth@childrensMN.org (A.W.); Cyndee.Daughtry@childrensMN.org (C.D.); Craig.Schulz@childrensMN.org (C.S.)
2 Department of Pediatrics, University of Minnesota Medical School, Minneapolis, MN 55455, USA
3 Georgetown University Medical Center, Washington, DC 20057, USA; james.giordano@georgetown.edu
4 Center for Spirituality & Healing, University of Minnesota, Minneapolis, MN 55455, USA
* Correspondence: Stefan.Friedrichsdorf@childrensMN.org

Academic Editor: Carl L. von Baeyer

Abstract: Primary pain disorders (formerly "functional pain syndromes") are common, under-diagnosed and under-treated in children and teenagers. This manuscript reviews key aspects which support understanding the development of pediatric chronic pain, points to the current pediatric chronic pain terminology, addresses effective treatment strategies, and discusses the evidence-based use of pharmacology. Common symptoms of an underlying pain vulnerability present in the three most common chronic pain disorders in pediatrics: primary headaches, centrally mediated abdominal pain syndromes, and/or chronic/recurrent musculoskeletal and joint pain. A significant number of children with repeated acute nociceptive pain episodes develop chronic pain in addition to or as a result of their underlying medical condition "chronic-on-acute pain." We provide description of the structure and process of our interdisciplinary, rehabilitative pain clinic in Minneapolis, Minnesota, USA with accompanying data in the treatment of chronic pain symptoms that persist beyond the expected time of healing. An interdisciplinary approach combining (1) rehabilitation; (2) integrative medicine/active mind-body techniques; (3) psychology; and (4) normalizing daily school attendance, sports, social life and sleep will be presented. As a result of restored function, pain improves and commonly resolves. Opioids are not indicated for primary pain disorders, and other medications, with few exceptions, are usually not first-line therapy.

Keywords: chronic pain; interdisciplinary treatment; children; adolescents; biopsychosocial; primary pain disorder; pediatric pain clinic

1. Introduction

Pediatric chronic pain is a significant problem with conservative estimates that posit 20% to 35% of children and adolescents affected by it worldwide [1–3]. Pain experienced in children's hospitals is known to be common, under-recognized, and under-treated, with more than 10% of hospitalized children showing features of chronic pain [4–7]. Although the majority of children reporting chronic pain are not greatly disabled by it [8], about 3% of pediatric chronic pain patients require intensive rehabilitation [9]. The total costs to society incurred by care for children and adolescents with moderate to severe chronic pain has been extrapolated to $19.5 billion annually in the USA [10]. For a recent systematic review of the etiology of chronic and recurrent pediatric pain not associated with disease, see King et al., 2011 [2].

The underlying pathophysiology of pain in children includes acute nociceptive pain (i.e., pain arising from the activation of peripheral nerve endings, including somatic and visceral pain), neuropathic pain (i.e., resulting from injury to, or dysfunction of, the somatosensory system), psycho-social-spiritual-emotional pain, total pain and/or the topic of this paper, chronic pain. Pain may originate from one, but more commonly involves a combination of these pathophysiologies. Commonly accepted definitions of chronic pain describe pain that persists for three months; however, the Rome IV criteria for functional abdominal pain disorders, for instance, typically require symptoms to be present and persist for at least two months [11]. Like many pediatric pain programs, we define chronic pain not necessarily by using arbitrary temporal parameters, but rather employ a more functional definition such as "pain that extends beyond the expected period of healing" and "hence lacks the acute warning function of physiological nociception" [12,13]. Simply put, pain lasting two months and 29 days does not necessarily change from "acute" to "chronic" once it merely extends to a period of three months in duration.

The 2012 American Pain Society Position Statement, "Assessment and Management of Children with Chronic Pain", indicates that chronic pain in children is the result of a dynamic integration of biological processes, psychological factors, and sociocultural variables, considered within a developmental trajectory [14]. Chronic pain includes persistent (ongoing) and recurrent (episodic) pain in children with underlying health conditions (e.g., inflammatory bowel disease, sickle cell disease, rheumatoid arthritis), and pain that is the disorder itself (e.g., primary headaches, centrally mediated abdominal pain syndrome, musculoskeletal pain, complex regional pain syndrome), with a significant number of children experiencing both entities, i.e., "chronic-on-acute" pain. Chronic pain affects the entire nervous system, and the term central sensitization, which is an increased central neural responsiveness to painful and non-painful stimuli, has been used to describe any central nervous system dysfunction or pathology that may contribute to the development or maintenance of many types of chronic pain [14,15].

Chronic childhood and adolescent pain is not only an issue of importance for the clinical care of pediatric patients, but also is a condition that exerts considerable bearing upon the medical, social and economic sectors. We believe that an improved understanding, definition and approach to treating chronic childhood and adolescent pain represent important steps toward both optimizing the clinical care of pediatric pain patients, and in this way, diminishing the overall negative impact of chronic pain on patients, medicine and society. In this light, and as an introduction to the Special Issue "Chronic and Recurrent Pain" in *Children* edited by L.S. Walker and C.L. von Baeyer [16], the aim of this paper is to highlight important key aspects in support of a fortified understanding of the development and expression of chronic pain in children and adolescents, such as pain catastrophizing and fear of pain. In addition, we aim to review the current pediatric chronic pain terminology and provide a brief description of the approach to assessing and treating chronic pain as practiced in our interdisciplinary pediatric pain clinic.

2. Children with Chronic Pain

2.1. Trajectory

Untreated chronic pain in children incurs a high risk for the subsequent development of pain and psychological disorders later in life. Seventeen percent of adult chronic pain patients reported a history of chronic pain in childhood or adolescence, with close to 80% indicating that the pain in childhood continued and persisted until adulthood [17]. In the USA, adults with chronic pain have a lower household income and higher risk of unemployment [18]. Studies of two birth cohorts from 1946 and 1958 showed that children with persistent abdominal pain and headaches go on to suffer more physical symptoms, anxiety and depression in adult life than healthy children [19–22]. A prospective study by Mulvaney and colleagues of 132 children with abdominal pain indicated long-term, high level risk of (adult) symptoms and impairment for a cluster of patients who did not have the most severe pain, but who had significantly more anxiety, depression, lower perceived self-worth, and more negative life events at baseline [23].

In another three-year prospective cohort study [24] involving 1336 children and teens in pain aged 11–14 years, Dunn et al. showed that 44% displayed a developmental trajectory for increased pain disorders and conditions, primarily presenting as headaches, back pain, abdominal pain and facial pain, and 12% presented with persistent pain. Individuals at highest risk to develop persistent pain were predominantly female, demonstrated the highest level of somatization and depression at both the start and end of the study period, and were least likely to be satisfied with their life. As well, research has shown that extra-intestinal somatic and depressive symptoms at the initial pediatric evaluation for functional abdominal pain were significant predictors of functional gastrointestinal disorders in adulthood [25]. Pediatric patients with functional abdominal pain exhibit long-term vulnerability to anxiety that begins in childhood and persists into late adolescence and early adulthood, even if abdominal pain resolves [26]. The National Longitudinal Study of Adolescent to Adult Health included more than 14,000 study participants and has shown that chronic pain in adolescence is associated with higher rates of mental health disorders reported in adulthood with anxiety (21.1% vs. 12.4% pain-free adolescents) and depressive disorders (24.5% vs. 14.1%) being most common [27]. Van Tilburg and colleagues analyzed data from a longitudinal study of a nationally representative sample of 9970 adolescents in the USA to show that adolescents with chronic pain and depression are at increased risk for both suicidal ideation and suicide attempt [28].

2.2. *Pain Catastrophizing and Fear of Pain*

The fear avoidance model of pain with an emphasis on the maladaptive behaviors that lead to activity avoidance has guided pediatric chronic pain research and clinical practice [29]. Certainly most, if not all, people seek to avoid pain. Fear of pain and subsequent exacerbation of its effects is common in both adults and children. Catastrophizing (or "Awfulizing") is a key mechanism by which the experience of pain can be exacerbated in children and adolescents. Catastrophizing represents a set of negative cognitive/emotional processes that include magnification (amplification of the significance of pain), rumination (anxious preoccupation with pain) and pessimism about pain sensations and feelings of helplessness when in pain. There is a significant body of research showing a correlation of children's pain behaviors and their (as well as their parents') extent of catastrophizing [30–32]. Pain reduction through distraction is delayed by catastrophizing [33], is associated with greater pain in children when either child or parent displays high pain catastrophizing [34]. Negative pain memory bias is advanced by parental (more than children's) pain catastrophizing and, in addition, expectations as well as cognitions of parents influence child pain memory formation [35].

Both physical and psychological dysfunction in pediatric chronic pain is modulated and upregulated by fear of pain [36]. Diminishing the fear of pain strongly correlates with positive functional outcomes in children with primary pain disorders [36]. Further, there is a robust positive association between pain-related fear and disability [37]. Consistent with the fear-avoidance model of chronic pain, these findings suggest that pain-related fear may be an important therapeutic target for approaches aimed at reducing pain-related disability.

2.3. *Time for a New Name: "Primary Pain Disorder"*

Many different chronic and recurrent pain syndromes in both adult and pediatric populations are now considered to be manifestations of an underlying vulnerability or pain spectrum condition, rather than being viewed as separate disorders [38]. Considerable evidence, especially from twin studies, points to a role of shared biological sensitivity, "pain vulnerability," "pain sensitivity," or "central sensitivity syndrome" [38–42]. Thus, conditions such as primary headaches (including tension headaches), centrally mediated abdominal pain syndromes, localized or widespread musculoskeletal pain (including "pain amplification syndrome," "non-cardiac chest pain," "costochondritis," "temporomandibular joint disorder," "juvenile fibromyalgia," etc.) are no longer regarded as separate entities with differing underlying pathophysiologies in need of different treatments. Instead, these conditions are now generally regarded as pain manifestations of the same underlying condition that present at varied locations.

The term primary pain disorder (formerly: functional pain syndrome) was first employed by Schechter in 2014 [43]. It describes a chronic pain disorder that cannot be explained by appropriate medical assessment(s) in terms of conventionally defined medical disease, as based on biochemical or structural abnormalities. A primary pain disorder is associated with significant disruption of everyday life and often leads to incapacitation. This disorder is not typically responsive to unimodal medical therapy, and attempts at such management can consume significant time, medical resources and finances. Persistent treatment failures can lead to pejorative implications such as patients perceiving that their pain is not organic and therefore not real or serious, and/or stigmatization (i.e., patients' symptoms may be characterized as fictitious or as evidence of malingering).

Toward advancing an improved understanding of primary pain disorder and its relation to chronic pain in children and adolescents, the following section presents a review of the three most prevalent symptoms, manifestations, and locations of a primary pain disorder (headaches, abdominal pain, and/or musculoskeletal pain).

3. Pain Manifestations and Locations of a Primary Pain Disorder

3.1. *Primary Headache: Tension Headaches and Migraines*

Traditionally, headaches were classified using a bimodal construct: tension headaches (infrequent episodic, frequent episodic, or chronic) versus migraines (with or without aura) [44]. In 2013 the International Headache Society (IHS) [45] classified "primary headaches" as migraines, tension-type headaches, trigeminal autonomic cephalalgias and "secondary headaches," e.g., a headache attributed to trauma or injury to the head, cranial or cervical vascular disorders, etc. Pediatric data supports the notion that childhood headaches are a continuum, rather than discrete entities [46,47]. Recent findings [48] suggest that "migraine" and "tension-type" headaches might not be separate diagnostic/disease entities, but rather represent a severity continuum for young adults 18–24 years of age who experience chronic headaches more than 3–4 days per week. Two cross-sectional studies [48] with more than 3400 headache patients revealed that those who are experiencing headaches at a younger age (18–24 years old) and with higher frequency (more than 15 headache days/month) displayed a unimodal distribution, suggesting the dimensional construct of a primary headache. Conversely, patients who experienced a lower frequency of headaches and were of older age showed bimodal headache distributions, which could be differentiated into "migraine" versus "tension-type" headache. In addition, pressure pain thresholds over the temporalis, masseter, and frontalis muscles in patients with headaches do not exhibit strong differences between migraine and tension headaches [49]. In other words, for pediatric patients who are headache-free most of the time and (only) experience episodic headaches, the "bimodal" classification of "tension-type" versus "migraines" continues to be clinically appropriate, as migraines (as opposed to tension-type) might be alleviated by a medication regimen [50–52] (see Section 5). On the other hand, for patients who present with chronic, daily headaches (or headaches that occur and persist more than 50% of the time) separation into "tension-type headaches" and "migraines" appears to be a less helpful distinction. For clinical signs that may require further workup of headache, see Table 1.

Medication overuse headaches (MOH) are not uncommon among pediatric patients with chronic headaches and usually occur when patients are taking analgesics (including acetaminophen, non-steroidal anti-inflammatory drugs (NSAIDs), or opioids), triptans, and/or ergotamine for more than 10–15 days/month (depending on medication class) [53–55]. Effective treatment requires a rapid discontinuation of medication [56]. In a case study of children and adolescents with daily or almost-daily headache concomitant with daily or almost-daily analgesic intake, Hering-Hanit et al. reported that a successful wean from analgesics was achieved without hospitalization or significant interference with daily life, and resulted in complete cessation of chronic daily headache in 25 of 26 patients [57].

Table 1. Headache warning signals requiring further workup, including neuroimaging.

- Focal or abnormal neurological signs, ataxia
- Papilledema (including rule out pseudotumor cerebri)
- Age < 3 years
- "Worst headache of my life"
- Progressive worsening headaches
- Ventriculoperitoneal-shunt
- Neurocutaneous syndrome
- Immunocompromised → Cerebrospinal fluid? (check with Infectious disease, oncology or transplant clinician)

Rule out: carbon monoxide toxicity; Obstructive sleep apnea.

3.2. Centrally Mediated Abdominal Pain Syndrome

In the 2016 revision of the Rome Criteria (now in its 4th iteration), the term "functional abdominal pain" has been replaced by "centrally mediated abdominal pain syndrome" (CAPS), which occurs as a result of central sensitization with disinhibition of pain signals, rather than increased peripheral afferent excitability [58]. For example, when compared to healthy peers, pre-adolescent girls with irritable bowel syndrome display impaired endogenous inhibition of somatic pain [59]. Adolescents with irritable bowel syndrome (IBS) symptoms are also more likely to experience widespread hyperalgesia [60]. CAPS in childhood and adolescence increases the risk for chronic primary pain disorder (abdominal pain, migraine/tension headache, and chronic musculoskeletal pain) in adulthood [61,62], and women with a pediatric history of functional abdominal pain display long-term vulnerability to pain [63]. For clinical warning signs that may require further workup of abdominal pain, see Table 2.

Table 2. Abdominal pain warning signals requiring further workup.

- Persistent right upper or right lower quadrant pain
- Pain that wakes child from sleep
- Dysphagia
- Arthritis
- Persistent vomiting
- Perirectal disease
- Gastrointestinal blood loss
- Involuntary weight loss
- Nocturnal diarrhea
- Deceleration of linear growth
- Unexplained fever

3.3. Musculoskeletal and Joint Pain

A systematic review by King et al. [2] reported that back pain is common in children and adolescents, with one-month prevalence rates ranging from 18% to 24% in samples of English and Swedish children [64,65]. Weekly or "at least weekly" back pain was reported in 9%–25% of patients [3,64,66].

Stanford et al. have shown that parent- and youth-reported anxiety/depression were predictive of start and end points of back pain trajectories [3]. Four studies reported a 9%–39% prevalence of musculoskeletal and/or limb pain in 3842 children and adolescents, depending on time period of reporting [67–70]. The relation between musculoskeletal/limb pain and athletic participation confounds findings in this area, as many participants reported that their pain was the result of a sports injury. The majority of the studies reported that musculoskeletal pain is more common in girls than in boys [2].

Diagnostic criteria for "fibromyalgia" are not validated in children and teenagers, and the term "widespread musculoskeletal pain" is more commonly used instead. For clinical warning signs that may require further workup in children presenting with musculoskeletal and/or joint pain, see Table 3.

Table 3. Musculoskeletal/joint pain warning signals requiring further workup.

- Arthralgia: Rubor, calor, edema
- Pain/stiffness in the morning
- Abnormal radiographic findings
- Pain at rest, relieved by activity
- Pain at night: Worsened by massage, analgesics ineffective
- Bony tenderness
- Poor growth
- Weight loss
- Abnormal blood results: Including complete blood count (CBC), C-reactive protein (CRP), erythrocyte sedimentation rate (ESR)

3.4. Orthostatic Dysfunction as Part of the Chronic Pain Picture: From "POTS" and "Autonomic Dysfunction", to "Chronic Lyme Disease"

During initial intake, more than 50% of our chronic pain patients reveal in their medical history that they experienced episodes of enigmatic symptoms of dizziness, fatigue, low energy, blurry vision, "blacking out," and/or tachycardia, which we usually interpret as a result of deconditioning; these symptoms are frequently exacerbated by anxiety. We nearly always see this as a result of fear of pain and deconditioning, and not as a unifying diagnosis of a medical condition.

In short, like the vast majority of pediatric pain centers, we do not support the notion that "post-orthostatic tachycardia syndrome" (POTS), "autonomic dysfunction," and/or "chronic Lyme disease" (i.e., diagnosis of persistent infection with *Borrelia burgdorferi* despite negative titers calling for long-term antibiotic treatment) [71] are either the underlying pathophysiology or a significant contributor of a primary pain disorder. In fact, in nearly all of our patients, the clinical symptoms of orthostatic dysfunction and other co-existing, enigmatic symptoms (following a reasonable negative workup) disappear during our rehabilitative pain program.

3.5. Conversion Disorder

An estimated 5%–10% of patients referred to our pain clinic display clinical signs of a conversion disorder, either singularly or more commonly in conjunction with a primary pain disorder. Conversion disorder is a condition, in which the patient may present with numbness, paralysis, blindness, inability to speak, and/or other neurologic symptoms that cannot be explained by medical evaluation and for which diagnostic testing does not reveal any physical cause [72,73]. Often, the patient presents with a debilitating symptom that begins suddenly, has a history of a psychological problem(s) that gets better after the symptom appears, and shows lack of concern that would usually occur with symptoms of such severity (e.g., a 12-year-old boy seen in our clinic who was not concerned by the fact that he could not bear any weight on his limb and had been in a wheelchair for eight months).

3.6. Children with Acute and Chronic Pain: Co-Existing Pain Entities Requiring Advanced Treatment Strategies

Primary pain disorders also co-exist, or can even be triggered by underlying organic disease, and pain symptoms do not necessarily represent inadequate treatment, flare-up, or recurrence. As previously mentioned, approximately 5% of children and teenagers in the general population have significant pain-related dysfunction [2]. As a result, we can expect that at least the same percentage of children with recurrent painful episodes, such as that occurring in sickle cell disease, inflammatory bowel disease, rheumatoid arthritis, congenital heart disease, or cancer, will display chronic pain features in addition (i.e., co-existance) to their underlying somatic pain episodes, and that pain is not necessarily caused by the organic disease itself.

The realization that a significant number of children with recurrent organic painful episodes whose pain proves to be complicated to treat, have what is known as "chronic-on-acute" disease, which may be potentially complicated even further by neuropathic and/or psycho-social-spiritual pain. Such pain is important, and we believe it has beneficial, clinical implications. Namely, it reduces over-investigation of the underlying organic disease, and over-treatment of pain (e.g., inappropriate long-term opioid administration). Clearly, repeated acute pain episodes increase the risk of significant pain-related dysfunction. For instance, chronic pain is significantly higher in survivors of childhood cancer than in their healthy siblings [74]. Chronic post-surgical pain (CPSP), potentially a transition from acute to chronic pain, has recently been described to occur in 12%–22% of children [75–77], and is possibly associated with parental catastrophizing [78].

In practical terms, for treatment of acute tissue injuries (such as new vaso-occlusive sickle cell disease or a flare-up of Crohn's disease with bloody diarrhea), short-term administration of opioids titrated to effect are in fact usually required for adequate analgesia as part of an advanced multimodal analgesic strategy [79,80]. However, as discussed below (in Section 5.3), in patients with chronic daily sickle-cell pain or chronic daily abdominal pain due to Crohn's disease that is in clinical remission, long-term daily administration of opioids would not be indicated.

4. Interdisciplinary Rehabilitative Pediatric Pain Program: Our Approach

Since 2006, our interdisciplinary rehabilitative pain clinic at Children's Hospitals and Clinics of Minnesota in Minneapolis, MN, USA, has been dedicated to the care of children and teenagers in pain. A multidisciplinary bio-psycho-social rehabilitation and functional restoration approach has been shown to effectively and efficiently improve function both in adults [81] and children/teenagers [82–86]. However, it remains unclear how long we can wait to send a child to a pain program, and it is also unknown at what point clinical deterioration begins. Adult meta-data show that wait times for chronic pain treatment of six months or longer are medically unacceptable and result in significant decreases in both health-related quality of life and psychological well-being [87]. Two-thirds of USA pediatricians felt it was not their primary responsibility to treat chronic pain [88]. The Pediatric Pain Screening Tool (PPST) was recently validated to assist clinicians stratifying their pediatric pain patients to appropriate interventions [89].

The three most commonly seen manifestations of a primary pain disorder in our pain clinic are (1) primary headache (tension headaches/migraines); (2) centrally mediated abdominal pain syndrome; and (3) chronic and recurrent musculoskeletal/joint pain, with the majority of patients having at least two of those symptoms. The frequency of these conditions is followed closely by the prevalence of Complex regional pain syndrome (CRPS) Type 1, with 11% of our patients presenting with this condition (See Table 6).

Consistent with the treatment approach of the majority of pediatric pain clinics in the USA and Canada [90], our clinic offers an interdisciplinary rehabilitative approach aiming at returning to normal function.

4.1. From Clinic Intake to the Exit Interview

In our clinic, children whose daily functioning is disrupted due to pain (e.g., are missing school, displaying poor sleep, withdrawing from social life and/or having been assessed with anxiety or depression) will be offered a 90-minute multidisciplinary intake (in the same room at the same time) with the patient/parents and a physical therapist, psychologist, social worker/family therapist and a pain physician or advanced nurse practitioner. Following this, the patient undergoes three individual evaluations: clinical examination, a physical therapy evaluation, and a psychological evaluation. Parents/caregivers meet separately with the social worker/family therapist for an evaluation of family factors that may impact the child's pain, including beliefs about pain and response to pain. Afterwards, the clinical team meets to discuss findings and suggest recommendations, while the family is given a short rest period/hiatus. Following the clinical team meeting, either the MD or NP meets with the patient and his or her family for a 60-minute exit interview to present and explain recommendations and treatment plan.

We found it most effective for a child with a primary pain disorder to return to normal function first, and as a result of such functional reintegration, to then subsequently focus upon decreasing pain subsequently. During the exit interview we reveal that we believe the child's pain to be "real," and establish the expectation that as a first step we work toward "life gets back to normal," and then as a result—"the pain gets better"—and not the other way around. For patients with a primary pain disorder, we set the expectation of becoming pain-free or mostly pain-free. We have found that this positive expectation represents something of a self-fulfilling prophecy, and data support that expectations predict chronic pain treatment outcomes [91]. In our clinic, only 16% of children at intake reported that they believed they could ever be pain-free. Upon exit interview at the end of the first visit, which represents the first formal intervention, 92% of children expressed the belief that they could, in fact, become pain-free.

We put great importance on demystifying the problem: pain has lost its warning signal, and using the affected body part does not result in greater harm. During the exit interview, we explain in age-appropriate language how the pain "is real," but "has lost its warning function". Using drawings on a flip-chart and age-appropriate examples, we then go into greater detail about the concept of pain transmission and important modalities to down-modulate pain (so-called "OFF-Switch" modulation) through activation of descending inhibiting pathways (DIP) from the "control-center" periaqueductal grey (PAG), which are engaged by (1) physical therapy/exercise and (2) integrative medicine/distraction. We also discuss up-regulation (so called "ON-switch" activation induced by the prefrontal cortex which worsens pain through stress, negative mood, anxiety, depression, school absenteeism, social withdrawal, insomnia, etc.) and which is mitigated by (3) psychological counseling; and (4) normalizing activities of daily life. We then discuss the need to target both shutting off the "ON-switch" and turning on the "OFF-switch" at the same time, explaining why all four modalities are offered concurrently in our clinic, and why these modalities might not have worked in the past, if and when administered separately.

4.2. Rehabilitative Pain Program Modalities

In order to enroll in our rehabilitative pain program, we expect children and their parents to participate in all (i.e., not just some) of the following five modalities.

4.2.1. Physical Therapy

Physical therapy and exercise are key modalities in the treatment of pediatric patients with primary pain disorder and/or CRPS [82,84–86,92–95]. Adolescents with chronic pain usually have a lower physical activity level [96] and physical activity has been shown to reduce the risk for depression in female adolescents [97]. In children and adolescents participating in a rehabilitative pain program, the rate of improvement in function was significantly more rapid than the decrease in pain [92].

In our clinic, a physical therapist (PT) facilitates restoration of movement and the reduction of pain. PTs develop an individualized treatment plan that is based on each patient's functional goals (e.g., returning to a sport or age-appropriate play activity). PTs who work with children with chronic pain utilize traditional therapeutic techniques (e.g., normalizing lost range of motion, strength, balance, etc.) along with more pain-specific interventions (e.g., graded motor imagery [98], pain-physiology education, etc.). The majority of chronic pain patients entering our clinic are found to be de-conditioned upon physical therapy evaluation. Clinically, many of our chronic pain patients place a high value on athletics, with the majority of patients participating in some form of sport. If pain disrupts physical activity, it likely also impacts patients' coping strategies as well as their socialization. Reasons we assert to be important to refer pediatric/adolescent pain patients to physical therapy are provided in Table 4.

The treatment goal we establish for and with our patients is to first return to function, and then to secondarily attempt to decrease pain as a result of this functional restoration.

The initial assessment goals include determining if any neuro-musculoskeletal factors contribute to pain, if any, and defining the patient's movement goals. Treatment goals are aimed at normalizing a patient's environmental interactions and engagements, and addressing and mitigating those neuro-musculoskeletal variables contributing to pain.

Table 4. Reasons to refer a pediatric chronic pain patient to physical therapy.

- Goals of returning to sport or activities
- Not participating in gym class
- Signs of weakness, poor balance, poor endurance, abnormal movement patterns, or poor posture, etc.
- Diagnoses associated with abnormal movement patterns or weakness: e.g., Ehlers–Danlos syndrome, complex regional pain syndrome (CRPS), centrally mediated abdominal pain syndrome (CAPS), chronic musculoskeletal pain, chronic headaches, etc.

4.2.2. Integrative Medicine: Active Mind-Body Techniques

Integrative modalities (sometimes referred to as complementary and alternative medicine) that have been described as effective in the management of pediatric pain include hypnosis, yoga, acupuncture, and massage [99–107]. Active mind-body techniques, such as guided imagery, hypnosis, biofeedback, yoga, and distraction each and all evoke pain modulation by engaging a number of mechanisms within the analgesic neuraxis. Techniques such as distraction and guided imagery appear to modulate the release of endogenous opioids from the periaqueductal and periventricular grey regions to disinhibit descending inhibitory pathways of the brainstem to suppress pain transmission in the dorsal horn of the spinal cord [108–112]. As well, distraction has been shown to increase activity of the orbitofrontal and perigenual anterior cingulate cortex, as well as periaqueductal grey and the posterior thalamus to modulate pain at the supraspinal level [113,114].

In our clinic, integrative and active mind-body techniques are taught to patients, or to the parents, when children are younger than school age, or cognitively impaired. Mind-body techniques focus on intervention strategies that integrate cognitive and emotional processes with physiological functions and experience in order to promote health. We expect all our patients (who are older than five years, and cognitively capable) to learn at least one active integrative medicine technique and incorporate this into their daily routine. Parents are offered training in the same techniques so that they can be aware of what their child is learning, and can reinforce practice as needed. We also expect our patients to learn in our clinic and practice daily at home or school at least one age-appropriate mind-body technique of relaxation and self-regulation. Modalities our patients have reported to be helpful include breathing strategies (e.g., diaphragmatic breathing, square breathing, and "snake"/slow exhale breathing), aromatherapy, biofeedback, progressive muscle relaxation, autogenic training, mindfulness, yoga, and/or self-hypnosis. In addition, we support and offer passive integrative modalities such as acupressure, acupuncture, and/or massage (as supplemental to, but not in place of, self-directed techniques).

4.2.3. Psychological Intervention

Anxiety, depressive, and behavioral disorders are early risk factors of chronic pain (rather than vice versa) [115]. At low levels of anxiety, higher pain is predictive of greater disability; however, highly anxious adolescents tend to function poorly regardless of level of pain [116]. Psychological treatments significantly reduce pain intensity that is reported by children and adolescents with headache, abdominal pain, and musculoskeletal/joint pain [117,118]. Cognitive behavioral therapy (CBT) led to significant improvements in pain coping, catastrophizing, and efficacy that were sustained over time in adolescents with chronic pain [119]. CBT has been shown to increase grey matter in the prefrontal cortex of patients with chronic pain, and this increase in prefrontal cortical grey matter has been associated with reduced pain catastrophizing [120].

In our clinic, psychological intervention is a routine part of our treatment approach, and serves to teach patients general coping skills and integrative medicine strategies, as well as help incorporate these into a daily routine to promote consistent practice, and to promote normalization of a patient's daily life. Most patients in our clinic experience psychological distress due to disrupted functioning, as secondary to pain, and not as a primary presenting concern. As such, our psychologists' role is to promote restoration of baseline functioning by teaching appropriate coping strategies and by targeting pain-related fears and catastrophizing that may disrupt normal cognitive and behavioral functions.

4.2.4. Normalizing Life: "The 4 S's": Sports, Social, Sleep and School

As previously discussed, we explain to our patients that "first your life gets back to normal, then your pain decreases—unfortunately it's not the other way around." We go on to explain "sometimes, pain may even increase, before it gets better." We explain that the "4 S's": sports, socialization, sleep and school need to return to normal parameters before pain resolution could or should be expected.

- Sports: As mentioned in the previous section addressing physical therapy, we place strong emphasis on restoring activity and returning patients to their normal regimen of physical activity, exercise and/or sports.
- Social: When adolescents with chronic pain do not perceive their friends as providing support, they tend to avoid social situations [121]. The social lives of the chronic pain patients in our clinic are commonly disrupted for a variety of reasons, including inability to keep up with peers, disruptions to sports/extra-curricular activities where social contacts occur, experience or fear of being teased because of pain ("you are faking it") or disability. In our clinic, the family therapist and psychologist work with the patient and his or her family to develop strategies and tactics to regain a balanced social life, provide validation of feeling misunderstood, and continuous medical reassurance that pain is physiologically mediated or "real".
- Sleep: The majority of children with chronic pain have sleep difficulties, including problems with sleep initiation, sleep maintenance, and/or early morning awakening [122]. These sleep problems tend to be persistent and are associated with negative impact for youths with chronic pain [123]. Treatment of insomnia in youths with chronic pain may lead to improvements in quality of life and reduction in healthcare cost. In our practice, the majority of patients' parents are successfully coached to assist their children in waking in the morning, having breakfast, attending to personal hygiene, and leaving the house in time to attend the first class at school. We encourage a "no nap" policy, and allow patients to "sleep in" one to two hours later (but no longer) on weekends. We expect that illuminated screens (e.g., television, computer monitors, smart phones, tablets, etc.) will not be used starting one hour before bedtime (or after bedtime), as studies have shown that the blue light emitted by such screens can interfere with melatonin production and/or release [124,125].

- School: Parental catastrophizing and protective responses to their child's pain predict school attendance rates and overall school performance [126]. Long-term scholastic impairment results in reduced occupational achievement, increased educational costs, and increased risk of developing psychiatric disorders (e.g., anxiety, depression) [127–129]. In our clinic, the child's social worker and psychologist work closely with the patient, parent, and school (if and when permission is granted) to develop a personalized school re-entry plan. Factors considered in developing a re-entry plan include possible learning concerns, stigmatization, teasing and/or bullying by peers, and secondary gain/special attention due to pain and/or disability behavior(s). We have found that with close communication, most schools are supportive of having students take time-limited breaks to practice integrative medicine strategies before returning to the classroom. We typically work with schools for informal accommodations, instead of pursuing an Individualized Education Plan (IEP) or a 504 plan (Section 504 of the USA Rehabilitation Act was developed to guarantee that a child with a disability as identified under the law who is attending an elementary or secondary educational institution will receive accommodations that insure equal capacity to access the learning environment and achieve academic success) to underscore our expectation that the student will return to baseline functioning without accommodation(s).

Parents are asked if they can consistently and successfully get their child/teenager to school regardless of the patient's report of their inability to go (due to chronic pain). The social worker helps the parent to develop a plan to insure their child's school attendance, inclusive of conjoining other family members to such tasks, if and as necessary to assist parents.

We usually do not support online school or home schooling for children who have attended a physical facility school prior to their pain.

4.2.5. Parent Coaching

Children with chronic pain often have a negative influence in and upon their family life, can pose a financial burden, both in direct and indirect costs incurred from healthcare utilization and lost wages due to parents taking time off work to care for the child, and the child in pain can exert considerable emotional toll on family members. Families of children with chronic pain generally have poorer family functioning, and pain-related disability is more consistently related to family functioning than pain intensity [130]. Studies have shown that mothers of children with chronic abdominal pain show pain bias when interpreting ambiguous emotional expressions, and such bias might possibly contribute to parenting behaviors that maintain or enhance the child's pain [131]. Children of parents with chronic pain have been shown to display poorer outcomes in health, as well as psychological and familial functioning [132], and show increased risk of developing anxiety and depression as teenagers [133].

Parents in our clinic tend to be hypervigilant and pay increased attention to their children's pain reports/behaviors, given that they commonly are asked to report on pain specifics and details during routine medical consults. As such, parents may accidentally reinforce their child's pain behaviors. It is our clinical experience that parents are often defensive about their role in (maintaining) their child's pain. Normalizing parental protectiveness is a helpful first step toward shifting parents' focus to attend to healthy, adaptive behaviors, and decreasing their attention to their child's pain behaviors. We often ask parents to focus on their child's functioning and ask about specific daily activities, instead of attending to pain-related disruptions of their child's functioning. Depending on the child's age and developmental level, we may encourage parents to actively model mind-body and integrative medicine strategies to help their child engage in active and appropriate coping.

Parents' experiences of/with chronic pain and disability can influence their children's pain beliefs and behaviors. Parents' pain experiences are openly addressed and discussed with both the child and parent(s). The social worker discusses how the patient's pain is different from the parent's disability and pain, and the expectation that the child can become pain-free. The message we seek to communicate is that there is no reason to believe that they will be disabled like their parent.

Parents are often taught some of the same skills that are taught to their child/teenager by the psychologist. The social worker does this in order to teach the parents how to calm themselves when their child is having a pain flare. The parent is encouraged to use such skills to avoid incurring emotional escalations when dealing with their child. We believe that the parent is in an ideal position to emotionally anchor their child and support the use of calming skills to reduce pain levels. It is also important to teach parents to gently remind their child that normalization of daily functioning must come first before pain starts to decrease, and that progress is measured initially by the patient's return to a normalized daily life for sports, social life, sleep and school. Indeed it is easy for both the patient and parent to lose sight of this when the child continues to experience and present with pain. While active engagement of the parent(s) is advocated when working with younger children, a different approach is used when the patient is a teenager. Teenagers are taught and encouraged to acquire, develop and employ such skills more independently, and to foster greater capabilities for independence in activities of daily living. It has been our experience that parents are usually motivated to change any maladaptive or deleterious behavior. Clearly, they are very distressed by both seeing their child in pain and not knowing how to help them. The skills provided by our approach give the parent focus and a set of tasks, which can reduce their sense of helplessness and decrease their catastrophizing, while concomitantly helping their child.

5. Medications

In our pediatric pain practice we commonly find medications as a sole therapy for primary pain disorders to be ineffective, especially if they are not accompanied by the aforementioned modalities of our rehabilitative pain program. Still, it is important to consider the validity and value of pharmacological interventions as part of an integrative approach to pediatric pain care. In this regards some pharmacological considerations are included below.

5.1. Basic Analgesics: Acetaminophen and Ibuprofen

For mild, acute pain (i.e., associated with tissue injury), acetaminophen and ibuprofen are the agents of choice [80]. No other NSAID has been sufficiently studied for efficacy and safety in the pediatric population so as to be recommended as an alternative to ibuprofen. Although there is evidence for the superior analgesic properties of ibuprofen versus acetaminophen, it is considered to be of limited value because the studies were mostly performed in acute pain settings and lack long-term safety data. Both acetaminophen and ibuprofen have potential toxicities. There are concerns about renal and gastrointestinal toxicity, and bleeding with ibuprofen and other NSAIDs, and risks of hepatotoxicity and acute overdose are associated with acetaminophen [80]. Celecoxib (a cyclooxygenase-2 (COX-2) enzyme inhibitor) might be considered, if classical NSAIDs are contraindicated (e.g., owing to bleeding risks, or gastrointestinal side effects). Celecoxib does not display less renal toxicity as compared to classic NSAIDs. Safety and efficacy have been established only in children two years of age or older with juvenile rheumatoid arthritis, and for a maximum of six months of treatment.

With the exception of ibuprofen's proven efficacy in reducing pain at the onset of a migraine episode [50–52], basic analgesics generally are not used to treat primary pain disorders in the absence of new tissue injury. As discussed earlier, daily use of analgesics in headache patients incurs significant risk of leading to medication overuse headaches ("rebound headaches").

Fast-Acting NSAID: Ibuprofen-Sodium

Data have shown that when compared to ibuprofen, ibuprofen-sodium produced significantly greater analgesia over 6 h, and required fewer re-medications than standard formulations [134]. In addition, 200 mg fast-acting ibuprofen (Numbers-needed-to-treat (NNT) 2.1; 95% confidence interval (CI) 1.9–2.4) was as effective as 400 mg standard ibuprofen (NNT 2.4; 95% CI 2.2–2.5), and produced a faster onset of analgesia. Meta-analysis showed that NSAID-salts display more rapid absorption, faster initial pain reduction, good overall analgesia in more patients at the same dose, and probably evoke longer-lasting analgesia, without reports of adverse events [135]. For example, in our practice, we suggest fast-acting ibuprofen plus acetaminophen as a first step, followed by a triptan, if ineffective, be utilized within 10 min of onset of a migraine attack. In the USA, ibuprofen-sodium is available over the counter for about $8–$10 for 80 tablets (containing 266 mg of ibuprofen sodium, which is the equivalent to 200 mg of standard ibuprofen).

5.2. Opioids

The Center for Disease Control and Prevention's recently published 2016 Guidelines for Prescribing Opioids for Chronic Pain [136] do not apply to children and teenagers [137] and encompass only "patients aged ≥18 years with chronic pain outside of palliative and end-of-life care." The guidelines state further that the "recommendations do not address the use of opioid pain medication in children or adolescents aged <18 years".

Opioids administered for primary pain disorders have low long-term efficacy, a poor safety profile, and commonly a worse clinical outcome [133–139]. Thus, opioids should not be administered to pediatric patients with primary pain disorders [43], i.e., chronic pain defined that extends beyond the expected time of healing and hence lacks the acute warning function of physiological nociception. Opioids may be more likely to cause more harm than benefit in the treatment of primary pain disorders, which include conditions such as tension-type/migraines headaches, chronic musculoskeletal pain, "chronic sickle cell pain" (pain that extends beyond the expected time of acute vaso-occlusive crisis) and centrally mediated abdominal pain syndrome. In our practice, we do not prescribe opioids for primary pain disorders in children or teenagers, as we consider them to be contraindicated. On the other hand, in persistent pain conditions (i.e., long-lasting and/or repetitive nociceptive pain caused by tissue injury, such as in children with junctional epidermolysis bullosa, osteogenesis imperfecta, or advanced metastasized bone tumors (e.g., Ewing sarcoma)) opioids are important and effective for long-term analgesic management.

5.3. Adjuvant Analgesics

Adjuvant analgesics (e.g., low-dose tricyclic antidepressants, gabapentinoids, α-agonists, melatonin, etc.) may serve as valuable adjuncts. Although commonly used for primary pain disorders, there is little evidence to support their use against pediatric pain. Most pediatric data for this heterogeneous class of medications is derived from neuropathic and acute pain conditions [138–144]. The most commonly prescribed adjuvant analgesics in our pain clinic are melatonin, lidocaine 5% patch, gabapentin, and low-dose amitriptyline (See Table 5).

For migraines, only ibuprofen and triptans are supported by sufficient evidence to engender use in pediatrics [50–52]. Medication to treat migraines in adolescents have a strong placebo effect, with pain relief at 2 h in the placebo arms of seven randomized controlled trials ranging from 53% to 57.5%. A meta-analysis of 21 randomized controlled trials (RCTs) of pediatric headache management [145] revealed that placebo decreased headache frequency from 5.6 to 2.9 headaches/month, and also most commonly used drugs had little to no evidence to support their use in children and adolescents. Drugs shown to be ineffective included clonidine, flunarizine, pizotifen, propranolol, valproate, and fluoxetine [145].

Table 5. Adjuvant analgesics used in pediatric pain management (Pain Medicine and Palliative Care, Children's Hospitals and Clinics of Minnesota) [79].

Class	Medication	Dose	Route of Administration	Comments/Side Effects (See Text for Further Details)
Tricyclic Antidepressants (TCA)	**Amitriptyline**	Starting dose 0.1 mg/kg QHS, usually slowly titrated up to 0.5 mg/kg (max. 20-25 mg)	PO	Tertiary amine TCA; stronger anticholinergic side effects (including sedation) than nortriptyline
	Nortriptyline	Starting dose 0.1 mg/kg QHS, usually titrated up to 0.5 mg/kg (max. 20-25 mg)	PO	Secondary amine TCA; anticholinergic side effects
Gabapentenoids	**Gabapentin**	Starting dose 2 mg/kg QHS, usually slowly titrated up to initial target dose of 6 mg/kg/dose TID (max. 300 mg/dose TID). Max. dose escalation to 24 mg/kg/dose TID (max. 1200 mg/dose TID)	PO	Slow dose increase required; side effects: ataxia, nystagmus, myalgia, hallucination, dizziness, somnolence, aggressive behaviors, hyperactivity, thought disorder, peripheral edema
	Pregabaline	Starting dose 0.3 mg/kg QHS, usually slowly titrated up to initial target dose of 1.5 mg/kg/dose BID (max. 75 mg/dose BID). Max. dose escalation to 6 mg/kg/dose BID (max. 300 mg/dose BID)	PO	Switch from gabapentin, if distressing side effects or inadequate analgesia. Side effects: ataxia, nystagmus, myalgia, hallucination, dizziness, somnolence, aggressive behaviors, hyperactivity, thought disorder, peripheral edema; Associated with weight gain
Sodium Channel Blocker/Local anesthetic	**Lidocaine 5%**	Max. of 4 patches (in patients > 50 kg) 12 h on/12 h off	Transdermal patch	Not for severe hepatic dysfunction
Alpha-Agonist	**Clonidine**	1–3 mcg/kg QHS to Q6h	PO/transdermal	
	Dexmedetomidine	Infusion: 0.3 mcg/kg/h; titrate to max. 2 mcg/kg/h	IV	
Hormone	**Melatonin**	0.06–0.2 mg/kg (max. 3–10 mg) QHS	PO	Sleep induction, use extended-release, if interrupted sleep, possible analgesic effect

QHS: every night at bedtime; PO: per os, oral administration; IV: intravenous administration; BID: bis in die, twice a day; TID: ter in die, three times a day; Q6h: every 6h.

5.4. Selective Serotonin Re-Uptake Inhibitors (SSRI)/Serotonin and Norepinephrine Reuptake Inhibitors (SNRI)

There is little evidence to support the use of SSRIs or SNRIs in children/teenagers with primary pain disorders. An over-quoted, uncontrolled open-label case series for example has claimed that 21 of 25 children with recurrent abdominal pain improved following SSRI treatment [146]. However, placebo effects were large with pediatric antidepressant trials in other settings, regression to the mean must be expected, and there might be inherent bias at play. Efficacy studies for duloxetine in pediatric pain patients are lacking. In our clinic practice, we add an SSRI (such as citalopram, sertraline, escitalopram) in addition to (not in substitution for) individual psychotherapy to the treatment regimen of some patients who present with an underlying mental health diagnosis of anxiety and/or depression.

5.5. Laxatives

Constipation is the most common diagnosis in children presenting with abdominal pain in the emergency room [147], and in our practice, we see a surprisingly large number of children with long-standing abdominal pain, who have constipation and/or overflow diarrhea despite having been seen by many clinicians and reports that they have tried many laxatives. In our practice, we nearly always employ a scheduled (not "as needed" or pro re nate "prn")) regimen of (1) "Mush" (stool softener such as lactulose or polyethylenglycol 3350); (2) "Push" (stimulant such as senna) and (3) "Uncorking" (glycerin suppository for children <4 years, and bisodacyl suppository for older children) if no stool has been evacuated in the previous 24 h. This regimen has proven to be highly effective in resolving constipation, thereby decreasing or resolving abdominal pain [148].

5.6. Multimodal ("Opioid-Sparing") Analgesia

Multimodal analgesia is an approach used to prevent and treat pain in children: multiple agents, interventions, rehabilitation, and psychological and integrative therapies often act synergistically to elicit more effective pediatric pain control with fewer side effects than a single analgesic or modality [149]. Multimodal analgesic therapy (versus opioids alone) has been shown to reduce the length of hospitalization in patients undergoing surgery [150].

Evidence-based, safe multimodal (i.e., opioid-sparing) analgesia may include one, several or all of the following approaches: pharmacology (e.g., simple analgesia and/or opioids and/or adjuvant analgesia), anesthetic interventions (e.g., neuroaxial analgesia, nerve blocks), rehabilitation (e.g., physical therapy, occupational therapy, sleep hygiene), psychological counseling (e.g., cognitive behavioral therapy), and age-appropriate positioning and integrative (non-pharmacological) therapies, such as breathing techniques, self-hypnosis, and distraction.

6. From Mechanism and Classifications to Practice: Obligations for Care

Taken together, the use of these approaches has been shown to be highly effective in treating primary pain disorder in our clinical experience. Our approach is based and built upon a growing body of information that is both revising extant concepts of pain and pain modulation, and exploring new approaches to the assessment and treatment of pain. To be sure, new insights and perspectives about mechanisms and categorizations of pain in general, and pediatric pain in particular, are indubitably important to provide better understanding of pathology and more precise nosology [151,152]. Large-scale initiatives, such as the ongoing, federally directed Brain Research through Advancing Innovative Neurotechnologies (BRAIN) [153], and precision medicine initiatives, are developing more finely grained approaches to research, which seek to better define the neurobiology and psychosocial aspects of pediatric pain. Such knowledge must be appreciated and employed for its practical utility toward improving diagnosis and treatment of the pain patient [154].

As we have stated previously, and reaffirm here: " ... we ... study pain so that we may unravel its mysteries and develop more and better ways of relieving pain...to restore and sustain ... living a life unencumbered by suffering" [155]. Understanding the bio-psychosocial dimensions of pain—as symptom, pathology and manifest illness—compels providing a more comprehensive and integrative approach to both assessment and treatment [156,157]. Such an approach entails the coordinated use of multiple disciplines, and engages both "high tech" and "low tech" means [158]. This enables both a more thorough evaluation of each patient's needs (in physiological, psychological and social dimensions), and more personalized, evidence-based intervention(s) to lessen or eradicate pain, and its manifest effects.

7. From Concepts to Practice: Our Experience at a Glimpse

Our interdisciplinary, rehabilitative pediatric pain clinic at Children's Minnesota has been seeing pediatric patients since 2006. Based on a 2007–2009 three-year prospective study (n = 145) and two chart reviews (2010 and 2014, n = 135) by Desai et al. [159,160] the majority (74%) of our new patients are female with an average age of 14 years (range ten-day-old infant to 17 years). The most common presenting conditions are listed in Table 6.

Table 6. Presenting or accompanying pain conditions: Initial intake at interdisciplinary pediatric pain clinic at Children's Minnesota.

- 74% Chronic or recurrent musculoskeletal pain
- 61% Primary headaches (tension-type/migraines)
- 38% CAPS
- 11% CRPS type I
- 26% Additional or accompanying underlying conditions, including

Avascular necrosis
Caffe's disease
Cerebral palsy/spasticity
Chiari-I-malformation with ventricular-peritoneal (VP) shunt
Chronic postsurgical pain
Conversion disorder
CRPS type 2
Erythromelalgi
Inflammatory bowel disease (Crohn's disease, ulcerative colitis)
Irritable bowel syndrome
Juvenile rheumatoid/idiopathic arthritis (JRA/JIA)
Malignancy
Muscular dystrophy
Penilodynia
Phantom limb pain
Progressive neurodegenerative/metabolic conditions incl. mitochondriopathies
Sickle cell disease
Vulvodynia

On average, our patients' pain began 2.4 years prior to intake and 57% of our patients had an immediate family member with chronic pain. On a pain scale 0–10, with 10 being the worst, our patients' average daily pain was rated 5.6/10 (worst: 8.8/10, least bad 3/10). A total of 75% of our pain patients also received a mental health diagnosis; 67% presented with anxiety (including general anxiety disorder, panic episodes, anxiety disorder not otherwise specified (NOS)), and 30% presented with depression (including major depression, and depressive disorder NOS) [160].

In reviewing our data from 2007 to 2009, 2010, and 2014, it appears that between 83% and 92% of new patients chose to follow-up with the rehabilitative treatment recommendations provided by our clinic after the initial intake. Of those, the majority (67%–79%) graduated successfully, (i.e., are pain-free or pain-free most of the time). Of the remaining, up to 26% were referred to additional and/or separate services (e.g., inpatient or outpatient psychiatry, eating disorder program, physical therapy/mental health provider closer to home) and of our most recent data review, 13% were still in treatment 6–12 months later [159]. The patients who successfully graduated had seen the physical therapist eight (mean; range 1–25) times, psychologist ten times (range 1–34), parents the family therapist/social four times (range 1–16), and the physician/nurse practitioner 2.5 times (range 1–7).

As previously noted, in our clinic at the first visit only 16% of children reported that they believed they could ever become pain-free. However, at the exit interview following the first visit, 92% of children asserted that they believed being pain-free was possible. The rehabilitative interdisciplinary treatment approach does not only seem to be effective for patients with primary pain disorders and CRPS, but also, in addition to other multimodal analgesia strategies, for the treatment of chronic-on-acute pain or chronic-on-neuropathic pain patients (see Section 3.6), indicating the significant overlap these conditions may have.

The work of our interdisciplinary team can be seen in a short movie, "Little Stars—Treating Chronic Pain in Children [161]."

8. Conclusions

Primary pain disorder (what was formerly known as "functional pain syndrome") is a common, under-diagnosed and under-treated condition in pediatric patients. Primary pain disorder occurs as a mechanistic vulnerability to multi-focal pain that can occur and be expressed at a number of bodily sites. Common symptoms of this underlying pain vulnerability include primary headache, centrally mediated abdominal pain syndrome, and chronic/recurrent musculoskeletal pain. A significant number of children with repeated acute nociceptive pain episodes develop chronic pain in addition to or as a result of their condition. Untreated chronic pediatric pain can increase the risk of pain, as well as physical and psychiatric disorders in adulthood. These findings reinforce the importance, if not obligation, to effectively address and treat pain in children and adolescents.

In our interdisciplinary pediatric pain management practice, we have shown that an integrative, multidisciplinary approach combining rehabilitation, complementary therapies (e.g., distraction, hypnosis, etc.), psychological counseling, and normalization of physical/sports activity, sleep, socialization, and school attendance—together with the prudent use of pharmacological agents—effectively mitigates and/or commonly resolves our patients' pain. Of note, however, is that opioids are not indicated for primary pain disorders, and other medications do not usually represent first-line therapy.

Further Resources for Clinicians and Patients

(1) Pediatric Pain Clinics in USA and Canada (American Pain Society): http://americanpainsociety.org/uploads/get-involved/PainClinicList_12_2015.pdf [162].
(2) Short Movie: Meet the Interdisciplinary Chronic Pain Clinic Team at Children's Minnesota: LittleStars TV https://www.youtube.com/watch?t=13&v=Bb1fHxfjdWI [161].
(3) Pain Bytes (Australia) [163].
(4) Persistent (Chronic) Pain 5-min video [164].
(5) Kiran Stordalen and Horst Rechelbacher Pediatric Pain, Palliative and Integrative Medicine Clinic Tour [165].
(6) Elliot Krane (TED-Talk) The mystery of chronic pain [166].
(7) The Department of Pain Medicine, Palliative Care, and Integrative Medicine, Children's Hospitals and Clinics of Minnesota [167].

Author Contributions: S.F. is primarily responsible for this review's conception, design and drafting of the text. All authors provided evaluation and revision of the manuscript, and have given final approval of the manuscript.

References

1. Goodman, J.E.; McGrath, P.J. The epidemiology of pain in children and adolescents: A review. *Pain* **1991**, *46*, 247–264. [CrossRef]
2. King, S.; Chambers, C.T.; Huguet, A.; MacNevin, R.C.; McGrath, P.J.; Parker, L.; MacDonald, A.J. The epidemiology of chronic pain in children and adolescents revisited: A systematic review. *Pain* **2011**, *152*, 2729–2738. [CrossRef] [PubMed]
3. Stanford, E.A.; Chambers, C.T.; Biesanz, J.C.; Chen, E. The frequency, trajectories and predictors of adolescent recurrent pain: A population-based approach. *Pain* **2008**, *138*, 11–21. [CrossRef] [PubMed]
4. Friedrichsdorf, S.J.; Postier, A.; Eull, D.; Weidner, C.; Foster, L.; Gilbert, M.; Campbell, F. Pain outcomes in a US children's hospital: A prospective cross-sectional survey. *Hosp. Pediatr.* **2015**, *5*, 18–26. [CrossRef] [PubMed]
5. Taylor, E.M.; Boyer, K.; Campbell, F.A. Pain in hospitalized children: A prospective cross-sectional survey of pain prevalence, intensity, assessment and management in a Canadian pediatric teaching hospital. *Pain Res. Manag.* **2008**, *13*, 25–32. [CrossRef] [PubMed]
6. Zhu, L.M.; Stinson, J.; Palozzi, L.; Weingarten, K.; Hogan, M.E.; Duong, S.; Carbajal, R.; Campbell, F.A.; Taddio, A. Improvements in pain outcomes in a Canadian pediatric teaching hospital following implementation of a multifaceted knowledge translation initiative. *Pain Res. Manag. J. Can. Pain Soc.* **2012**, *17*, 173–179. [CrossRef]
7. Stevens, B.J.; Harrison, D.; Rashotte, J.; Yamada, J.; Abbott, L.K.; Coburn, G.; Stinson, J.; Le May, S. Pain assessment and intensity in hospitalized children in canada. *J. Pain* **2012**, *13*, 857–865. [CrossRef] [PubMed]
8. Huguet, A.; Miro, J. The severity of chronic pediatric pain: An epidemiological study. *J. Pain* **2008**, *9*, 226–236. [CrossRef] [PubMed]
9. Hechler, T.; Dobe, M.; Zernikow, B. Commentary: A worldwide call for multimodal inpatient treatment for children and adolescents suffering from chronic pain and pain-related disability. *J. Pediatr. Psychol.* **2010**, *35*, 138–140. [CrossRef] [PubMed]
10. Groenewald, C.B.; Essner, B.S.; Wright, D.; Fesinmeyer, M.D.; Palermo, T.M. The economic costs of chronic pain among a cohort of treatment-seeking adolescents in the United States. *J. Pain* **2014**, *15*, 925–933. [CrossRef] [PubMed]
11. Hyams, J.S.; di Lorenzo, C.; Saps, M.; Shulman, R.J.; Staiano, A.; van Tilburg, M. Functional disorders: Children and adolescents. *Gastroenterology* **2016**. [CrossRef]
12. Turk, D.; Okifuji, A. Pain terms and taxonomies of pain. In *Bonica's Management of Pain*; Bonica, J., Loeser, J., Chapman, C., Turk, D., Butler, S., Eds.; Lippincott Williams & Wilkins: Philadelphia, PA, USA, 2001.
13. Treede, R.D.; Rief, W.; Barke, A.; Aziz, Q.; Bennett, M.I.; Benoliel, R.; Cohen, M.; Evers, S.; Finnerup, N.B.; First, M.B.; et al. A classification of chronic pain for ICD-11. *Pain* **2015**, *156*, 1003–1007. [CrossRef] [PubMed]
14. Force, A.P.S.P.C.P.T. Assessment and Management of Children with Chronic Pain. A Position Statement from the American Pain Society. Available online: http://americanpainsociety.org/uploads/get-involved/pediatric-chronic-pain-statement.pdf (accessed on 7 December 2016).
15. Woolf, C.J. Central sensitization: Implications for the diagnosis and treatment of pain. *Pain* **2011**, *152*, S2–S15. [CrossRef] [PubMed]
16. Special Issue "Chronic and Recurrent Pain". Available online: http://www.mdpi.com/journal/children/special_issues/chronic_pain (accessed on 7 December 2016).
17. Hassett, A.L.; Hilliard, P.E.; Goesling, J.; Clauw, D.J.; Harte, S.E.; Brummett, C.M. Reports of chronic pain in childhood and adolescence among patients at a tertiary care pain clinic. *J. Pain* **2013**, *14*, 1390–1397. [CrossRef] [PubMed]
18. Johannes, C.B.; Le, T.K.; Zhou, X.; Johnston, J.A.; Dworkin, R.H. The prevalence of chronic pain in United States adults: Results of an internet-based survey. *J. Pain* **2010**, *11*, 1230–1239. [CrossRef] [PubMed]

19. Hotopf, M.; Mayou, R.; Wadsworth, M.; Wessely, S. Psychosocial and developmental antecedents of chest pain in young adults. *Psychosom. Med.* **1999**, *61*, 861–867. [CrossRef] [PubMed]
20. Hotopf, M.; Carr, S.; Mayou, R.; Wadsworth, M.; Wessely, S. Why do children have chronic abdominal pain, and what happens to them when they grow up? Population based cohort study. *BMJ* **1998**, *316*, 1196–1200. [CrossRef] [PubMed]
21. Jones, G.T.; Silman, A.J.; Power, C.; Macfarlane, G.J. Are common symptoms in childhood associated with chronic widespread body pain in adulthood? Results from the 1958 British birth cohort study. *Arthritis Rheum.* **2007**, *56*, 1669–1675. [CrossRef] [PubMed]
22. Power, C.; Elliott, J. Cohort profile: 1958 British birth cohort (National Child Development Study). *Int. J. Epidemiol.* **2006**, *35*, 34–41. [CrossRef] [PubMed]
23. Mulvaney, S.; Lambert, E.W.; Garber, J.; Walker, L.S. Trajectories of symptoms and impairment for pediatric patients with functional abdominal pain: A 5-year longitudinal study. *J. Am. Acad. Child Adolesc. Psychiatry* **2006**, *45*, 737–744. [CrossRef] [PubMed]
24. Dunn, K.M.; Jordan, K.P.; Mancl, L.; Drangsholt, M.T.; Le Resche, L. Trajectories of pain in adolescents: A prospective cohort study. *Pain* **2011**, *152*, 66–73. [CrossRef] [PubMed]
25. Horst, S.; Shelby, G.; Anderson, J.; Acra, S.; Polk, D.B.; Saville, B.R.; Garber, J.; Walker, L.S. Predicting persistence of functional abdominal pain from childhood into young adulthood. *Clin. Gastroenterol. Hepatol.* **2014**, *12*, 2026–2032. [CrossRef] [PubMed]
26. Shelby, G.D.; Shirkey, K.C.; Sherman, A.L.; Beck, J.E.; Haman, K.; Shears, A.R.; Horst, S.N.; Smith, C.A.; Garber, J.; Walker, L.S. Functional abdominal pain in childhood and long-term vulnerability to anxiety disorders. *Pediatrics* **2013**, *132*, 475–482. [CrossRef] [PubMed]
27. Noel, M.; Groenewald, C.B.; Beals-Erickson, S.E.; Gebert, J.T.; Palermo, T.M. Chronic pain in adolescence and internalizing mental health disorders: A nationally representative study. *Pain* **2016**, *157*, 1333–1338. [CrossRef] [PubMed]
28. Van Tilburg, M.A.; Spence, N.J.; Whitehead, W.E.; Bangdiwala, S.; Goldston, D.B. Chronic pain in adolescents is associated with suicidal thoughts and behaviors. *J. Pain* **2011**, *12*, 1032–1039. [CrossRef] [PubMed]
29. Fisher, E.; Palermo, T.M. Goal pursuit in youth with chronic pain. *Children* **2016**, *3*, 36. [CrossRef] [PubMed]
30. Cunningham, N.R.; Lynch-Jordan, A.; Barnett, K.; Peugh, J.; Sil, S.; Goldschneider, K.; Kashikar-Zuck, S. Child pain catastrophizing mediates the relation between parent responses to pain and disability in youth with functional abdominal pain. *J. Pediatr. Gastroenterol. Nutr.* **2014**, *59*, 732–738. [CrossRef] [PubMed]
31. Lynch-Jordan, A.M.; Kashikar-Zuck, S.; Szabova, A.; Goldschneider, K.R. The interplay of parent and adolescent catastrophizing and its impact on adolescents' pain, functioning, and pain behavior. *Clin. J. Pain* **2013**, *29*, 681–688. [CrossRef] [PubMed]
32. Williams, S.E.; Blount, R.L.; Walker, L.S. Children's pain threat appraisal and catastrophizing moderate the impact of parent verbal behavior on children's symptom complaints. *J. Pediatr. Psychol.* **2011**, *36*, 55–63. [CrossRef] [PubMed]
33. Campbell, C.M.; Witmer, K.; Simango, M.; Carteret, A.; Loggia, M.L.; Campbell, J.N.; Haythornthwaite, J.A.; Edwards, R.R. Catastrophizing delays the analgesic effect of distraction. *Pain* **2010**, *149*, 202–207. [CrossRef] [PubMed]
34. Birnie, K.A.; Chambers, C.T.; Chorney, J.; Fernandez, C.V.; McGrath, P.J. Dyadic analysis of child and parent trait and state pain catastrophizing in the process of Children's Pain Communication. *Pain* **2016**, *157*, 938–948. [CrossRef] [PubMed]
35. Noel, M.; Rabbitts, J.A.; Tai, G.G.; Palermo, T.M. Remembering pain after surgery: A longitudinal examination of the role of pain catastrophizing in children's and parents' recall. *Pain* **2015**, *156*, 800–808. [CrossRef] [PubMed]
36. Simons, L.E.; Kaczynski, K.J.; Conroy, C.; Logan, D.E. Fear of pain in the context of intensive pain rehabilitation among children and adolescents with neuropathic pain: Associations with treatment response. *J. Pain* **2012**, *13*, 1151–1161. [CrossRef] [PubMed]
37. Zale, E.L.; Lange, K.L.; Fields, S.A.; Ditre, J.W. The relation between pain-related fear and disability: A meta-analysis. *J. Pain* **2013**, *14*, 1019–1030. [CrossRef] [PubMed]
38. Von Baeyer, C.L.; Champion, G.D. Commentary: Multiple pains as functional pain syndromes. *J. Pediatr. Psychol.* **2011**, *36*, 433–437. [CrossRef] [PubMed]

39. Kindler, L.L.; Bennett, R.M.; Jones, K.D. Central sensitivity syndromes: Mounting pathophysiologic evidence to link fibromyalgia with other common chronic pain disorders. *Pain Manag. Nurs.* **2011**, *12*, 15–24. [CrossRef] [PubMed]
40. Williams, F.M.; Spector, T.D.; MacGregor, A.J. Pain reporting at different body sites is explained by a single underlying genetic factor. *Rheumatology* **2010**, *49*, 1753–1755. [CrossRef] [PubMed]
41. Mayer, E.A.; Bushnell, M.C. *Functional Pain Syndromes: Presentation and Pathophysiology*; IASP Press: Seattle, WA, USA, 2009.
42. Burri, A.; Ogata, S.; Vehof, J.; Williams, F. Chronic widespread pain: Clinical comorbidities and psychological correlates. *Pain* **2015**, *156*, 1458–1464. [CrossRef] [PubMed]
43. Schechter, N.L. Functional pain: Time for a new name. *JAMA Pediatr.* **2014**, *168*, 693–694. [CrossRef] [PubMed]
44. McAbee, G.N.; Morse, A.M.; Assadi, M. Pediatric aspects of headache classification in the international classification of headache disorders-3 (ichd-3 beta version). *Curr. Pain Headache Rep.* **2016**, *20*, 7. [CrossRef] [PubMed]
45. Headache Classification Committee of the International Headache Society. The International Classification of Headache Disorders, 3rd Edition (Beta Version). *Cephalalgia Int. J. Headache* **2013**, *33*, 629–808.
46. Viswanathan, V.; Bridges, S.J.; Whitehouse, W.; Newton, R.W. Childhood headaches: Discrete entities or continuum? *Dev. Med. Child Neurol.* **1998**, *40*, 544–550. [CrossRef] [PubMed]
47. Zebenholzer, K.; Wober, C.; Kienbacher, C.; Wober-Bingol, C. Migrainous disorder and headache of the tension-type not fulfilling the criteria: A follow-up study in children and adolescents. *Cephalalgia Int. J. Headache* **2000**, *20*, 611–616. [CrossRef]
48. Turner, D.P.; Smitherman, T.A.; Black, A.K.; Penzien, D.B.; Porter, J.A.; Lofland, K.R.; Houle, T.T. Are migraine and tension-type headache diagnostic types or points on a severity continuum? An exploration of the latent taxometric structure of headache. *Pain* **2015**, *156*, 1200–1207. [CrossRef] [PubMed]
49. Andersen, S.; Petersen, M.W.; Svendsen, A.S.; Gazerani, P. Pressure pain thresholds assessed over temporalis, masseter, and frontalis muscles in healthy individuals, patients with tension-type headache, and those with migraine—A systematic review. *Pain* **2015**, *156*, 1409–1423. [CrossRef] [PubMed]
50. Sun, H.; Bastings, E.; Temeck, J.; Smith, P.B.; Men, A.; Tandon, V.; Murphy, D.; Rodriguez, W. Migraine therapeutics in adolescents: A systematic analysis and historic perspectives of triptan trials in adolescents. *JAMA Pediatr.* **2013**, *167*, 243–249. [CrossRef] [PubMed]
51. Silver, S.; Gano, D.; Gerretsen, P. Acute treatment of paediatric migraine: A meta-analysis of efficacy. *J. Paediatr. Child Health* **2008**, *44*, 3–9. [CrossRef] [PubMed]
52. Damen, L.; Bruijn, J.K.; Verhagen, A.P.; Berger, M.Y.; Passchier, J.; Koes, B.W. Symptomatic treatment of migraine in children: A systematic review of medication trials. *Pediatrics* **2005**, *116*, e295–e302. [CrossRef] [PubMed]
53. Sun-Edelstein, C.; Bigal, M.E.; Rapoport, A.M. Chronic migraine and medication overuse headache: Clarifying the current international headache society classification criteria. *Cephalalgia Int. J. Headache* **2009**, *29*, 445–452. [CrossRef] [PubMed]
54. Bigal, M.E.; Tepper, S.J.; Sheftell, F.D.; Rapoport, A.M.; Lipton, R.B. Chronic daily headache: Correlation between the 2004 and the 1988 international headache society diagnostic criteria. *Headache* **2004**, *44*, 684–691. [CrossRef] [PubMed]
55. Limmroth, V.; Katsarava, Z.; Fritsche, G.; Przywara, S.; Diener, H.C. Features of medication overuse headache following overuse of different acute headache drugs. *Neurology* **2002**, *59*, 1011–1014. [CrossRef] [PubMed]
56. MacGregor, E.A.; Steiner, T.J.; Davies, P.T.G. *Guidelines for All Healthcare Professionals in the Diagnosis and Management of Migraine, Tension-Type, Cluster and Medication-Overuse Headache*, 3rd ed. (1st revision). Available online: http://www.nhsgrampian.org/neurology/files/2010_BASH_Guidelines.pdf (accessed on 7 December 2016).
57. Hering-Hanit, R.; Gadoth, N.; Cohen, A.; Horev, Z. Successful withdrawal from analgesic abuse in a group of youngsters with chronic daily headache. *J. Child Neurol.* **2001**, *16*, 448–449. [CrossRef] [PubMed]
58. Keefer, L.; Drossman, D.A.; Guthrie, E.; Simren, M.; Tillisch, K.; Olden, K.; Whorwell, P.J. Centrally mediated disorders of gastrointestinal pain. *Gastroenterology* **2016**. [CrossRef] [PubMed]

59. Williams, A.E.; Heitkemper, M.; Self, M.M.; Czyzewski, D.I.; Shulman, R.J. Endogenous inhibition of somatic pain is impaired in girls with irritable bowel syndrome compared with healthy girls. *J. Pain* **2013**, *14*, 921–930. [CrossRef] [PubMed]
60. Stabell, N.; Stubhaug, A.; Flaegstad, T.; Mayer, E.; Naliboff, B.D.; Nielsen, C.S. Widespread hyperalgesia in adolescents with symptoms of irritable bowel syndrome: Results from a large population-based study. *J. Pain* **2014**, *15*, 898–906. [CrossRef] [PubMed]
61. Walker, L.S.; Dengler-Crish, C.M.; Rippel, S.; Bruehl, S. Functional abdominal pain in childhood and adolescence increases risk for chronic pain in adulthood. *Pain* **2010**, *150*, 568–572. [CrossRef] [PubMed]
62. Dengler-Crish, C.M.; Horst, S.N.; Walker, L.S. Somatic complaints in childhood functional abdominal pain are associated with functional gastrointestinal disorders in adolescence and adulthood. *J. Pediatr. Gastroenterol. Nutr.* **2011**, *52*, 162–165. [CrossRef] [PubMed]
63. Dengler-Crish, C.M.; Bruehl, S.; Walker, L.S. Increased wind-up to heat pain in women with a childhood history of functional abdominal pain. *Pain* **2011**, *152*, 802–808. [CrossRef] [PubMed]
64. Petersen, S.; Bergstrom, E.; Brulin, C. High prevalence of tiredness and pain in young schoolchildren. *Scand. J. Public Health* **2003**, *31*, 367–374. [CrossRef] [PubMed]
65. Watson, K.D.; Papageorgiou, A.C.; Jones, G.T.; Taylor, S.; Symmons, D.P.; Silman, A.J.; Macfarlane, G.J. Low back pain in schoolchildren: Occurrence and characteristics. *Pain* **2002**, *97*, 87–92. [CrossRef]
66. Kristjansdottir, G. Prevalence of self-reported back pain in school children: A study of sociodemographic differences. *Eur. J. Pediatr.* **1996**, *155*, 984–986. [CrossRef] [PubMed]
67. Smedbraten, B.K.; Natvig, B.; Rutle, O.; Bruusgaard, D. Self-reported bodily pain in schoolchildren. *Scand. J. Rheumatol.* **1998**, *27*, 273–276. [PubMed]
68. Brun Sundblad, G.M.; Saartok, T.; Engstrom, L.M. Prevalence and co-occurrence of self-rated pain and perceived health in school-children: Age and gender differences. *Eur. J. Pain* **2007**, *11*, 171–180. [CrossRef] [PubMed]
69. Vahasarja, V. Prevalence of chronic knee pain in children and adolescents in Northern Finland. *Acta Paediatr.* **1995**, *84*, 803–805. [CrossRef] [PubMed]
70. Mikkelsson, M.; Salminen, J.J.; Kautiainen, H. Non-specific musculoskeletal pain in preadolescents. Prevalence and 1-year persistence. *Pain* **1997**, *73*, 29–35. [CrossRef]
71. Centers for Disease Control and Prevention. Post-Treatment Lyme Disease Syndrome. Available online: http://www.cdc.gov/lyme/postlds/ (accessed on 7 December 2016).
72. U.S. National Library of Medicine. Conversion Disorder. Available online: https://medlineplus.gov/ency/article/000954.htm (accessed on 7 December 2016).
73. Cottencin, O. Conversion disorders: Psychiatric and psychotherapeutic aspects. *Neurophysiol. Clin.* **2014**, *44*, 405–410. [CrossRef] [PubMed]
74. Lu, Q.; Krull, K.R.; Leisenring, W.; Owen, J.E.; Kawashima, T.; Tsao, J.C.; Zebrack, B.; Mertens, A.; Armstrong, G.T.; Stovall, M.; et al. Pain in long-term adult survivors of childhood cancers and their siblings: A report from the childhood cancer survivor study. *Pain* **2011**, *152*, 2616–2624. [CrossRef] [PubMed]
75. Fortier, M.A.; Chou, J.; Maurer, E.L.; Kain, Z.N. Acute to chronic postoperative pain in children: Preliminary findings. *J. Pediatr. Surg.* **2011**, *46*, 1700–1705. [CrossRef] [PubMed]
76. Page, M.G.; Stinson, J.; Campbell, F.; Isaac, L.; Katz, J. Identification of pain-related psychological risk factors for the development and maintenance of pediatric chronic postsurgical pain. *J. Pain Res.* **2013**, *6*, 167–180. [CrossRef] [PubMed]
77. Sieberg, C.B.; Simons, L.E.; Edelstein, M.R.; DeAngelis, M.R.; Pielech, M.; Sethna, N.; Hresko, M.T. Pain prevalence and trajectories following pediatric spinal fusion surgery. *J. Pain* **2013**, *14*, 1694–1702. [CrossRef] [PubMed]
78. Rabbitts, J.A.; Zhou, C.; Groenewald, C.B.; Durkin, L.; Palermo, T.M. Trajectories of postsurgical pain in children: Risk factors and impact of late pain recovery on long-term health outcomes after major surgery. *Pain* **2015**, *156*, 2383–2389. [CrossRef] [PubMed]
79. Friedrichsdorf, S.J. Prevention and treatment of pain in hospitalized infants, children, and teenagers: From myths and morphine to multimodal analgesia. In Proceedings of the Pain 2016: Refresher Courses, 16th World Congress on Pain, Yokohama, Japan, 23–30 September 2016; International Association for the Study of Pain, IASP Press: Washington, DC, USA, 2016; pp. 309–319.

80. World Health Organization. WHO-Principles of Acute Pain Management for Children. Available online: http://apps.who.int/iris/bitstream/10665/44540/1/9789241548120_Guidelines.pdf (accessed on 7 December 2016).
81. Guzman, J.; Esmail, R.; Karjalainen, K.; Malmivaara, A.; Irvin, E.; Bombardier, C. Multidisciplinary bio-psycho-social rehabilitation for chronic low back pain. *Cochrane Database Syst. Rev.* **2002**. [CrossRef]
82. Logan, D.E.; Carpino, E.A.; Chiang, G.; Condon, M.; Firn, E.; Gaughan, V.J.; Hogan, M.; Leslie, D.S.; Olson, K.; Sager, S.; et al. A day-hospital approach to treatment of pediatric complex regional pain syndrome: Initial functional outcomes. *Clin. J. Pain* **2012**, *28*, 766–774. [CrossRef] [PubMed]
83. Hechler, T.; Ruhe, A.K.; Schmidt, P.; Hirsch, J.; Wager, J.; Dobe, M.; Krummenauer, F.; Zernikow, B. Inpatient-based intensive interdisciplinary pain treatment for highly impaired children with severe chronic pain: Randomized controlled trial of efficacy and economic effects. *Pain* **2014**, *155*, 118–128. [CrossRef] [PubMed]
84. Eccleston, C.; Malleson, P.N.; Clinch, J.; Connell, H.; Sourbut, C. Chronic pain in adolescents: Evaluation of a programme of interdisciplinary cognitive behaviour therapy. *Arch. Dis. Child* **2003**, *88*, 881–885. [CrossRef] [PubMed]
85. Maynard, C.S.; Amari, A.; Wieczorek, B.; Christensen, J.R.; Slifer, K.J. Interdisciplinary behavioral rehabilitation of pediatric pain-associated disability: Retrospective review of an inpatient treatment protocol. *J. Pediatr. Psychol.* **2010**, *35*, 128–137. [CrossRef] [PubMed]
86. Palermo, T.M.; Scher, M.S. Treatment of functional impairment in severe somatoform pain disorder: A case example. *J. Pediatr. Psychol.* **2001**, *26*, 429–434. [CrossRef] [PubMed]
87. Lynch, M.E.; Campbell, F.; Clark, A.J.; Dunbar, M.J.; Goldstein, D.; Peng, P.; Stinson, J.; Tupper, H. A systematic review of the effect of waiting for treatment for chronic pain. *Pain* **2008**, *136*, 97–116. [CrossRef] [PubMed]
88. Thompson, L.A.; Knapp, C.A.; Feeg, V.; Madden, V.L.; Shenkman, E.A. Pediatricians' management practices for chronic pain. *J. Palliat. Med.* **2010**, *13*, 171–178. [CrossRef] [PubMed]
89. Simons, L.E.; Smith, A.; Ibagon, C.; Coakley, R.; Logan, D.E.; Schechter, N.; Borsook, D.; Hill, J.C. Pediatric pain screening tool: Rapid identification of risk in youth with pain complaints. *Pain* **2015**, *156*, 1511–1518. [CrossRef] [PubMed]
90. Society, A.P. Pediatric Chronic Pain Programs by State/Province. Available online: http://americanpainsociety.org/uploads/get-involved/PainClinicList_12_2015.pdf (accessed on 7 December 2016).
91. Cormier, S.; Lavigne, G.L.; Choiniere, M.; Rainville, P. Expectations predict chronic pain treatment outcomes. *Pain* **2016**, *157*, 329–338. [CrossRef] [PubMed]
92. Lynch-Jordan, A.M.; Sil, S.; Peugh, J.; Cunningham, N.; Kashikar-Zuck, S.; Goldschneider, K.R. Differential changes in functional disability and pain intensity over the course of psychological treatment for children with chronic pain. *Pain* **2014**, *155*, 1955–1961. [CrossRef] [PubMed]
93. Sherry, D.D.; Wallace, C.A.; Kelley, C.; Kidder, M.; Sapp, L. Short- and long-term outcomes of children with complex regional pain syndrome type I treated with exercise therapy. *Clin. J. Pain* **1999**, *15*, 218–223. [CrossRef] [PubMed]
94. Odell, S.; Logan, D.E. Pediatric pain management: The multidisciplinary approach. *J. Pain Res.* **2013**, *6*, 785–790. [CrossRef] [PubMed]
95. Lee, B.H.; Scharff, L.; Sethna, N.F.; McCarthy, C.F.; Scott-Sutherland, J.; Shea, A.M.; Sullivan, P.; Meier, P.; Zurakowski, D.; Masek, B.J.; et al. Physical therapy and cognitive-behavioral treatment for complex regional pain syndromes. *J. Pediatr.* **2002**, *141*, 135–140. [CrossRef] [PubMed]
96. Wilson, A.C.; Palermo, T.M. Physical activity and function in adolescents with chronic pain: A controlled study using actigraphy. *J. Pain* **2012**, *13*, 121–130. [CrossRef] [PubMed]
97. Jerstad, S.J.; Boutelle, K.N.; Ness, K.K.; Stice, E. Prospective reciprocal relations between physical activity and depression in female adolescents. *J. Consult. Clin. Psychol.* **2010**, *78*, 268–272. [CrossRef] [PubMed]
98. Bowering, K.J.; O'Connell, N.E.; Tabor, A.; Catley, M.J.; Leake, H.B.; Moseley, G.L.; Stanton, T.R. The effects of graded motor imagery and its components on chronic pain: A systematic review and meta-analysis. *J. Pain* **2013**, *14*, 3–13. [CrossRef] [PubMed]
99. Bussing, A.; Ostermann, T.; Ludtke, R.; Michalsen, A. Effects of yoga interventions on pain and pain-associated disability: A meta-analysis. *J. Pain* **2012**, *13*, 1–9. [CrossRef] [PubMed]

100. Evans, S.; Moieni, M.; Taub, R.; Subramanian, S.K.; Tsao, J.C.; Sternlieb, B.; Zeltzer, L.K. Iyengar Yoga for young adults with rheumatoid arthritis: Results from a mixed-methods pilot study. *J. Pain Symptom Manag.* **2010**, *39*, 904–913. [CrossRef] [PubMed]
101. Vas, J.; Santos-Rey, K.; Navarro-Pablo, R.; Modesto, M.; Aguilar, I.; Campos, M.A.; Aguilar-Velasco, J.F.; Romero, M.; Parraga, P.; Hervas, V.; et al. Acupuncture for fibromyalgia in primary care: A randomised controlled trial. *Acupunct. Med.* **2016**, *34*, 257–266. [CrossRef] [PubMed]
102. Verkamp, E.K.; Flowers, S.R.; Lynch-Jordan, A.M.; Taylor, J.; Ting, T.V.; Kashikar-Zuck, S. A survey of conventional and complementary therapies used by youth with juvenile-onset fibromyalgia. *Pain Manag. Nurs.* **2013**, *14*, e244–e250. [CrossRef] [PubMed]
103. Friedrichsdorf, S.; Kuttner, L.; Westendorp, K.; McCarty, R. *Integrative Pediatric Palliative Care*; Oxford University Press: Oxford, UK, 2010.
104. Kuttner, L.; Friedrichsdorf, S.J. Hypnosis and palliative care. In *Therapeutic Hypnosis with Children and Adolescents*, 2nd ed.; Crown House Publishing Limited: Bethel, CT, USA, 2013; pp. 491–509.
105. Hunt, K.; Ernst, E. The evidence-base for complementary medicine in children: A critical overview of systematic reviews. *Arch. Dis. Child.* **2011**, *96*, 769–776. [CrossRef] [PubMed]
106. Evans, S.; Tsao, J.C.; Zeltzer, L.K. Complementary and alternative medicine for acute procedural pain in children. *Altern. Ther. Health Med.* **2008**, *14*, 52–56. [PubMed]
107. Richardson, J.; Smith, J.E.; McCall, G.; Pilkington, K. Hypnosis for procedure-related pain and distress in pediatric cancer patients: A systematic review of effectiveness and methodology related to hypnosis interventions. *J. Pain Symptom Manag.* **2006**, *31*, 70–84. [CrossRef] [PubMed]
108. Hemington, K.S.; Coulombe, M.A. The periaqueductal gray and descending pain modulation: Why should we study them and what role do they play in chronic pain? *J. Neurophysiol.* **2015**, *114*, 2080–2088. [CrossRef] [PubMed]
109. Valet, M.; Sprenger, T.; Boecker, H.; Willoch, F.; Rummeny, E.; Conrad, B.; Erhard, P.; Tolle, T.R. Distraction modulates connectivity of the cingulo-frontal cortex and the midbrain during pain—An FMRI analysis. *Pain* **2004**, *109*, 399–408. [CrossRef] [PubMed]
110. Tracey, I.; Ploghaus, A.; Gati, J.S.; Clare, S.; Smith, S.; Menon, R.S.; Matthews, P.M. Imaging attentional modulation of pain in the periaqueductal gray in humans. *J. Neurosci.* **2002**, *22*, 2748–2752. [PubMed]
111. Derbyshire, S.W.; Osborn, J. Modeling pain circuits: How imaging may modify perception. *Neuroimaging Clin. N. Am.* **2007**, *17*, 485–493. [CrossRef] [PubMed]
112. Bingel, U.; Wanigasekera, V.; Wiech, K.; Ni Mhuircheartaigh, R.; Lee, M.C.; Ploner, M.; Tracey, I. The effect of treatment expectation on drug efficacy: Imaging the analgesic benefit of the opioid remifentanil. *Sci. Transl. Med.* **2011**, *3*, 70ra14. [CrossRef] [PubMed]
113. Yu, R.; Gollub, R.L.; Spaeth, R.; Napadow, V.; Wasan, A.; Kong, J. Disrupted functional connectivity of the periaqueductal gray in chronic low back pain. *Neuroimage Clin.* **2014**, *6*, 100–108. [CrossRef] [PubMed]
114. Giordano, J. The neurobiology of nociceptive and anti-nociceptive systems. *Pain Phys.* **2005**, *8*, 277–290.
115. Tegethoff, M.; Belardi, A.; Stalujanis, E.; Meinlschmidt, G. Comorbidity of mental disorders and chronic pain: Chronology of onset in adolescents of a national representative cohort. *J. Pain* **2015**, *16*, 1054–1064. [CrossRef] [PubMed]
116. Cohen, L.L.; Vowles, K.E.; Eccleston, C. The impact of adolescent chronic pain on functioning: Disentangling the complex role of anxiety. *J. Pain* **2010**, *11*, 1039–1046. [CrossRef] [PubMed]
117. Palermo, T.M.; Eccleston, C.; Lewandowski, A.S.; Williams, A.C.; Morley, S. Randomized controlled trials of psychological therapies for management of chronic pain in children and adolescents: An updated meta-analytic review. *Pain* **2010**, *148*, 387–397. [CrossRef] [PubMed]
118. Eccleston, C.; Palermo, T.M.; Williams, A.C.; Lewandowski Holley, A.; Morley, S.; Fisher, E.; Law, E. Psychological therapies for the management of chronic and recurrent pain in children and adolescents. *Cochrane Database Syst. Rev.* **2014**. [CrossRef]
119. Kashikar-Zuck, S.; Sil, S.; Lynch-Jordan, A.M.; Ting, T.V.; Peugh, J.; Schikler, K.N.; Hashkes, P.J.; Arnold, L.M.; Passo, M.; Richards-Mauze, M.M.; et al. Changes in pain coping, catastrophizing, and coping efficacy after cognitive-behavioral therapy in children and adolescents with juvenile fibromyalgia. *J. Pain* **2013**, *14*, 492–501. [CrossRef] [PubMed]

120. Seminowicz, D.A.; Shpaner, M.; Keaser, M.L.; Krauthamer, G.M.; Mantegna, J.; Dumas, J.A.; Newhouse, P.A.; Filippi, C.G.; Keefe, F.J.; Naylor, M.R. Cognitive-behavioral therapy increases prefrontal cortex gray matter in patients with chronic pain. *J. Pain* **2013**, *14*, 1573–1584. [CrossRef] [PubMed]
121. Forgeron, P.A.; McGrath, P.; Stevens, B.; Evans, J.; Dick, B.; Finley, G.A.; Carlson, T. Social information processing in adolescents with chronic pain: My friends don't really understand me. *Pain* **2011**, *152*, 2773–2780. [CrossRef] [PubMed]
122. Palermo, T.M.; Wilson, A.C.; Lewandowski, A.S.; Toliver-Sokol, M.; Murray, C.B. Behavioral and psychosocial factors associated with insomnia in adolescents with chronic pain. *Pain* **2011**, *152*, 89–94. [CrossRef] [PubMed]
123. Palermo, T.M.; Law, E.; Churchill, S.S.; Walker, A. Longitudinal course and impact of insomnia symptoms in adolescents with and without chronic pain. *J. Pain* **2012**, *13*, 1099–1106. [CrossRef] [PubMed]
124. Letter, H.H. Blue Light Has a Dark Side. Available online: http://www.health.harvard.edu/staying-healthy/blue-light-has-a-dark-side (accessed on 7 December 2016).
125. Gooley, J.J.; Chamberlain, K.; Smith, K.A.; Khalsa, S.B.; Rajaratnam, S.M.; van Reen, E.; Zeitzer, J.M.; Czeisler, C.A.; Lockley, S.W. Exposure to room light before bedtime suppresses melatonin onset and shortens melatonin duration in humans. *J. Clin. Endocrinol. Metab.* **2011**, *96*, E463–E472. [CrossRef] [PubMed]
126. Logan, D.E.; Simons, L.E.; Carpino, E.A. Too sick for school? Parent influences on school functioning among children with chronic pain. *Pain* **2012**, *153*, 437–443. [CrossRef] [PubMed]
127. Bernstein, G.A.; Hektner, J.M.; Borchardt, C.M.; McMillan, M.H. Treatment of school refusal: One-year follow-up. *J. Am. Aca. Child Adolesc. Psychiatry* **2001**, *40*, 206–213. [CrossRef] [PubMed]
128. King, N.J.; Bernstein, G.A. School refusal in children and adolescents: A review of the past 10 years. *J. Am. Aca. Child Adolesc. Psychiatry* **2001**, *40*, 197–205. [CrossRef] [PubMed]
129. Evans, L.D. Functional school refusal subtypes: Anxiety, avoidance, malingering. *Psychol. Sch.* **2000**, *37*, 183–191. [CrossRef]
130. Lewandowski, A.S.; Palermo, T.M.; Stinson, J.; Handley, S.; Chambers, C.T. Systematic review of family functioning in families of children and adolescents with chronic pain. *J. Pain* **2010**, *11*, 1027–1038. [CrossRef] [PubMed]
131. Liossi, C.; White, P.; Croome, N.; Hatira, P. Pain-related bias in the classification of emotionally ambiguous facial expressions in mothers of children with chronic abdominal pain. *Pain* **2012**, *153*, 674–681. [CrossRef] [PubMed]
132. Higgins, K.S.; Birnie, K.A.; Chambers, C.T.; Wilson, A.C.; Caes, L.; Clark, A.J.; Lynch, M.; Stinson, J.; Campbell-Yeo, M. Offspring of parents with chronic pain: A systematic review and meta-analysis of pain, health, psychological, and family outcomes. *Pain* **2015**, *156*, 2256–2266. [CrossRef] [PubMed]
133. Kaasboll, J.; Lydersen, S.; Indredavik, M.S. Psychological symptoms in children of parents with chronic pain-the hunt study. *Pain* **2012**, *153*, 1054–1062. [CrossRef] [PubMed]
134. Peloso, P.M. Faster, higher, stronger: To the gold medal podium? *Pain* **2014**, *155*, 4–5. [CrossRef] [PubMed]
135. Moore, R.A.; Derry, S.; Straube, S.; Ireson-Paine, J.; Wiffen, P.J. Faster, higher, stronger? Evidence for formulation and efficacy for ibuprofen in acute pain. *Pain* **2014**, *155*, 14–21. [CrossRef] [PubMed]
136. Dowell, D.; Haegerich, T.M.; Chou, R. Cdc guideline for prescribing opioids for chronic pain—United States, 2016. *MMWR Recomm. Rep.* **2016**, *65*, 1–49. [CrossRef] [PubMed]
137. Schechter, N.L.; Walco, G.A. The potential impact on children of the CDC guideline for prescribing opioids for chronic pain: Above all, do no harm. *JAMA Pediatr.* **2016**, *170*, 425–426. [CrossRef] [PubMed]
138. Friedrichsdorf, S.J.; Nugent, A.P. Management of neuropathic pain in children with cancer. *Curr. Opin. Support. Palliat. Care* **2013**, *7*, 131–138. [CrossRef] [PubMed]
139. Vidor, L.P.; Torres, I.L.; Custodio de Souza, I.C.; Fregni, F.; Caumo, W. Analgesic and sedative effects of melatonin in temporomandibular disorders: A double-blind, randomized, parallel-group, placebo-controlled study. *J. Pain Symptom Manag.* **2013**, *46*, 422–432. [CrossRef] [PubMed]
140. Schwertner, A.; Conceicao Dos Santos, C.C.; Costa, G.D.; Deitos, A.; de Souza, A.; de Souza, I.C.; Torres, I.L.; da Cunha Filho, J.S.; Caumo, W. Efficacy of melatonin in the treatment of endometriosis: A phase II, randomized, double-blind, placebo-controlled trial. *Pain* **2013**, *154*, 874–881. [CrossRef] [PubMed]
141. Finnerup, N.B.; Attal, N.; Haroutounian, S.; McNicol, E.; Baron, R.; Dworkin, R.H.; Gilron, I.; Haanpaa, M.; Hansson, P.; Jensen, T.S.; et al. Pharmacotherapy for neuropathic pain in adults: A systematic review and meta-analysis. *Lancet Neurol.* **2015**, *14*, 162–173. [CrossRef]

142. Hauer, J.M.; Solodiuk, J.C. Gabapentin for management of recurrent pain in 22 nonverbal children with severe neurological impairment: A retrospective analysis. *J. Palliat. Med.* **2015**, *18*, 453–456. [CrossRef] [PubMed]
143. Edwards, L.; DeMeo, S.; Hornik, C.D.; Cotten, C.M.; Smith, P.B.; Pizoli, C.; Hauer, J.M.; Bidegain, M. Gabapentin use in the neonatal intensive care unit. *J. Pediatr.* **2016**, *169*, 310–312. [CrossRef] [PubMed]
144. Derry, S.; Wiffen, P.J.; Moore, R.A.; Quinlan, J. Topical lidocaine for neuropathic pain in adults. *Cochrane Database Syst. Rev.* **2014**, *7*. [CrossRef]
145. El-Chammas, K.; Keyes, J.; Thompson, N.; Vijayakumar, J.; Becher, D.; Jackson, J.L. Pharmacologic treatment of pediatric headaches: A meta-analysis. *JAMA Pediatr.* **2013**, *167*, 250–258. [CrossRef] [PubMed]
146. Campo, J.V.; Perel, J.; Lucas, A.; Bridge, J.; Ehmann, M.; Kalas, C.; Monk, K.; Axelson, D.; Birmaher, B.; Ryan, N.; et al. Citalopram treatment of pediatric recurrent abdominal pain and comorbid internalizing disorders: An exploratory study. *J. Am. Acad. Child. Adolesc. Psychiatry* **2004**, *43*, 1234–1242. [CrossRef] [PubMed]
147. Caperell, K.; Pitetti, R.; Cross, K.P. Race and acute abdominal pain in a pediatric emergency department. *Pediatrics* **2013**, *131*, 1098–1106. [CrossRef] [PubMed]
148. Friedrichsdorf, S.J.; Drake, R.; Webster, L.M. Gastrointestinal symptoms. In *Textbook of Interdisciplinary Pediatric Palliative Care*; Elsevier/Saunders: Philadelphia, PA, USA, 2011; pp. 311–334.
149. Friedrichsdorf, S.J. Cancer pain management in children. In *Anaesthesia, Intensive Care, and Pain Management for the Cancer Patient*; Farquhar-Smith, P., Wigmore, T., Eds.; Oxford University Press: Oxford, UK; New York, NY, USA, 2011; pp. 215–227.
150. Michelson, J.D.; Addante, R.A.; Charlson, M.D. Multimodal analgesia therapy reduces length of hospitalization in patients undergoing fusions of the ankle and hindfoot. *Foot Ankle Int.* **2013**, *34*, 1526–1534. [CrossRef] [PubMed]
151. Giordano, J. The neuroscience of pain, and the neuroethics of pain care. *Neuroethics* **2009**, *3*, 89–94. [CrossRef]
152. Giordano, J. Pain research: Can paradigmatic revision bridge the demands of medicine, scientific philosophy and ethics? *Pain Phys.* **2004**, *7*, 407–410.
153. Jorgenson, L.A.; Newsome, W.T.; Anderson, D.J.; Bargmann, C.I.; Brown, E.N.; Deisseroth, K.; Donoghue, J.P.; Hudson, K.L.; Ling, G.S.; MacLeish, P.R.; et al. The brain initiative: Developing technology to catalyse neuroscience discovery. *Philos. Trans. R. Soc. Lond. Ser. B Biol. Sci.* **2015**, *370*. [CrossRef] [PubMed]
154. Giordano, J.; Schatman, M.E. Pain medicine from "bench to bedside": Bridging the disconnect(s) between research and clinical care. *J. Humanit. Sci. Healthc.* **2011**, *1*, 22–40.
155. Giordano, J. *Pain: Mind, Meaning, and Medicine*; PPM Press: Glen Falls, PA, USA, 2009; p. 48.
156. Giordano, J. Maldynia: Chronic pain as illness, and the need for complementarity in pain care. *Forsch. Komplement.* **2008**, *15*, 277–281. [CrossRef] [PubMed]
157. Giordano, J. Pain and suffering: Körper and leib, and the telos of pain care. *Philos. Psychiatry Psychol.* **2013**, *19*, 279–283.
158. Giordano, J.; Benedikter, R.; Boswell, M.V. Pain medicine, biotechnology and market effects: Tools, tekne and moral responsibility. *J. Ethics Biol. Eng. Med.* **2010**, *1*, 135–142. [CrossRef]
159. Desai, K.; Daughtree, C.; Friedrichsdorf, S.J. An interdisciplinary pain clinic: A year in review (poster). In Proceedings of the 10th International Forum on Pediatric Pain (IFPP), White Point Beach Resort, Hunts Point, NS, Canada, 1–4 October 2015.
160. Friedrichsdorf, S.J.; Postier, A.; Eull, D.; Gilbert, M.; Desai, K.; Gibbon, C.; Flood, A. Interdisciplinary pediatric outpatient pain clinic: Improvement in pain, function and predictors of successful graduation. Unpublished work. 2016.
161. "Little Stars—Treating Chronic Pain in Children". Available online: https://www.youtube.com/watch?t=13&v=Bb1fHxfjdWI (accessed on 7 December 2016).
162. Pediatric Pain Clinics in USA and Canada (American Pain Society). Available online: http://americanpainsociety.org/uploads/get-involved/PainClinicList_12_2015.pdf (accessed on 7 December 2016).
163. Pain Bytes (Australia). Available online: http://www.aci.health.nsw.gov.au/chronic-pain/painbytes (accessed on 7 December 2016).
164. Persistent (Chronic) Pain 5-min video[164]. Available online: https://www.youtube.com/watch?v=RWMKucuejIs (accessed on 7 December 2016).

165. Kiran Stordalen and Horst Rechelbacher Pediatric Pain, Palliative and Integrative Medicine Clinic Tour. Available online: https://vimeo.com/122654881 (accessed on 7 December 2016).
166. Elliot Krane (TED-Talk) The mystery of chronic pain. Available online: https://www.youtube.com/watch?v=J6--CMhcCfQ (accessed on 7 December 2016).
167. The Department of Pain Medicine, Palliative Care, and Integrative Medicine, Children's Hospitals and Clinics of Minnesota. Available online: https://www.childrensmn.org/painpalliativeintegrativemed (accessed on 7 December 2016).

11

Enhanced Brain Responses to Pain-Related Words in Chronic Back Pain Patients and their Modulation by Current Pain

Alexander Ritter [1,2,†], Marcel Franz [1,†], Christian Puta [3], Caroline Dietrich [1], Wolfgang H. R. Miltner [1] and Thomas Weiss [1,*]

1 Department of Biological and Clinical Psychology, Friedrich Schiller University of Jena, Am Steiger 3, Haus 1, Jena D-07743, Germany; alexander.ritter@uni-jena.de (A.R.); marcel.franz@uni-jena.de (M.F.); caroline.dietrich@uni-jena.de (C.D.); wolfgang.miltner@uni-jena.de (W.H.R.M.)

2 Section of Neurological Rehabilitation, Hans–Berger Department of Neurology at Jena University Hospital, Erlanger Allee 101, Jena D-07747, Germany

3 Department of Sports Medicine and Health Promotion, Friedrich Schiller University of Jena, Wöllnitzer Str. 42, Jena D-07749, Germany; christian.puta@uni-jena.de

* Correspondence: Thomas.Weiss@uni-jena.de

† These authors contributed equally to this work.

Academic Editor: Robert J. Gatchel

Abstract: Previous functional magnetic resonance imaging (fMRI) studies in healthy controls (HC) and pain-free migraine patients found activations to pain-related words in brain regions known to be activated while subjects experience pain. The aim of the present study was to identify neural activations induced by pain-related words in a sample of chronic back pain (CBP) patients experiencing current chronic pain compared to HC. In particular, we were interested in how current pain influences brain activations induced by pain-related adjectives. Subjects viewed pain-related, negative, positive, and neutral words; subjects were asked to generate mental images related to these words during fMRI scanning. Brain activation was compared between CBP patients and HC in response to the different word categories and examined in relation to current pain in CBP patients. Pain-related words vs. neutral words activated a network of brain regions including cingulate cortex and insula in subjects and patients. There was stronger activation in medial and dorsolateral prefrontal cortex (DLPFC) and anterior midcingulate cortex in CPB patients than in HC. The magnitude of activation for pain-related vs. negative words showed a negative linear relationship to CBP patients' current pain. Our findings confirm earlier observations showing that pain-related words activate brain networks similar to noxious stimulation. Importantly, CBP patients show even stronger activation of these structures while merely processing pain-related words. Current pain directly influences on this activation.

Keywords: chronic back pain; semantic processing; current pain; fMRI

---

1. Introduction

Processing and perceptual evaluation of noxious events and their underlying neural substrates are strongly modulated by psychological variables such as attention [1–4], emotion [5–10], expectation [11,12], and learning [13,14]. Furthermore, several studies indicate that environmental semantic and visual pain-related cues can induce activity in structures of the brain that process, among others, nociceptive information [15–17] even when no noxious stimulus is applied [18,19]. Based on Hebb's concept of cell assemblies, it can be assumed that whenever we experience pain, its semantic and emotional representations are activated simultaneously with neural structures that process noxious events and constitute the experience of pain [20,21]. Consequently, words that are used to describe pain-related experiences were found to alter pain itself [22,23], and to activate brain structures engaged in the processing of noxious stimuli, e.g., anterior cingulate cortex, insula, secondary somatosensory cortex (SII), prefrontal cortex, and parietal cortex [24,25].

It has been shown that chronic back pain (CBP) patients differ from healthy controls (HC) in structural [26], functional [27,28], and neurochemical brain parameters [29,30]. In CBP patients, pain is a common everyday experience and pain has been expressed hundreds of times throughout the course of chronic pain development. It was suggested that CBP patients as chronic pain sufferers should have developed a strong pain network and a strong link of this network to their lexicon of pain terms. Accordingly, chronic pain patients exhibit larger event-related potentials (ERPs) to painful stimuli [31], larger late ERP amplitudes when noxious stimuli were primed by pain-related words [14], and stronger blood oxygenation level dependent (BOLD) responses even when pain was not attended [32–34]. Furthermore, chronic pain patients showed larger late ERP magnitudes in response to pain-related words and rated such words more negatively than neutral words, indicating that pain-related words draw similar attention and information processing as if an actually painful stimulus would have been processed [35]. In summary, the processing of pain-related words leads to enhanced behavioral and neuronal responses even when semantic processing is precluded from conscious access.

The present study aimed to extend previous findings by investigating the processing of pain-related words in CBP patients with actually ongoing (current) back pain. It was expected that the presence of current pain would activate the brain regions important for the analysis of pain and, thereby, enhance the processing of pain-related words. These assumptions lead to the following hypotheses: H1—CBP patients exhibit different valence, arousal, and pain relevance to pain-related words compared to HC; H2—CBP patients vs. HC show a stronger activation during the processing of pain-related than non-pain-related word categories and to negative words; and H3—There is a linear relationship between the strength of current pain and the measured BOLD response during the processing of pain-related words in CBP patients.

2. Materials and Methods

2.1. Patients and Controls

Participants of this study were recruited by advertisement at the university or by personal contact. Thirteen patients with CBP (2 men; 23–56 years old, mean age = 44.3 years) and thirteen pain-free HC (2 men; 24–58 years old, mean age = 46.5 years), matched for gender, age, and education, participated in this study as paid volunteers. Sociodemographic and clinical characteristics of participants are summarized in Table 1. The CBP patients have been examined by physicians and met the following criteria: (1) minimum duration of low back pain: for 6 months; (2) pain classified as 'non-specific low back pain' (no indication for nerve root problems and radiation to foot or toes, numbness and/or paraesthesia; straight leg raising test caused no leg pain); (3) magnetic resonance imaging (MRI) of the spine only indicated age-related wear and tear but no spinal disorders or disc pathology; (4) no psychiatric disorders, no disease associated to small fiber pathology (e.g., diabetes mellitus), no other chronic disorder; (5) no use of medication (except contraceptive) for at least 48 h prior to the experiment (requested before scanning). All participants were native German speakers and right-handed as assessed by the Edinburgh Handedness Inventory (EHI) [36]. None of the healthy controls reported former subacute or chronic pain episodes (longer than one month), any neurological, psychiatric or other chronic disorder. Because depression may alter the processing of pain-related words [37], depressive symptoms were assessed with a German version of the Beck Depression Inventory-II (BDI-II) [38]. For the assessment of catastrophizing thoughts and persuasions, all subjects completed the Pain Catastrophizing Scale (PCS, [39]; German version: [40]). In accordance with the

Declaration of Helsinki, written informed consent was obtained from each participant before the study, and the Ethics Committee of the Friedrich Schiller University approved the experiment.

Table 1. Demographic and clinical characteristics as well as behavioral data of chronic back pain patients (CBP) and healthy controls (HC).

	CBP	HC			
Sex					
Male/Female	2/11	2/11			
Age **(in years)**	44.31 ± 12.15	46.46 ± 10.19			
Range	23–56	24–58			
Pain history					
6–12 months	N = 2	N = 0			
2–5 years	N = 4	N = 0			
>5 years	N = 7	N = 0			
Pain intensity			*t*	*df*	*p*
Mean pain intensity (VAS [a] recent 4 weeks)	3.31 ± 1.83	0.09 ± 0.30	5.72	10.53	<0.001
Strongest pain (VAS recent 4 weeks)	5.14 ± 1.85	0.27 ± 0.90	6.27	12.76	<0.001
Current pain (VAS post scanning)	1.72 ± 1.34	0.05 ± 0.15	4.15	10.25	0.002
BDI [b] score	7.77 ± 5.13	2.62 ± 1.76	3.50	12.12	0.004
Pain Catastrophizing Scale (PCS)	14.08 ± 6.11	11.82 ± 7.04	0.61	24	0.550
Rumination	5.46 ± 3.46	5.09 ± 3.27	0.12	24	0.905
Helplessness	4.85 ± 3.11	4.00 ± 2.61	0.49	24	0.632
Magnification	3.77 ± 2.32	2.73 ± 2.19	0.98	24	0.351
Task difficulty [c]	1.38 ± 1.50	1.38 ± 1.50	0	24	1
			χ^2		
Correct word categorization [d]	15.66 ± 0.79	15.45 ± 1.65	0.04	1	0.865

Note: Values are mean ± SD; [a] Visual Analogue Scale (VAS): 0 = "no pain", 10 = "strongest pain imaginable"; [b] BDI = Beck Depression Inventory; [c] Visual Analogue Scale (VAS): 0 = "very easy", 10 = "very difficult"; [d] correct categorizations out of 16 judgments.

2.2. Verbal Stimuli

Verbal stimuli included pain-related and non-pain-related negative, neutral, and positive adjectives. In a pilot study, 40 words were selected, and rated for valence, arousal, and pain relevance. Pain-related adjectives, affectively negative adjectives, and positive adjectives were matched for arousal. In addition, pain-related and negative adjectives were also matched for valence. Furthermore, word categories were matched according to the number of syllables and frequency in German language (COSMAS II database, http://www.ids-mannheim.de/cosmas2/). For a more detailed description of stimulus selection and the stimulus set, see Richter, Eck, Straube, Miltner and Weiss [32].

2.3. Experimental Procedure

Examples of each word category were presented while participants were familiarized with the experimental procedure prior to the experiment. A video beamer projected the stimuli onto a screen mounted on the head coil of the MRI scanner. The experimental design is displayed in Figure 1. Subjects were instructed to focus on the semantics of the words by generating a mental image of a situation associated with the word. To increase compliance, subjects were told that they would be asked for examples of their imaginations after the experiment. All subjects were able to associate appropriate mental images to the words. For example, neutral word "traubenförmig" ("aciniform") was frequently associated with wine grapes and positive word "wärmend" ("warming") was commonly associated with an oven. Word stimuli were presented in 16 blocks (4 blocks of each word category). Each block consisted of five words (belonging to one word category); each word was displayed for 4.1 s and was followed by a blank screen for 0.1 s. Each block was followed by a delay phase in which a fixation cross was presented for 11 s and a subsequent interval of 7 s. During this interval, subjects were requested to choose the correct word category from two categories presented (e.g., A = pain-related, B = negative). Subjects responded by a MRI-compatible button response box fixed below their right hand. After the selection, a fixation cross was presented for 13 s. Each word was presented twice throughout the experiment. The order of the words within each block and the order of blocks were pseudo-randomized with the restriction that the same word category was not presented twice in succession. The whole fMRI run lasted 14 min.

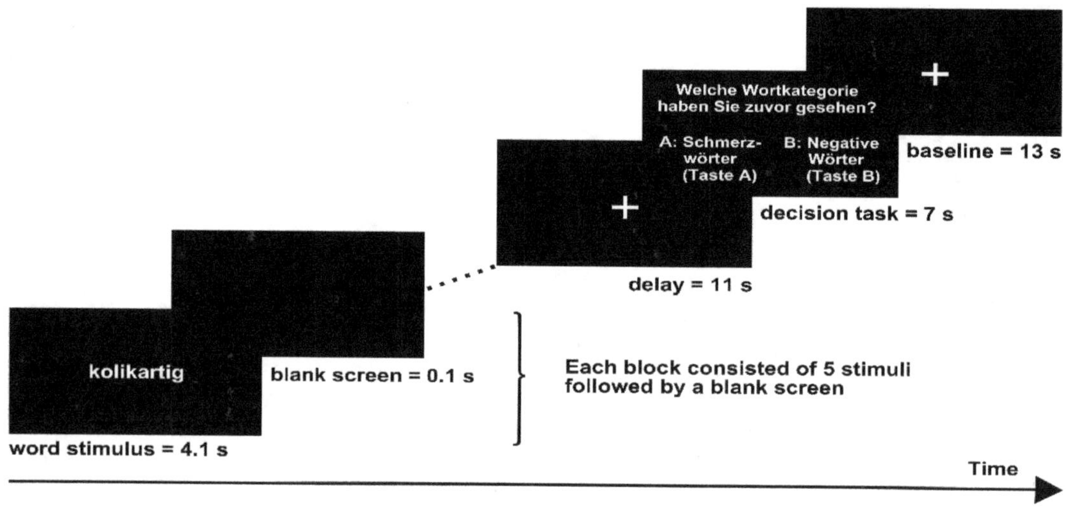

Figure 1. Stimulus protocol.

After the scanning session, participants rated the mean valence, arousal, and pain relevance of each word category on a 10-point numerical rating scale (NRS), with 0 = "negative/no arousal/not relevant", and 10 = "positive/maximum arousal/highly relevant". Following the scanning procedure, all subjects also rated their current back pain on a VAS (visual analogue scale, = "no pain", 10 = "worst pain imaginable"). The pain ratings were obtained at the end of the experiment to avoid any mutual influence between the rating of words and the pain rating. Furthermore, a rating of task difficulty was requested using a VAS (0 = "very easy", 10 = "very difficult"). During the study, we introduced the vividness of imagination scale [41] measuring emotional imagination, i.e., the ability to create emotional scenarios in mind. Higher ratings are associated with enhanced vividness of imagination.

2.4. *Analysis of Behavioral Data*

All statistical calculations were carried out using IBM SPSS Statistics 19 (IBM, Armonk, NY, USA). Normal distribution of behavioral data was determined by Kolmogorov-Smirnov Test. Levene's test was applied to assess the equality of variances across the two groups. Variables were statistically analyzed using Student's t- test if they were distributed normally; otherwise, χ^2-tests were applied. Welch's t-test was used for variables with unequal variances across groups. Differences between CBP patients and HC were evaluated for the ratings of arousal, valence, pain relevance, and vividness of imagination of word material [41].

To test differences of word category between patients and HC, separate two-way repeated measurements ANOVAs for mixed experimental design (between-subject factor Group and within-subject factor Word Category) were conducted. We considered values of $p < 0.05$ to be statistically significant.

2.5. *fMRI-Data Acquisition and Analysis*

MRI was obtained by a 3-Tesla magnetic resonance scanner (Tim Trio, Siemens, Medical Systems, Erlangen, Germany). For fMRI, 305 volumes were recorded using a T2* weighted echo-planar sequence (time to echo (TE) = 30 ms, flip angle = 90°, matrix = 64 × 64, field of view (FOV) = 192 mm, scan repeat time (TR) = 2.8 s). Each volume was comprised of 40 axial slices (thickness = 3 mm, no gap, in-plane resolution = 3 × 3 mm) parallel to the intercommissural plane (AC–PC-plane). Additionally, a high-resolution T1-weighted anatomical volume was obtained based on 192 slices with TE = 5 ms, matrix = 256 × 256 mm and resolution = 1 × 1 × 1 mm. Imaging data were pre-processed and analyzed using BrainVoyagerQX, Version 2.8 (Brain Innovation, Maastricht, The Netherlands) and NeuroElf V0.9 (Jochen Weber, SCAN Unit, Columbia University, New York City, NY, USA, http://www.neuroelf.net).

All volumes were realigned to the first volume in order to minimize the effects of head movements on data analysis. Further data pre-processing comprised spatial (6 mm full-width half-maximum isotropic Gaussian kernel) as well as temporal smoothing (high pass filter: 3 cycles per run). Anatomical and functional images were co-registered and normalized to the Talairach space [42]. Statistical analysis of fMRI-data was performed by multiple linear regression of the signal time course at each voxel. The expected blood oxygen level-dependent (BOLD) signal change for each event type (predictor) was modeled by a canonical hemodynamic response function (modified gamma function). A random-effects General Linear Model was used to identify associated brain activity in all acquired slices. To balance between type I and type II errors, we tested whether the detected clusters survived a correction for multiple comparisons. We used the approach as implemented in Brain Voyager which is based on a 3D extension of the randomization procedure described by Forman and colleagues [43,44]. First, voxel-level threshold was set at $p < 0.05$ (uncorrected). Threshold maps were then submitted to a correction for multiple comparisons for each contrast. The correction criterion was based on the estimate of the map's spatial smoothness and on a Monte Carlo simulation (1000 iterations) for estimating cluster-level false-positive rates. The minimum cluster size threshold yielding a cluster level false-positive rate of 1% was applied to the statistical maps of each contrast [45]. All clusters reported in this article survived this control of multiple comparisons. Main effects were analyzed for the contrast between pain-related words vs. baseline (hypothesis 1; H1). Separate interaction analyses including the factor Group were performed for the relevant contrasts between word categories according to H2: pain-related (weighted 3 times according to the other word categories) vs. all other word categories (negative, neutral, and positive words) and pain-related vs. negative words. For the comparison between CBP patients and HC, the variance of depression (BDI-II) served as covariate in the General Linear Model.

In the next step, we analyzed correlations between VAS pain ratings after the scanning procedure with the relevant differences of parameter estimates (difference: pain vs. negative) for the group of the CBP patients only (HC were excluded because they had no pain, so there is no variance in these parameters allowing a correlative analysis) according to H3. Voxel-level threshold was set at $p < 0.01$ (uncorrected). The map was submitted to a correction for multiple comparisons (see above). After 1000 iterations, the minimum cluster size threshold yielding a cluster level false-positive rate of 1% was applied to the statistical maps.

3. Results

3.1. Questionnaire and Behavioral Data

Questionnaire data. On average, CBP patients reported significantly higher current pain ratings (M = 1.69, SD = 1.36) than healthy controls (HC) (M = 0.04, SD = 0.14), *Welch's* t (12.25) = 4.34, $p < 0.001$ (Table 1). In addition, total BDI-2 scores of CBP patients (M = 7.77, SD = 5.13) were significantly higher than those of HC (M = 2.62, SD = 1.76), *Welch's* $t(14.78) = 3.424$, $p = .004$ (Table 1). According to BDI-scores, only one patient expressed a clinically meaningful depression (score of 20; [38]). Since results remained essentially unchanged after exclusion of this subject, we kept this subject in all further analyses. BDI showed no linear relationship to VAS ratings for current pain ($r(26) = 0.353$, $p = 0.77$). fMRI group differences were calculated with BDI II values as a covariate. There was no significant difference between groups in pain catastrophizing according to the Pain Catastrophizing Scale (PCS; Table 1).

H1: Behavioral Effects of Group and Word Category

During the experiment, all participants categorized the words properly (M_{CBP} = 15.66 and M_{HC} = 15.45 correct out of 16 judgments, see Table 1). ANOVA results of the differences between CBP patients' and HC subjects' ratings (regarding post-scanning arousal, valence, and pain relevance) of the word categories are depicted in Figure 2.

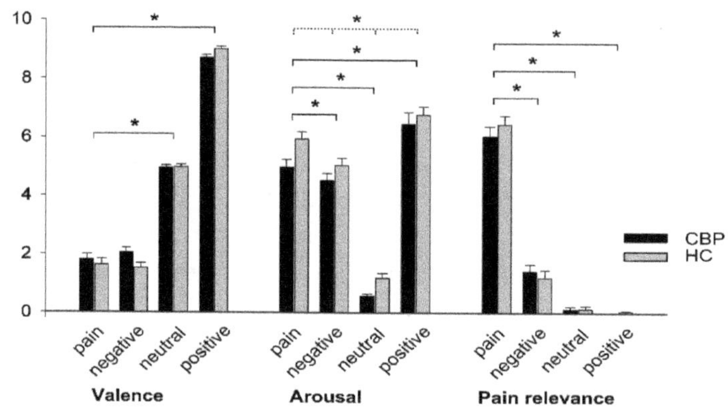

Figure 2. Mean ratings (standard errors) of valence, arousal, and pain relevance of each word category for CBP patients and HC. Valence (0 = "negative"; 10 = "positive"), arousal (0 = "no arousal"; 10 = "maximal arousal"), and pain relevance (0 = "not relevant"; 10 = "highly relevant"). Asterisks (*) indicate significant contrasts of Word Category (black line) and significant main effects of Group (dotted line).

Valence: Valence of word categories was rated differently as indicated by a significant main effect of Word Category ($F_{3, 54} = 940.31$, $p < 0.001$, $\eta^2 = 0.981$). Contrasts were performed by comparing the pain-related word category to the remaining categories: This analysis revealed significant contrasts for neutral vs. pain-related words ($F_{1, 18} = 315.49$, $p < 0.001$, $\eta^2 = 0.946$) and positive vs. pain-related words ($F_{1, 18} = 1803.89$, $p < 0.001$, $\eta^2 = 0.990$). The contrast negative vs. pain-related words were not significant ($F_{1, 18} = 0.139$, $p = 0.714$, $\eta^2 = 0.008$) indicating similar valence of these word categories. No significant main effect of Group ($F_{1, 18} = 494$, $p = 0.491$, $\eta^2 = 0.027$) and no significant interaction of Word Category*Group ($F_{3, 54} = 2.41$, $p = 0.077$, $\eta^2 = 0.118$) was observed on any valence rating.

Arousal: Mauchly's test indicated that the assumption of sphericity was violated for the main effect of Word Category, ($\chi^2(5) = 11.66$, $p = 0.040$). Therefore, degrees of freedom were corrected using the Greenhouse–Geisser estimate of sphericity ($\varepsilon = 0.67$). As expected, there was a significant main effect of the factor Word Category on arousal ratings ($F_{2.02, 36.35} = 181.14$, $p < 0.001$, $\eta^2 = 0.910$), with pain-related words being rated as more arousing than neutral words ($F_{1, 18} = 505.98$, $p < 0.001$, $\eta^2 = 0.966$). A significant contrast was observed for the comparison between pain-related and positive words ($F_{1, 18} = 13.32$, $p = 0.002$, $\eta^2 = 0.425$) as well as between pain-related and negative words ($F_{1, 18} = 11.87$, $p = 0.003$). Likewise, there was a significant main effect of Group on arousal ratings ($F_{1, 18} = 13.26$, $p = 0.002$, $\eta^2 = 0.424$) with CBP patients showing lower arousal ratings than HC. No significant interaction Word Category × Group was observed ($F_{2.02, 36.35} = 0.53$, $p = 0.597$, $\eta^2 = 0.028$).

Pain Relevance: Mauchly's test indicated that the assumption of sphericity was violated for the main effect of Word Category, ($\chi^2(5) = 25.57$, $p < 0.001$). Therefore, degrees of freedom were corrected using Greenhouse–Geisser estimate of sphericity ($\varepsilon = 0.65$). A repeated measure ANOVA confirmed the effect of Word Category on the rating scores of pain relevance ($F_{1.94, 34.85} = 413.15$, $p < 0.001$, $\eta^2 = 0.958$). Contrasts of the factor Word Category confirmed that pain-related words were rated as more pain relevant than negative ($F_{1, 18} = 487.09$, $p < 0.001$, $\eta^2 = 0.947$), neutral ($F_{1, 18} = 763.58$, $p < 0.001$, $\eta^2 = 0.977$), and positive words ($F_{1, 18} = 714.04$, $p < 0.001$, $\eta^2 = 0.975$). There was no significant main effect of Group ($F_{1, 18} = 0.13$, $p = 0.722$, $\eta^2 = 0.007$) and no significant interaction between Word Category × Group ($F_{1.94, 34.85} = 0.83$, $p = 0.440$, $\eta^2 = 0.044$).

There was also no significant main effect of Vividness of Imagination ($F_{3,36} = 1.626$, $p = 0.2$, $\eta^2 = 0.119$) between word categories and no significant interaction Word Category × Group ($F_{3,36} = 0.463$, $p = 0.71$, $\eta^2 = 0.037$). Average vividness ratings for both groups were 5.58 for neutral words, 5.85 for positive words, 5.65 for negative words and 5.19 for pain-related words. Higher ratings are associated with enhanced vividness of imagination. These data show that both groups were similarly able to generate the requested emotive images associated with the presented words.

3.2. Imaging

CBP patients and HC showed activations in a similar network of brain regions in response to viewing pain-related words vs. a fixation cross (baseline). This network includes—among others—the striate and extrastriate cortex of the occipital lobe extending into the fusiform gyrus, widely distributed activations in the frontal lobe bilaterally, bilateral activations of the supplementary motor area (SMA) and pre-SMA, the primary motor cortex (MI) and the anterior cingulate cortex (ACC) (Supplementary Materials Table S1). These activations are in line with previous research [32,34].

3.2.1. H2: Effects of Group and Word Category

The interaction between Group and Word category (pain-related vs. negative words) revealed increased activations in CBP patients in the medial prefrontal cortex (mPFC), the anterior midcingulate cortex (aMCC), and in the dorsolateral prefrontal cortex (DLPFC; Figure 3A and Table 2). These results are in line with H2. For separate main effects of word category (pain-related words versus negative words), see Supplementary Materials Tables S3 and S4.

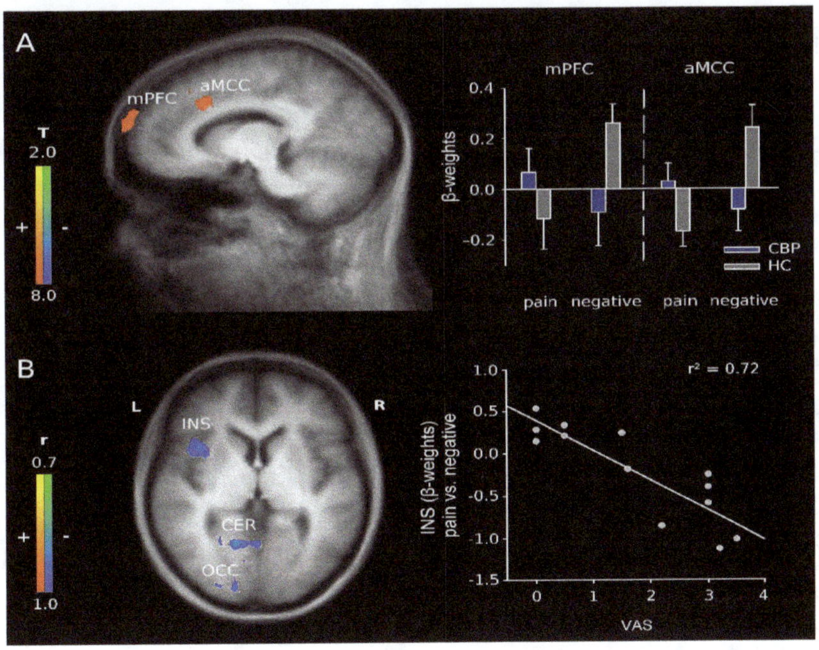

Figure 3. (**A**) activation maps illustrating the interaction between group (CBP patients vs. HC) and word category (pain-related vs. negative adjectives) with activations in the medial prefrontal cortex (mPFC) and anterior midcingular cortex (aMCC) including the dorsolateral prefrontal cortex (DLPFC); x = −10. Right: schematic overview of the β-weights for the aforementioned structures; mean + Standard Error; and (**B**) correlation of current pain (VAS) with the differences in parameter estimates for the contrast pain-related vs. negative adjectives in CBP patients in insula (INS), cerebellum (CER) and occipital cortex (OCC); z = 4. Activations are superimposed on a Talairach template (average of all subjects). Right: correlation plot for the relation of current pain (VAS) and differences in parameter estimates for the contrast pain-related vs. negative adjectives for the anterior insula.

Table 2. Activations to pain-related versus negative words in the comparison between CBP patients and HC.

x	y	z	Cluster Size	*t*-Value	Brain Region	Laterality	Brodmann Area
−20	13	35	76	4.92	anterior cingulate cortex/ dorsolateral prefrontal cortex	R/L	32
−10	−76	64	54	3.97	medial prefrontal cortex	L	10

Listed are clusters of activation with an uncorrected cluster threshold of $p < 0.05$. Talairach coordinates are provided for the maxima of the respective cluster. The corresponding neuroanatomical regions, the Brodmann areas, and the laterality (L, left; R, right) are described.

We also tested the interaction between Group and Word category for pain-related words and all other word categories [32,34]. This comparison revealed activations in the subgenual anterior cingulate cortex (sACC), the MCC, the posterior cingulate cortex (PCC), bilaterally in the posterior insula, the primary somatosensory cortex (SI) and MI, the fusiform gyrus, the posterior parietal cortex, the mPFC, and in the limbic parahippocampal gyrus (Supplementary Materials Table S2). These results confirm H2.

3.2.2. H3: Correlation Analyses of Word Category in CBP Patients

To test whether the current pain affects the processing of adjectives (H3), a correlation analysis between ratings (VAS) of current pain and the differences in activation between pain-related vs. negative words was performed for the group of CBP patients. We found clusters of negatively correlated activity in several regions including MI and the anterior insula (Figure 3B and Table 3).

Table 3. Correlations between current pain ratings (VAS) and the differences in activation between pain-related vs. negative words in CBP patients.

x	y	z	Cluster Size	*r*-Value	Brain Region	Laterality	Brodmann Area
39	13	2	48	−0.83	insula	R	13/44
45	−65	21	56	−0.84	medial temporal cortex	R	39
−16	−62	−11	108	−0.84	cerebellum	L	
5	−87	18	193	−0.88	occipital cortex	R	17/18/23
−43	−15	41	40	−0.90	precentral cortex (MI)	L	4
−4	−77	39	106	−0.91	parietal cortex/occipital cortex	L	19/7
14	−55	−8	211	−0.96	cerebellum	R	19

Listed are clusters of activation with an uncorrected cluster threshold of $p < 0.01$. Talairach coordinates are provided for the maxima of the respective cluster. The corresponding neuroanatomical regions, the Brodmann areas, and the laterality (L, left; R, right) are described.

4. Discussion

The present fMRI study revealed several important results. Firstly, our results support previous findings [32,34] that showed an increase of activation during the processing of pain-related words in several regions of the brain including parts of brain areas that also become activated when exposed to painful stimuli. Secondly, patients suffering from CBP showed stronger activations than HC for pain-related vs. other word categories in several brain structures including the insula and parts of the cingulate cortex. Thirdly, data revealed linear relationships between patients' current pain and brain activations in CBP patients in a variety of brain structures that are known to be involved in the processing of pain. Behavioral data showed only one effect including factor Group, i.e., a main effect of Group on arousal.

4.1. H1: Behavioral Effects of Group and Word Category

Behavioral data show the only effect including factor Group as main effect or interaction for arousal evoked by the different word categories. This effect results from lower arousal ratings in CBP patients compared to HC. There are several reasons that might account for this effect as well as for the absence of significant differences with respect to valence and pain relevance. First, in our sample, CBP patients had relatively low chronic back pain. We discuss this point extensively in Section 4.4 (Study Limitations). Second, ratings of CBP were especially low when the experiment took place. This has previously been reported and might result from distraction and excitement along with the scanning procedure [2,46]. Third, these partly unexpected behavioral results might be due to the permanent exposure to CBP and CBP-related stimuli that the patients suffer from. As a result, habituation to pain-related stimuli may have taken place. Fifth, we also have to take into account that pain-related words were well matched with the other word categories, but they were not specific for CBP; instead, they were referred to pain in general. This might have lowered the impact on our patients specifically suffering from CBP. Nevertheless, there were clear main effects of factor Word Category demonstrating that the expected valence and arousal were specific for each of the word categories. This might serve as a manipulation check of the stimulus material. Moreover, as there were no interaction effects of Word Category × Group on valence, arousal, or pain relevance, these effects could not account for the fMRI results.

4.2. H2: Effects of Group and Word Category

CBP patients showed stronger activations than HC during the processing of pain-related words vs. negative words in the medial prefrontal cortex and in a cluster including the aMCC and the DLPFC. In comparison, HC showed stronger brain activation during the processing of negative words and lower brain activation to pain-related words in these structures. Thus, a general difference in processing of pain-related verbal material was observed in CBP patients. Frontal lobe activity during the experience of pain was regularly observed and is generally linked to attention and cognitive processes [47,48]. The mPFC was found to be activated whenever contextual information was used to guide behavior [49]. This structure additionally exerts top-down pain modulation when cognitively demanding tasks interfere with the pain sensation [12,50–52]. Thus, activity in the mPFC seems to be strongly modulated during expectation of painful events [12]. In the sense of a priming mechanism, the pain-associated adjectives might have pre-activated a network of structures that were associated with the neuromatrix of pain in the past as a larger neural network. Thus, the cluster including the face area of M1 might be pre-activated due to painful facial expressions [53,54] according to current pain. In a broader sense, similar priming effects have also been shown for action verbs and activation of the sensorimotor cortex [55–57]. In the sense of such a priming mechanism and as the mPFC is involved in the recall of recent and remote memory traces [58], we suggest that the processing of painful words is associated with pain-related memories in CBP patients. The DLPFC is known to mediate the cognitive dimension of pain [18,59–62]. In previous studies, a stronger activation of the DLPFC was found in response to pain-related words as well [32,34]. In the present study, the activation in DLPFC is stronger in CBP patients than in HC, presumably, because these patients are prone to perceive pain more frequently and more seriously than HC. Activity of the aMCC has repeatedly been found for the subjective experience of pain [63]. More specifically, the aMCC seems to integrate pain processing and motor function [64,65]. Thus, structures that are commonly activated when CBP patients are exposed to current painful stimuli seem to be equally activated by words that indicate or connote pain.

In line with previous findings [32], the interaction between pain-related and other word categories revealed enhanced activation in several brain regions including sACC, the aMCC, the ventral posterior cingulate gyrus, the fusiform gyrus, the parahippocampal gyrus, and the posterior insula. Most of these brain areas are implicated in the experience of pain. For example, sACC is involved in the processing of emotional aspects of pain [66], but also in the processing of anxiety and stress [67]. The stronger activation of this structure in CBP patients suggests that pain-related words bear an elevated level of emotional salience and increased stress relatively to non-pain-related words of negative valence for CBP sufferers. It thus might be that their attention is more frequently focused on potential painful threats in the environment.

4.3. H3: Relationship to Current Pain

The correlation between current pain (VAS) and differences in activation between pain-related vs. negative words revealed negative correlations in MI and the anterior insula. This is in contrast to our hypothesis H3, i.e., we only found structures where the difference in activation between pain-related and negative words correlated negatively with VAS, but no structure with a positive linear correlation. This result might be due to several reasons. One possible explanation might be that current pain results in a constant activation of these structures. With fMRI, it is not possible to demonstrate this activation as the statistics belong to differences. However, if a pre-activation exists, then the activation of these structures by pain-related words might become less efficient due to pre-activation. Thus, the anterior insula might be pre-activated as a result of current pain due to its significance for the processing of salience information [17,68], which is a core feature of pain [15]. An alternative interpretation might result from the pain-inhibiting pain effect [69,70]. It is well known that two pain stimuli interact by different mechanisms influencing each other [52]. In this sense, chronic pain might result in a lower activation to a pain-related stimulus, even when this stimulus is a pain-related word.

4.4. Study Limitations

One limitation of the present study is its relative small number of participants. Strict inclusion criteria and exact matching of participants' gender and age in both groups made recruitment difficult. However, even in this rather small sample of 13 subjects per group, we revealed significant differences in fMRI activations. Another important limitation of our study is that the CBP patients showed a comparatively low CBP intensity and a relatively low tendency to pain catastrophizing. These characteristics of our CBP patients might result from our inclusion criteria that were already at the advertisement, namely the request not to use any medication (beside contraceptive) 48 h prior to the experiment. This might have deterred more seriously affected CBP patients from participating in our experiment. This limitation is not only important with respect to explaining part of the behavioral results, but it should also be taken into account for the generalizability of the fMRI results. Nevertheless, the magnitudes of pain intensity ratings differed highly significantly from HC. In addition, CBP patients were significantly more depressed than HC, indicating an impairment of everyday life due to chronic pain states. Therefore, in the sense of generalizability, we would expect that our results rather underestimate the effect of CBP. Another limitation is that fMRI group differences were calculated using depression (BDI values) as covariates. Furthermore, our subjects were requested to attend to the presented words and to produce images in their mind with respect to these words. However, we were not able to control whether subjects fulfilled the requests. Future research might investigate whether the present results will remain stable when subjects do not attend or are not requested to imagine related scenes, as well as when CBP patients are more affected than those patients of our sample.

5. Conclusions

In summary, the present results revealed that CBP patients compared to HC show enhanced activations to pain-related words in brain structures commonly activated while processing painful events and while processing words with strong associations to pain. Thus, processing of verbal pain-related information is emphasized and particularly meaningful for chronic pain sufferers. However, as differences in brain activations to verbal expressions of pain vs. negative words became smaller, the stronger the current pain was in the CBP patients. These results are in accordance with the associative network theory [56], indicating a significant and systematic interplay between word and pain processing that is enhanced during chronic pain states.

Acknowledgments: This study was supported by the German Federal Ministry of Education and Research BMBF (01EC1003).

Author Contributions: Thomas Weiss designed the experiment, Alexander Ritter, Thomas Weiss, Marcel Franz, Caroline Dietrich, Christian Puta and Wolfgang H. R. Miltner wrote the manuscript. Alexander Ritter and Marcel Franz analyzed the data.

Abbreviations

The following abbreviations are used in this manuscript:

CBP	chronic back pain
HC	healthy control
fMRI	functional magnetic resonance imaging
BOLD	blood oxygen level-dependent
DLPFC	dorsolateral prefrontal cortex
ERP	event-related potential
VAS	visual analogue scale
NRS	numerical rating scale
mPFC	medial prefrontal cortex
INS	insula
CER	cerebellum
OCC	occipital cortex
SMA	supplementary motor area
MI	primary motor cortex
ACC	anterior cingulate cortex
PCC	posterior cingulate cortex
MCC	midcingular cortex
sACC	subgenual anterior cingulate cortex
aMCC	anterior midcingulate cortex

References

1. Kenntner-Mabiala, R.; Weyers, P.; Pauli, P. Independent effects of emotion and attention on sensory and affective pain perception. *Cogn. Emot.* **2007**, *21*, 1615–1629. [CrossRef]
2. Villemure, C.; Slotnick, B.M.; Bushnell, M.C. Effects of odors on pain perception: Deciphering the roles of emotion and attention. *Pain* **2003**, *106*, 101–108. [CrossRef]
3. Seminowicz, D.A.; Davis, K.D. Interactions of pain intensity and cognitive load: The brain stays on task. *Cereb. Cortex* **2007**, *17*, 1412–1422. [CrossRef] [PubMed]
4. Valet, M.; Sprenger, T.; Boecker, H.; Willoch, F.; Rummeny, E.; Conrad, B.; Erhard, P.; Tolle, T.R. Distraction modulates connectivity of the cingulo-frontal cortex and the midbrain during pain—An FMR1 analysis. *Pain* **2004**, *109*, 399–408. [CrossRef] [PubMed]
5. Loggia, M.L.; Mogil, J.S.; Bushnell, M.C. Empathy hurts: Compassion for another increases both sensory and affective components of pain perception. *Pain* **2008**, *136*, 168–176. [CrossRef] [PubMed]
6. Rainville, P.; Bao, Q.V.H.; Chretien, P. Pain-related emotions modulate experimental pain perception and autonomic responses. *Pain* **2005**, *118*, 306–318. [CrossRef] [PubMed]
7. Godinho, F.; Magnin, M.; Frot, M.; Perchet, C.; Garcia-Larrea, L. Emotional modulation of pain: Is it the sensation or what we recall? *J. Neurosci.* **2006**, *26*, 11454–11461. [CrossRef] [PubMed]
8. Decety, J.; Jackson, P.L.; Brunet, E.; Meltzoff, A.N. Empathy examined through the neural mechanisms involved in imagining how I feel versus how you feel pain. *Neuropsychologia* **2006**, *44*, 752–761.
9. Kenntner-Mabiala, R.; Pauli, P. Affective modulation of brain potentials to painful and nonpainful stimuli. *Psychophysiology* **2005**, *42*, 559–567. [CrossRef] [PubMed]
10. Singer, T.; Seymour, B.; O'Doherty, J.; Kaube, H.; Dolan, R.J.; Frith, C.D. Empathy for pain involves the affective but not sensory components of pain. *Science* **2004**, *303*, 1157–1162. [CrossRef] [PubMed]

11. Coghill, R.C.; Koyama, T.; McHaffie, J.G.; Laurienti, P.J. The subjective experience of pain: Where expectations become reality. *Proc. Natl. Acad. Sci. USA* **2005**, *102*, 12950–12955.
12. Wager, T.D.; Rilling, J.K.; Smith, E.E.; Sokolik, A.; Casey, K.L.; Davidson, R.J.; Kosslyn, S.M.; Rose, R.M.; Cohen, J.D. Placebo-induced changes in fMRI in the anticipation and experience of pain. *Science* **2004**, *303*, 1162–1167. [CrossRef] [PubMed]
13. Miltner, W.H.R.; Braun, C.; Arnold, M.; Witte, H.; Taub, E. Coherence of gamma-band eeg activity as a basis for associative learning. *Nature* **1999**, *397*, 434–436. [CrossRef] [PubMed]
14. Weiss, T.; Miltner, W.H.R.; Dillmann, J. The influence of semantic priming on event-related potentials to painful laser-heat stimuli in migraine patients. *Neurosci. Lett.* **2003**, *340*, 135–138. [CrossRef]
15. Iannetti, G.D.; Hughes, N.P.; Lee, M.C.; Mouraux, A. Determinants of laser-evoked EEG responses: Pain perception or stimulus saliency? *J. Neurophysiol.* **2008**, *100*, 815–828. [CrossRef] [PubMed]
16. Iannetti, G.D.; Mouraux, A. From the neuromatrix to the pain matrix (and back). *Exp. Brain Res.* **2010**, *205*, 1–12. [CrossRef] [PubMed]
17. Legrain, V.; Iannetti, G.D.; Plaghki, L.; Mouraux, A. The pain matrix reloaded: A salience detection system for the body. *Prog. Neurobiol.* **2011**, *93*, 111–124. [CrossRef] [PubMed]
18. Apkarian, A.V.; Bushnell, M.C.; Treede, R.D.; Zubieta, J.K. Human brain mechanisms of pain perception and regulation in health and disease. *Eur. J. Pain* **2005**, *9*, 463–484. [CrossRef] [PubMed]
19. Melzack, R. From the gate to the neuromatrix. *Pain* **1999**, S121–S126. [CrossRef]
20. Bower, G.H. Mood and memory. *Am. Psychol.* **1981**, *36*, 129–148. [CrossRef] [PubMed]
21. Hebb, D.O. *The Organization of Behavior: A Neuropsychological Theory*; Wiley: New York, NY, USA, 1949; p. 335.
22. Dutt-Gupta, J.; Bown, T.; Cyna, A.M. Effect of communication on pain during intravenous cannulation: A randomized controlled trial. *Br. J. Anaesth.* **2007**, *99*, 871–875. [CrossRef] [PubMed]
23. Ott, J.; Aust, S.; Nouri, K.; Promberger, R. An everyday phrase may harm your patients the influence of negative words on pain during venous blood sampling. *Clin. J. Pain* **2012**, *28*, 324–328. [CrossRef] [PubMed]
24. Gu, X.; Han, S. Neural substrates underlying evaluation of pain in actions depicted in words. *Behav. Brain Res.* **2007**, *181*, 218–223. [CrossRef] [PubMed]
25. Osaka, N.; Osaka, M.; Morishita, M.; Kondo, H.; Fukuyama, H. A word expressing affective pain activates the anterior cingulate cortex in the human brain: An fMRI study. *Behav. Brain Res.* **2004**, *153*, 123–127. [CrossRef] [PubMed]
26. Apkarian, A.V.; Sosa, Y.; Sonty, S.; Levy, R.M.; Harden, R.N.; Parrish, T.B.; Gitelman, D.R. Chronic back pain is associated with decreased prefrontal and thalamic gray matter density. *J. Neurosci.* **2004**, *24*, 10410–10415. [CrossRef] [PubMed]
27. Flor, H.; Braun, C.; Elbert, T.; Birbaumer, N. Extensive reorganization of primary somatosensory cortex in chronic back pain patients. *Neurosci. Lett.* **1997**, *224*, 5–8. [CrossRef]
28. Baliki, M.N.; Chialvo, D.R.; Geha, P.Y.; Levy, R.M.; Harden, R.N.; Parrish, T.B.; Apkarian, A.V. Chronic pain and the emotional brain: Specific brain activity associated with spontaneous fluctuations of intensity of chronic back pain. *J. Neurosci.* **2006**, *26*, 12165–12173. [CrossRef] [PubMed]
29. Wand, B.M.; Parkitny, L.; O'Connell, N.E.; Luomajoki, H.; McAuley, J.H.; Thacker, M.; Moseley, G.L. Cortical changes in chronic low back pain: Current state of the art and implications for clinical practice. *Man. Ther.* **2011**, *16*, 15–20. [CrossRef] [PubMed]
30. Siddall, P.J.; Stanwell, P.; Woodhouse, A.; Somorjai, R.L.; Dolenko, B.; Nikulin, A.; Bourne, R.; Himmelreich, U.; Lean, C.; Cousins, M.J.; et al. Magnetic resonance spectroscopy detects biochemical changes in the brain associated with chronic low back pain: A preliminary report. *Anesth. Analg.* **2006**, *102*, 1164–1168. [CrossRef] [PubMed]
31. Lutzenberger, W.; Flor, H.; Birbaumer, N. Enhanced dimensional complexity of the eeg during memory for personal pain in chronic pain patients. *Neurosci. Lett.* **1997**, *226*, 167–170. [CrossRef]
32. Richter, M.; Eck, J.; Straube, T.; Miltner, W.H.R.; Weiss, T. Do words hurt? Brain activation during the processing of pain-related words. *Pain* **2010**, *148*, 198–205. [CrossRef] [PubMed]
33. Simon, D.; Craig, K.D.; Miltner, W.H.R.; Rainville, P. Brain responses to dynamic facial expressions of pain. *Pain* **2006**, *126*, 309–318. [CrossRef] [PubMed]
34. Eck, J.; Richter, M.; Straube, T.; Miltner, W.H.R.; Weiss, T. Affective brain regions are activated during the processing of pain-related words in migraine patients. *Pain* **2011**, *152*, 1104–1113. [CrossRef] [PubMed]

35. Flor, H.; Knost, B.; Birbaumer, N. Processing of pain- and body-related verbal material in chronic pain patients: Central and peripheral correlates. *Pain* **1997**, *73*, 413–421. [CrossRef]
36. Oldfield, R.C. Assessment and analysis of handedness - edinburgh inventory. *Neuropsychologia* **1971**, *9*, 97–113. [CrossRef]
37. Nikendei, C.; Dengler, W.; Wiedemann, G.; Pauli, P. Selective processing of pain-related word stimuli in subclinical depression as indicated by event-related brain potentials. *Biol. Psychol.* **2005**, *70*, 52–60. [CrossRef] [PubMed]
38. Hautzinger, M.; Kühner, C.; Keller, F. *Bdi-ii Beck-Depressions-Inventar*; Harcourt Test Services: Frankfurt, Germany, 2006.
39. Sullivan, M.J.L.; Bishop, S.R.; Pivik, J. The pain catastrophizing scale: Development and validation. *Psychol. Assess.* **1995**, *7*, 524–532. [CrossRef]
40. Meyer, K.; Sprott, H.; Mannion, A.F. Cross-cultural adaptation, reliability, and validity of the german version of the pain catastrophizing scale. *J. Psychosom. Res.* **2008**, *64*, 469–478. [CrossRef] [PubMed]
41. Guy, M.E.; Mccarter, R.E. Scale to measure emotive imagery. *Percept. Mot. Skill* **1978**, *46*, 1267–1274. [CrossRef]
42. Talairach, J.; Tournoux, P. *Coplanar Stereotaxic atlas of the Human Brain*; Thieme: Stuttgart, Germany, 1988.
43. Forman, S.D.; Cohen, J.D.; Fitzgerald, M.; Eddy, W.F.; Mintun, M.A.; Noll, D.C. Improved assessment of significant activation in functional magnetic-resonance-imaging (fmri)—Use of a cluster-size threshold. *Magn. Reson. Med.* **1995**, *33*, 636–647. [CrossRef] [PubMed]
44. Goebel, R.; Esposito, F.; Formisano, E. Analysis of functional image analysis contest (FIAC) data with brainvoyager QX: From single-subject to cortically aligned group general linear model analysis and self-organizing group independent component analysis. *Hum. Brain Mapp.* **2006**, *27*, 392–401. [CrossRef] [PubMed]
45. Straube, T.; Schmidt, S.; Weiss, T.; Mentzel, H.J.; Miltner, W.H.R. Sex differences in brain activation to anticipated and experienced pain in the medial prefrontal cortex. *Hum. Brain Mapp.* **2009**, *30*, 689–698. [CrossRef] [PubMed]
46. Bantick, S.J.; Wise, R.G.; Ploghaus, A.; Clare, S.; Smith, S.M.; Tracey, I. Imaging how attention modulates pain in humans using functional MRI. *Brain* **2002**, *125*, 310–319. [CrossRef] [PubMed]
47. Bornhovd, K.; Quante, M.; Glauche, V.; Bromm, B.; Weiller, C.; Buchel, C. Painful stimuli evoke different stimulus-response functions in the amygdala, prefrontal, insula and somatosensory cortex: A single-trial fMRI study. *Brain* **2002**, *125*, 1326–1336. [CrossRef] [PubMed]
48. Tolle, T.R.; Kaufmann, T.; Siessmeier, T.; Lautenbacher, S.; Berthele, A.; Munz, F.; Zieglgansberger, W.; Willoch, F.; Schwaiger, M.; Conrad, B.; et al. Region-specific encoding of sensory and affective components of pain in the human brain: A positron emission tomography correlation analysis. *Ann. Neurol.* **1999**, *45*, 40–47. [CrossRef]
49. Euston, D.R.; Gruber, A.J.; McNaughton, B.L. The role of medial prefrontal cortex in memory and decision making. *Neuron* **2012**, *76*, 1057–1070. [CrossRef] [PubMed]
50. Bingel, U.; Schoell, E.; Buchel, C. Imaging pain modulation in health and disease. *Curr. Opin. Neurol.* **2007**, *20*, 424–431. [CrossRef] [PubMed]
51. Petrovic, P.; Ingvar, M. Imaging cognitive modulation of pain processing. *Pain* **2002**, *95*, 1–5. [CrossRef]
52. Tracey, I.; Mantyh, P.W. The cerebral signature and its modulation for pain perception. *Neuron* **2007**, *55*, 377–391. [CrossRef] [PubMed]
53. Kunz, M.; Chen, J.I.; Lautenbacher, S.; Vachon-Presseau, E.; Rainville, P. Cerebral regulation of facial expressions of pain. *J. Neurosci.* **2011**, *31*, 8730–8738. [CrossRef] [PubMed]
54. Kunz, M.; Lautenbacher, S.; LeBlanc, N.; Rainville, P. Are both the sensory and the affective dimensions of pain encoded in the face? *Pain* **2012**, *153*, 350–358. [CrossRef] [PubMed]
55. Pulvermuller, F. Brain embodiment of syntax and grammar: Discrete combinatorial mechanisms spelt out in neuronal circuits. *Brain Lang.* **2010**, *112*, 167–179. [CrossRef] [PubMed]
56. Pulvermuller, F.; Fadiga, L. Active perception: Sensorimotor circuits as a cortical basis for language. *Nat. Rev. Neurosci.* **2010**, *11*, 351–360. [CrossRef] [PubMed]
57. Pulvermuller, F. Brain reflections of words and their meaning. *Trends Cogn. Sci.* **2001**, *5*, 517–524. [CrossRef]
58. Hugues, S.; Garcia, R. Reorganization of learning-associated prefrontal synaptic plasticity between the recall of recent and remote fear extinction memory. *Learn. Mem.* **2007**, *14*, 520–524. [CrossRef] [PubMed]

59. Brighina, F.; De Tommaso, M.; Giglia, F.; Scalia, S.; Cosentino, G.; Puma, A.; Panetta, M.; Giglia, G.; Fierro, B. Modulation of pain perception by transcranial magnetic stimulation of left prefrontal cortex. *J. Headache Pain* **2011**, *12*, 185–191. [CrossRef] [PubMed]
60. Lorenz, J.; Minoshima, S.; Casey, K.L. Keeping pain out of mind: The role of the dorsolateral prefrontal cortex in pain modulation. *Brain* **2003**, *126*, 1079–1091. [CrossRef] [PubMed]
61. Ung, H.; Brown, J.E.; Johnson, K.A.; Younger, J.; Hush, J.; Mackey, S. Multivariate classification of structural MRI data detects chronic low back pain. *Cereb. Cortex* **2014**, *24*, 1037–1044. [CrossRef] [PubMed]
62. Bushnell, M.C.; Ceko, M.; Low, L.A. Cognitive and emotional control of pain and its disruption in chronic pain. *Nat. Rev. Neurosci.* **2013**, *14*, 502–511. [CrossRef] [PubMed]
63. Shackman, A.J.; Salomons, T.V.; Slagter, H.A.; Fox, A.S.; Winter, J.J.; Davidson, R.J. The integration of negative affect, pain and cognitive control in the cingulate cortex. *Nat. Rev. Neurosci.* **2011**, *12*, 154–167. [CrossRef] [PubMed]
64. Misra, G.; Coombes, S.A. Neuroimaging evidence of motor control and pain processing in the human midcingulate cortex. *Cereb. Cortex* **2015**, *25*, 1906–1919. [CrossRef] [PubMed]
65. Peyron, R.; Faillenot, I.; Mertens, P.; Laurent, B.; Garcia-Larrea, L. Motor cortex stimulation in neuropathic pain. Correlations between analgesic effect and hemodynamic changes in the brain. A pet study. *Neuroimage* **2007**, *34*, 310–321. [CrossRef] [PubMed]
66. Vogt, B.A. Pain and emotion interactions in subregions of the cingulate gyrus. *Nat. Rev. Neurosci.* **2005**, *6*, 533–544. [CrossRef] [PubMed]
67. Peyron, R.; Laurent, B.; Garcia-Larrea, L. Functional imaging of brain responses to pain. A review and meta-analysis (2000). *Neurophysiol. Clin.* **2000**, *30*, 263–288. [CrossRef]
68. Wiech, K.; Lin, C.S.; Brodersen, K.H.; Bingel, U.; Ploner, M.; Tracey, I. Anterior insula integrates information about salience into perceptual decisions about pain. *J. Neurosci.* **2010**, *30*, 16324–16331. [CrossRef] [PubMed]
69. Diers, M.; Koeppe, C.; Diesch, E.; Stolle, A.M.; Holzl, R.; Schiltenwolf, M.; van Ackern, K.; Flor, H. Central processing of acute muscle pain in chronic low back pain patients: An EEG mapping study. *J. Clin. Neurophysiol.* **2007**, *24*, 76–83. [CrossRef] [PubMed]
70. Reinert, A.; Treede, R.; Bromm, B. The pain inhibiting pain effect: An electrophysiological study in humans. *Brain Res.* **2000**, *862*, 103–110. [CrossRef]

12

Early Changes in Pain Acceptance Predict Pain Outcomes in Interdisciplinary Treatment for Chronic Pain

Thomas Probst [1,*], Robert Jank [1], Nele Dreyer [2], Stefanie Seel [2], Ruth Wagner [3], Klaus Hanshans [3], Renate Reyersbach [3], Andreas Mühlberger [2], Claas Lahmann [4] and Christoph Pieh [1]

1 Department for Psychotherapy and Biopsychosocial Health, Danube University Krems, 3500 Krems, Austria
2 Institute for Psychology, Regensburg University, 93053 Regensburg, Germany
3 Hospital Barmherzige Brüder, 93049 Regensburg, Germany
4 Department of Psychosomatic Medicine and Psychotherapy, University Medical Center Freiburg, Faculty of Medicine, University of Freiburg, 79106 Freiburg, Germany
* Correspondence: thomas.probst@donau-uni.ac.at

Abstract: Studies have shown that pain acceptance is associated with a better pain outcome. The current study explored whether changes in pain acceptance in the very early treatment phase of an interdisciplinary cognitive-behavioral therapy (CBT)-based treatment program for chronic pain predict pain outcomes. A total of 69 patients with chronic, non-malignant pain (at least 6 months) were treated in a day-clinic for four-weeks. Pain acceptance was measured with the Chronic Pain Acceptance Questionnaire (CPAQ), pain outcomes included pain intensity (Numeric Rating Scale, NRS) as well as affective and sensory pain perception (Pain Perception Scale, SES-A and SES-S). Regression analyses controlling for the pre-treatment values of the pain outcomes, age, and gender were performed. Early changes in pain acceptance predicted pain intensity at post-treatment measured with the NRS (B = −0.04 (SE = 0.02); T = −2.28; $p = 0.026$), affective pain perception at post-treatment assessed with the SES-A (B = −0.26 (SE = 0.10); T = −2.79; $p = 0.007$), and sensory pain perception at post-treatment measured with the SES-S (B = −0.19 (SE = 0.08); T = −2.44; $p = 0.017$). Yet, a binary logistic regression analysis revealed that early changes in pain acceptance did not predict clinically relevant pre-post changes in pain intensity (at least 2 points on the NRS). Early changes in pain acceptance were associated with pain outcomes, however, the impact was beneath the threshold defined as clinically relevant.

Keywords: chronic pain; pain acceptance; early change; interdisciplinary pain treatment

---

1. Introduction

Chronic pain (CP) is a serious clinical problem [1]. In the United States, more than 100 million people suffer from CP and the annual costs for the society range between $560 and $635 billion [2]. As the presence of pain affects all aspects of an individual's functioning, an interdisciplinary approach incorporating the knowledge and skills of different healthcare providers is essential [3].

Interdisciplinary treatments for CP are based on the bio-psycho-social model of pain [4]. Such interdisciplinary treatments are conducted by a multi-professional team and address biological factors (e.g., medication, exercise), psychological factors (e.g., cognitions, emotions), as well as social factors (e.g., family, work) [4]. Several studies on CP showed that such interdisciplinary interventions are efficacious in randomized controlled trials [5,6] as well as effective under the conditions of routine care [7,8].

Psychotherapy is a central component in interdisciplinary pain treatments and cognitive-behavioral therapy (CBT) is the most often used [9]. Several meta-analyses and reviews have evaluated the efficacy of CBT for patients with CP [10]. A Cochrane review [11] revealed that CBT had statistically significant but small effects on pain and disability. The effects on mood and catastrophizing were moderate. These effects were compared with treatment-as-usual and wait-list control conditions. An integrative review of Knoerl et al. reported that CBT reduced pain intensity in 43% of the trials [12].

Another psychotherapeutic approach for the treatment of CP is Acceptance and Commitment Therapy (ACT; [13]). Acceptance and Commitment Therapy is a contextual form of CBT. Recent reviews reported that ACT is beneficial for patients with CP [14,15]. The ACT aims at increasing psychological flexibility (PF) and decreasing its counterpart psychological inflexibility [13,16]. While psychological inflexibility is associated with psychological problems or even psychiatric symptoms, PF is defined as the capacity to be in conscious and open contact with one's thoughts and feelings, and to behave according to one's values and goals [17]. Psychological flexibility consists of six core components (acceptance, cognitive defusion, self as a context, committed action, values, contact with the present moment) [18]. In the context of CP, pain acceptance is central to PF. Pain acceptance refers to the degree to which a patient is willing to live with pain or decides to get on with life despite pain. The Chronic Pain Acceptance Questionnaire (CPAQ; [19]) is a psychometrically sound instrument to operationalize pain acceptance and consists of a total scale and the following two subscales: Activity engagement and pain willingness. Activity engagement refers to the performance of personally valued activities, even in the presence of pain. Pain willingness refers to the willingness to give up attempts to control or avoid pain. Several studies on ACT for CP found that improvements in pain acceptance are associated with better pain outcomes [20–22]. Yet, two other studies suggest that pain acceptance is a change mechanism in other treatments as well and no ACT specific treatment process. These studies investigated whether improvements in pain acceptance are correlated with pain outcomes in interdisciplinary CBT-based treatments. Baranoff et al. [23] reported that pre-post improvements in pain acceptance were associated with improvements in almost all outcomes at the end of an interdisciplinary CBT-based treatment for CP. In another study on interdisciplinary CBT-based treatment for CP, Akerblom et al. [9] found that pain acceptance was not related to the outcome pain intensity but that it was the strongest mediator for the other outcome measures. These studies showed that improvements in pain acceptance play a crucial role for pain outcomes in different therapeutic approaches for CP. Baranoff et al. as well as Akerblom et al. assessed pain acceptance at pre-treatment, post-treatment, and at follow-up, but not during the interdisciplinary CBT-based treatment. To extend these previous findings, pain acceptance was monitored during interdisciplinary CBT-based treatment for CP in this project. The aim of the current study was to evaluate whether changes of pain acceptance in the very early treatment phase (first week) predict pain outcomes at post-treatment. We hypothesized that such early changes related to PF are predictors of pain outcomes at post-treatment, since early changes of variables related to psychological inflexibility (e.g., catastrophizing, depression, anxiety) have already been shown to be predictors of changes in pain and interference [24–27].

2. Materials and Method

2.1. Measurements

2.1.1. Pain Acceptance

Pain acceptance was measured with the Chronic Pain Acceptance Questionnaire (CPAQ [19,28]). The CPAQ consists of 20 items and has satisfactorily psychometric properties [19,28,29]. For the present study, only the total score of the CPAQ was analyzed. In the sample of the current study, the internal consistency at pre-treatment was Cronbachs Alpha $\alpha = 0.87$. Higher CPAQ scores indicate higher pain acceptance. Early changes in pain acceptance were operationalized as the difference between the CPAQ scores after the first treatment week and the CPAQ scores at the beginning of treatment. Differences were calculated so that more positive differences indicate more improvements in pain acceptance.

2.1.2. Pain Outcomes

Pain was measured with (1) an 11-point Numerical Rating Scale (NRS) and (2) the Pain Perception Scale. The NRS is a common self-rating instrument to measure pain intensity in patients with CP from 0 (no pain) to 10 (worst imaginable pain). The psychometric properties of the NRS have been investigated in several studies [30,31]. In the current study, self-ratings on average pain intensity were investigated. The Pain Perception Scale (SES) has 28 items and measures affective and sensory pain perception [32]. Both scales showed good internal consistencies in our sample at pre-treatment, with Cronbachs Alpha $\alpha = 0.93$ for the affective pain perception scale (SES-A) and Cronbachs $\alpha = 0.88$ for the sensory pain perception scale (SES-S). The pre-treatment and post-treatment scores of the NRS and SES were analyzed in the current study.

2.2. *Study Sample*

All patients taking part in the interdisciplinary CBT-based treatment for CP at the Hospital Barmherzige Brüder, Regensburg (Germany) between June 2014 and November 2015 were asked to participate in the study. During this time interval, N = 69 patients with CP were treated in a day-clinic setting for four weeks and all of them gave written informed consent to partake in this study. All patients suffered from chronic, non-malignant pain according to the ICD-10 diagnosis "chronic pain disorder with somatic and psychological factors (F45.41)". Of the patients, 36.2% had a comorbid depression diagnosis, 50.7% fulfilled the criteria for at least one comorbid psychiatric disorder.

2.3. *Intervention*

The interdisciplinary treatment was performed according to the pain treatment program "Marburger Schmerzbewältigungsprogramm" [33]. It is a CBT-based program for CP. The patients received treatment for four weeks. Each week treatment lasted from 8:00 a.m. to 4:00 p.m. between Monday and Thursday as well as from 08:00 a.m. to 01:15 p.m. at Friday. The treatment consisted of individual treatment as well as group therapy (closed groups; up to 8 patients per group). The interdisciplinary pain treatment was performed by a team of physicians, psychologists, physical therapists, occupational therapists, and social workers. The CBT component focused mainly on psychoeducation, the bio-psycho-social pain model, relaxation training, and directing the attention towards positive experiences in group sessions and individual sessions. The CBT-based group sessions took part four times per week, and the individual sessions once a week.

2.4. *Statistical Analysis*

All analyses were conducted with SPSS25. To evaluate pre-post changes of pain outcomes (NRS; SES-A; SES-S), we conducted paired t-tests and calculated effect sizes (d) according to the following formula: $(M_{prä} - M_{post})/SD_{prä}$. Effect sizes are interpreted as follows: $d \geq 0.20$ small effect, $d \geq 0.50$ medium effect, $d \geq 0.80$ large effect. Linear regression analyses (method selection "enter") were performed to address the research question whether early changes in pain acceptance predict pain outcomes at post-treatment. One linear regression model was performed for each pain outcome, i.e., either the NRS at post-treatment, or the SES-A at post-treatment, or the SES-S at post-treatment were the dependent variable. As predictors, we added early changes in pain acceptance, the pre-treatment scores of the respective pain outcome variable (to control for pre-treatment values), age, and gender. Moreover, a logistic regression analysis (method selection "enter") was performed to evaluate whether early changes in pain acceptance during the first treatment week predict clinically relevant changes in pain intensity from pre- to post-treatment (≥ 2 points improvement on the NRS from pre- to post-treatment) [34]. The dichotomized NRS (0 = pre-post NRS improvement < 2 points; 1 = pre-post NRS improvement ≥ 2 points) was the dependent variable, and predictors were early changes in pain acceptance, age, and gender. We included age and gender in the regression models, since they have been shown to influence pain outcomes in previous studies [35,36]. Moreover, Pearson correlation coefficients were calculated between the measures at pre-treatment to investigate potential overlap between the measures. The significance level was set at $p < 0.05$ and the statistical tests were performed two-tailed. Missing data were replaced by the average of the time series.

2.5. Ethical Consideration

The Ethics Committee of the University Clinic Regensburg approved the materials and methods for this study. All patients gave written informed consent.

3. Results

The sample comprised N = 69 patients with CP (49 females), who were on average M = 52.62 (standard deviation (SD) = 9.78) years old. The participants gave written informed consent to participate in the study, but during the study, some patients did not fill in the measures or dropped out from treatment. Table 1 shows how many patients filled in the applied measures.

Table 1. Number of patients filling in the questionnaires. N = 69.

Measure	Number of Patients Filling in the Measure N (%)
NRS pre-treatment	66 (96%)
NRS post-treatment	53 (77%)
SES-A pre-treatment	61 (88%)
SES-A post-treatment	52 (75%)
SES-S pre-treatment	62 (90%)
SES-S post-treatment	50 (72%)
CPAQ pre-treatment	52 (75%)
CPAQ after first treatment week	61 (88%)

Note: NRS = Numeric Rating Scale; SES-A = Affective Pain Perception Scale; SES-S = Sensory Pain Perception Scale; CPAQ = Chronic Pain Acceptance Questionnaire.

The correlations between the measures at pre-treatment are presented in Table 2. Pain intensity was positively correlated with affective pain perception (r = 0.56; $p < 0.001$) and with sensory pain perception (r = 0.25; $p = 0.040$). Affective and sensory pain perception were also positively correlated (r = 0.57; $p < 0.001$). Significantly negative correlations emerged between pain intensity and pain acceptance (r = −0.27; $p = 0.025$) as well as between affective pain perception and pain acceptance (r = −0.48; $p < 0.001$).

Table 2. Correlations between the measures at pre-treatment. N = 69.

		SES-A	SES-S	CPAQ
NRS	r	0.56	0.25	−0.27
	p-value	<0.001	0.040	0.025
SES-A	r		0.57	−0.48
	p-value		<0.001	<0.001
SES-S	r			−0.23
	p-value			0.061

Note: NRS = Numeric Rating Scale; SES-A = Affective Pain Perception Scale; SES-S = Sensory Pain Perception Scale.

Results of the analyses evaluating pre-post changes of the pain outcomes are presented in Table 3. Pain intensity improved ($t(68) = 5.82$; $p < 0.001$) with a large effect size of d = 0.81, affective pain perception improved ($t(68) = 4.43$; $p < 0.001$) with a medium effect size of d = 0.60, and sensory pain perception improved ($t(68) = 3.26$; $p = 0.002$) with a small effect size of d = 0.41.

Table 3. Pre–post changes in pain outcomes. N = 69.

	Pre-Treatment M (SD)	Post-Treatment M (SD)	Statistics	Effect Size
Pain intensity (NRS)	6.33 (1.62)	4.97 (1.65)	$t(68) = 5.82; p < 0.001$	d = 0.84
Affective Pain Perception (SES-A)	35.90 (9.60)	30.12 (10.21)	$t(68) = 4.43; p < 0.001$	d = 0.60
Sensory Pain Perception (SES-S)	31.94 (8.64)	28.38 (8.02)	$t(68) = 3.26; p = 0.002$	d = 0.41

Note: NRS = Numeric Rating Scale; SES-A = Affective Pain Perception Scale; SES-S = Sensory Pain Perception Scale; SD = standard deviation.

Three linear regression analysis were conducted to evaluate if early changes in pain acceptance predict the pain outcomes (NRS, SES-A, SES-S) at post-treatment. As can be seen in Table 4, early changes in pain acceptance were negatively correlated with the three pain outcomes. This means that early improvements in pain acceptance were associated with more favorable pain outcomes (i.e., less pain intensity, less affective pain perception, and less sensory pain perception at post-treatment), since higher values on the NRS, SES-A, and SES-S indicate more severe pain, whereas more positive CPAQ difference scores indicate larger early improvements in pain acceptance.

Table 4. Results of the multiple regression analyses testing early changes in pain acceptance as predictors of pain outcomes. N = 69.

	Unstandardized Coefficients B (SE)	Standardized Coefficients Beta	T	*p*-Value
Pain intensity (NRS)				
(Constant)	3.31 (1.21)		2.74	0.008
Early changes in pain acceptance (CPAQ)	−0.04 (0.02)	−0.27	−2.28	0.026
NRS pre-treatment	0.34 (0.12)	0.33	2.81	0.007
Age	−0.01 (0.02)	−0.06	−0.46	0.648
Gender	0.07 (0.43)	0.02	0.17	0.869
Affective Pain Perception (SES-A)				
(Constant)	22.45 (7.03)		3.20	0.002
Early changes in pain acceptance (CPAQ)	−0.26 (0.10)	−0.31	−2.79	0.007
SES-A pre-treatment	0.41 (0.11)	0.38	3.66	0.001
Age	−0.17 (0.11)	−0.16	−1.48	0.145
Gender	1.74 (2.43)	0.08	0.72	0.476
Sensory Pain Perception (SES-S)				
(Constant)	23.53 (6.21)		3.79	<0.001
Early changes in pain acceptance (CPAQ)	−0.19 (0.08)	−0.28	−2.44	0.017
SES-S pre-treatment	0.35 (0.10)	0.38	3.50	0.001
Age	−0.10 (0.09)	−0.12	−1.10	0.276
Gender	−0.53 (1.95)	−0.03	−0.27	0.787

Note: NRS = Numeric Rating Scale; SES-A = Affective Pain Perception Scale; SES-S = Sensory Pain Perception Scale; CPAQ = Chronic Pain Acceptance Questionnaire; SE = standard error.

Outcome pain intensity (NRS): R^2 was 0.17 ($F(4, 64) = 3.34$, $p = 0.015$). Early changes in pain acceptance predicted pain intensity at post-treatment (B = −0.04 (standard error (SE) = 0.02); T = −2.28; $p = 0.026$) when statistically controlling for pain intensity at pre-treatment (B = 0.34 (SE = 0.12); T = 2.81; $p = 0.007$), age (B = −0.01 (SE = 0.02); T = −0.46; $p = 0.648$), and gender (B = 0.07 (SE = 0.43); T = 0.17; $p = 0.869$).

Outcome affective pain perception (SES-A): R^2 reached 0.31 ($F(4, 64) = 7.27$, $p < 0.001$). Affective pain perception at post-treatment was predicted by early changes in pain acceptance (B = −0.26 (SE = 0.10); T = −2.79; $p = 0.007$) when statistically controlling for affective pain perception at pre-treatment (B = 0.41 (SE = 0.11); T = 3.66; $p = 0.001$), age (B = −0.17 (SE = 0.11); T = −1.48; $p = 0.145$), and gender (B = 1.74 (SE = 2.43); T = 0.72; $p = 0.476$).

Outcome sensory pain perception (SES-S): R^2 amounted to 0.27 ($F(4, 64) = 5.91$, $p < 0.001$). When statistically controlling for sensory pain perception at pre-treatment (B = 0.35 (SE = 0.10); T = 3.50; $p = 0.001$), age (B = −0.10 (SE = 0.09); T = −1.10; $p = 0.276$), and gender (B = −0.53 (SE = 1.95); T = −0.27; $p = 0.787$), sensory pain perception at post-treatment was predicted by early changes in pain acceptance (B = −0.19 (SE = 0.08); T = −2.44; $p = 0.017$).

For the outcome pain intensity, we calculated how many patients show a clinically relevant improvement from pre- to post-treatment of at least 2 points on the NRS [34]. N = 31 (45%) improved at least 2 points from pre- to post-treatment and N = 38 (55%) did not. A logistic regression analysis was performed to investigate whether early changes in pain acceptance predict clinically relevant pre-post changes in pain intensity. The results of this logistic regression (−2 Log-Likelihood = 90.77; Cox and Snell R-Quadrat = 0.06; Nagelkerkes R-Quadrat = 0.08) showed that early changes in pain acceptance do not predict clinically significant NRS changes (Exp(B) = 1.04; 95% confidence interval (CI): 0.99; 1.09; $p = 0.157$) when controlling for age (Exp(B) = 1.03; 95% CI: 0.98; 1.09; $p = 0.304$) and gender (Exp(B) = 1.07; 95% CI: 0.36; 3.25; $p = 0.900$).

4. Discussion

This study evaluated whether early changes in pain acceptance predict pain outcomes at the end of an interdisciplinary CBT-based treatment for CP. As pain outcomes, we evaluated pain intensity, affective pain perception, and sensory pain perception. The results showed that early changes in pain acceptance within the first treatment week were associated with less pain intensity, less affective pain perception, and less sensory pain perception at the end of an interdisciplinary pain program. However, clinically relevant changes in pain intensity from pre- to post-treatment were not predicted by early changes in pain acceptance.

Our results extend past research on pain acceptance in interdisciplinary CBT-based treatments for CP [9,23], which showed that changes in pain acceptance are associated with outcomes. Yet, the previous studies did not investigate pain acceptance in the early treatment phase. With regard to the pain outcome pain intensity, our results appear to be in contrast to another study [9] where the outcome pain intensity was not correlated with changes in pain acceptance. One explanation could be that Akerblom et al. [9] analyzed pre-post changes in pain acceptance, whereas we investigated early changes in pain acceptance during the first treatment week. It might be that the outcome pain intensity is predicted by early changes in pain acceptance but not by pre-post changes in pain acceptance. This speculation receives some support from pain studies showing that different predictors of the outcome can be found in the early and late treatment phase [24–27].

When interpreting our results, it should be kept in mind that pain acceptance is no explicit treatment target in CBT-based treatments. We can only speculate about the factors influencing early changes in pain acceptance. Possibly, non-specific common factors like the therapeutic alliance or hope might be associated with early changes in pain acceptance as these common factors have been discussed to play a role in the early phase of psychotherapy [37,38], but this needs to be further studied in the area of pain. It should also be kept in mind that some of the pain outcome measures (NRS, SES-A) were significantly correlated with the pain acceptance measure at pre-treatment. Therefore, the correlation between changes in pain acceptance and changes in pain intensity as well as changes in affective pain perception may be overstated. There are several further shortcomings to discuss. Although the external validity/generalizability of the results is positively influenced by the conditions of routine practice, the following points limit the generalizability. All patients had the ICD-10 diagnosis "chronic pain disorder with somatic and psychological factors (F45.41)" and it remains unclear how early changes in pain acceptance influence pain outcomes in patients with other forms of pain. The representativeness is further reduced by the rather small sample size (N = 69) as well as the relatively large amount of missing data. The sample is, for example, too small for a sound investigation of moderators between early changes in pain acceptance and pain outcomes. Future larger studies could include age and gender as moderators and investigate whether the effect of early changes in pain acceptance on pain outcomes interacts with age and gender. Besides CP, more than half of the patients had various, especially psychiatric diagnoses. Another limitation is that the diagnoses were made by the clinic team, but not with a structured or standardized clinical interview. Due to the naturalistic design we did not calculate a power analysis ahead of the study. We replaced missing data by the average of the time series. This approach leads to an overestimation of the effect compared to replacing missing post-treatment data with the pre-treatment values. Other strategies to handle missing data (e.g., Expectation-Maximization algorithm) might lead to different results. Furthermore, regression analysis does not allow drawing causal inferences and the internal validity of the results is rather low. A randomized controlled trial comparing a condition including a component to increase pain acceptance in the early treatment phase and a condition excluding this component would produce results of higher internal validity. Based on our results, one would expect that pain outcomes are better in the condition with the component to increase pain acceptance in the early treatment phase. A further limitation is that we only included pain acceptance as process variable. The inclusion of more process variables (e.g., pain catastrophizing) would have allowed to investigate whether early changes in one process variable are more or less important predictors of pain outcomes than early changes in other process variables. Another shortcoming is that pain intensity and pain perception were the solely outcomes in the current study and other outcomes such as functioning or patient satisfaction should also be integrated to evaluate treatments for CP [39]. Pain acceptance might also be an important outcome in treatments for CP and we analyzed pain acceptance as a process measure only. Furthermore, our results rely on self-report data and complementary assessments of more objective pain outcomes (e.g., quantitative sensory testing) would be welcome in future studies. Moreover, our definition of early change should be discussed in more detail. We investigated difference scores within the first week to investigate early changes in pain acceptance. The first treatment week might a suitable time frame to study early changes, but other studies defined the change from pre- to mid-treatment [25,26], or the change from pre-treatment to the third treatment week [24,40] as early change. It should also be mentioned that there are several other approaches to operationalize change rate [41] such as deviations from expected recovery curves [40], sudden gains [42] reliable change [43] or the method of percent of improvement [44]. Finally, we only investigated how early changes in pain acceptance influence the short-term outcome at the end of the interdisciplinary treatment for CP, but we do not know how the long-term outcome is predicted by early changes of pain acceptance due to the lack of follow-up assessments.

5. Conclusions

Early changes in pain acceptance are associated with continuous pain outcomes, but not with clinically relevant improvements in pain intensity.

Author Contributions: Conceptualization, T.P. and A.M..; methodology, T.P.; software, T.P., R.J., N.D. and S.S.; validation, A.M., C.L. and C.P.; formal analysis, T.P. and R.J.; investigation, N.D. and S.S.; resources, R.W., K.H., R.R., A.M. and C.P.; data curation, N.D. and S.S.; writing—original draft preparation, T.P. and R.J.; writing—review and editing, T.P. and C.P.; visualization, T.P.; supervision, T.P., A.M., C.L. and C.P.; project administration, T.P., N.D., S.S., R.W., K.H., R.R. and A.M.

Acknowledgments: The data underlying the findings of the study are available from the corresponding author upon request.

References

1. Gereau, R.W.; Sluka, K.A.; Maixner, W.; Savage, S.R.; Price, T.J.; Murinson, B.B.; Sullivan, M.D.; Fillingim, R.B. A pain research agenda for the 21st century. *J. Pain* **2014**, *15*, 1203–1214. [CrossRef] [PubMed]
2. Gaskin, D.J.; Richard, P. The economic costs of pain in the United States. *J. Pain* **2014**, *13*, 715–724. [CrossRef] [PubMed]

3. Interdisciplinary Pain Management. Available online: http://americanpainsociety.org/uploads/about/position-statements/interdisciplinary-white-paper.pdf (accessed on 31 May 2019).
4. Gatchel, R.J.; McGeary, D.D.; McGeary, C.A.; Lippe, B. Interdisciplinary chronic pain management: Past, present, and future. *Am. Psychol.* **2014**, *69*, 119–130. [CrossRef] [PubMed]
5. Kamper, S.J.; Apeldoorn, A.T.; Chiarotto, A.; Smeets, R.J.; Ostelo, R.W.; Guzman, J.; van Tulder, M.W. Multidisciplinary biopsychosocial rehabilitation for chronic low back pain. *Cochrane Database Syst. Rev.* **2014**, *9*, CD000963. [CrossRef] [PubMed]
6. Guzman, J.; Esmail, R.; Karjalainen, K.; Malmivaara, A.; Irvin, E.; Bombardier, C. Multidisciplinary rehabilitation for chronic low back pain: Systematic review. *BMJ* **2001**, *322*, 1511. [CrossRef] [PubMed]
7. Pieh, C.; Neumeier, S.; Loew, T.; Altmeppen, J.; Angerer, M.; Busch, V.; Lahmann, C. Effectiveness of a multimodal treatment program for somatoform pain disorder. *Pain Pract.* **2014**, *14*, E146–E151. [CrossRef] [PubMed]
8. Preis, M.A.; Vogtle, E.; Dreyer, N.; Seel, S.; Wagner, R.; Hanshans, K.; Reyersbach, R.; Pieh, C.; Muhlberger, A.; Probst, T. Long-term outcomes of a multimodal day-clinic treatment for chronic pain under the conditions of routine care. *Pain Res. Manag.* **2018**, *2018*, 9472104. [CrossRef]
9. Akerblom, S.; Perrin, S.; Rivano Fischer, M.; McCracken, L.M. The mediating role of acceptance in multidisciplinary cognitive-behavioral therapy for chronic pain. *J. Pain.* **2015**, *16*, 606–615. [CrossRef]
10. Ehde, D.M.; Dillworth, T.M.; Turner, J.A. Cognitive-behavioral therapy for individuals with chronic pain: Efficacy, innovations, and directions for research. *Am. Psychol.* **2014**, *69*, 153–166. [CrossRef]
11. Williams, A.C.; Eccleston, C.; Morley, S. Psychological therapies for the management of chronic pain (excluding headache) in adults. *Cochrane Database Syst. Rev.* **2012**, *11*, CD007407. [CrossRef]
12. Knoerl, R.; Lavoie Smith, E.M.; Weisberg, J. Chronic pain and cognitive behavioral therapy: An integrative review. *West. J. Nurs. Res.* **2016**, *38*, 596–628. [CrossRef] [PubMed]
13. Hayes, S.C. Acceptance and commitment therapy, relational frame theory, and the third wave of behavioral and cognitive therapies. *Behav. Ther.* **2016**, *47*, 869–885. [CrossRef] [PubMed]
14. Hughes, L.S.; Clark, J.; Colclough, J.A.; Dale, E.; McMillan, D. Acceptance and commitment therapy (ACT) for chronic pain: A systematic review and meta-analyses. *Clin. J. Pain.* **2017**, *33*, 552–568. [CrossRef] [PubMed]
15. Veehof, M.M.; Trompetter, H.R.; Bohlmeijer, E.T.; Schreurs, K.M. Acceptance- and mindfulness-based interventions for the treatment of chronic pain: A meta-analytic review. *Cogn. Behav. Ther.* **2016**, *45*, 5–31. [CrossRef] [PubMed]
16. Hayes, S.C.; Luoma, J.B.; Bond, F.W.; Masuda, A.; Lillis, J. Acceptance and commitment therapy: Model, processes and outcomes. *Behav. Res. Ther.* **2006**, *44*, 1–25. [CrossRef]
17. McCracken, L.M.; Morley, S. The psychological flexibility model: A basis for integration and progress in psychological approaches to chronic pain management. *J. Pain.* **2014**, *15*, 221–234. [CrossRef]
18. Hayes, S.C.; Strosahl, K.D.; Wilson, K.G. *Acceptance and commitment therapy: The Process and Practice of Mindful Change*, 2nd ed.; Guilford Publications: New York, NY, USA, 2011.
19. McCracken, L.M.; Vowles, K.E.; Eccleston, C. Acceptance of chronic pain: Component analysis and a revised assessment method. *Pain* **2004**, *107*, 159–166. [CrossRef]
20. Cederberg, J.T.; Cernvall, M.; Dahl, J.; von Essen, L.; Ljungman, G. Acceptance as a mediator for change in acceptance and commitment therapy for persons with chronic pain? *Int. J. Behav. Med.* **2016**, *23*, 21–29. [CrossRef]
21. Vowles, K.E.; McCracken, L.M. Acceptance and values-based action in chronic pain: A study of treatment effectiveness and process. *J. Consult. Clin. Psychol.* **2008**, *76*, 397–407. [CrossRef]
22. Lin, J.; Klatt, L.I.; McCracken, L.M.; Baumeister, H. Psychological flexibility mediates the effect of an online-based acceptance and commitment therapy for chronic pain: An investigation of change processes. *Pain* **2018**, *159*, 663–672. [CrossRef]
23. Baranoff, J.; Hanrahan, S.J.; Kapur, D.; Connor, J.P. Acceptance as a process variable in relation to catastrophizing in multidisciplinary pain treatment. *Eur. J. Pain.* **2013**, *17*, 101–110. [CrossRef]
24. Bergbom, S.; Boersma, K.; Linton, S.J. Both early and late changes in psychological variables relate to treatment outcome for musculoskeletal pain patients at risk for disability. *Behav. Res. Ther.* **2012**, *50*, 726–734. [CrossRef] [PubMed]

25. Wideman, T.H.; Adams, H.; Sullivan, M.J. A prospective sequential analysis of the fear-avoidance model of pain. *Pain* **2009**, *145*, 45–51. [CrossRef] [PubMed]
26. Burns, J.W.; Glenn, B.; Bruehl, S.; Harden, R.N.; Lofland, K. Cognitive factors influence outcome following multidisciplinary chronic pain treatment: A replication and extension of a cross-lagged panel analysis. *Behav. Res. Ther.* **2003**, *41*, 1163–1182. [CrossRef]
27. Burns, J.W.; Kubilus, A.; Bruehl, S.; Harden, R.N.; Lofland, K. Do changes in cognitive factors influence outcome following multidisciplinary treatment for chronic pain? A cross-lagged panel analysis. *J. Consult. Clin. Psychol.* **2003**, *71*, 81–91. [CrossRef] [PubMed]
28. Nilges, P.; Köster, B.; Schmidt, C.O. Schmerzakzeptanz – Konzept und Überprüfung einer deutschen Fassung des Chronic Pain Acceptance Questionnaire. *Der Schmerz* **2007**, *21*, 57–67. [CrossRef] [PubMed]
29. Reneman, M.F.; Dijkstra, A.; Geertzen, J.H.; Dijkstra, P.U. Psychometric properties of Chronic Pain Acceptance Questionnaires: A systematic review. *Eur. J. Pain* **2010**, *14*, 457–465. [CrossRef]
30. Jensen, M.P.; Turner, J.A.; Romano, J.M.; Fisher, L.D. Comparative reliability and validity of chronic pain intensity measures. *Pain* **1999**, *83*, 157–162. [CrossRef]
31. Ferreira-Valente, M.A.; Pais-Ribeiro, J.L.; Jensen, M.P. Validity of four pain intensity rating scales. *Pain* **2011**, *152*, 2399–2404. [CrossRef]
32. Geissner, E. Die Schmerzempfindungsskala SES–Ein differenziertes und veränderungssensitives Verfahren zur Erfassung chronischer und akuter Schmerzen. *Rehabilitation* **1995**, *34*, 35–43.
33. Basler, H.-D. *Psychologische Therapie bei Kopf- und Rückenschmerzen: Das Marburger Schmerzbewältigungsprogramm zur Gruppen- und Einzeltherapie*, 1st ed.; Quintessenz; MMV, Medizin-Verl.: München, Germany, 1998.
34. Farrar, J.T.; Young, J.P., Jr.; LaMoreaux, L.; Werth, J.L.; Poole, R.M. Clinical importance of changes in chronic pain intensity measured on an 11-point numerical pain rating scale. *Pain* **2001**, *94*, 149–158. [CrossRef]
35. Pieh, C.; Altmeppen, J.; Neumeier, S.; Loew, T.; Angerer, M.; Lahmann, C. Gender differences in outcomes of a multimodal pain management program. *Pain* **2012**, *153*, 197–202. [CrossRef] [PubMed]
36. Buchner, M.; Neubauer, E.; Zahlten-Hinguranage, A.; Schiltenwolf, M. Age as a predicting factor in the therapy outcome of multidisciplinary treatment of patients with chronic low back pain—a prospective longitudinal clinical study in 405 patients. *Clin. Rheumatol.* **2007**, *26*, 385–392. [CrossRef] [PubMed]
37. Lambert, M.J. Early response in psychotherapy: Further evidence for the importance of common factors rather than "placebo effects". *J. Clin. Psychol.* **2005**, *61*, 855–869. [CrossRef] [PubMed]
38. Ilardi, S.S.; Craighead, W.E. The role of nonspecific factors in cognitive-behavior therapy for depression. *Clin. Psychol-Sci. Pr.* **1994**, *1*, 138–155. [CrossRef]
39. Dworkin, R.H.; Turk, D.C.; Farrar, J.T.; Haythornthwaite, J.A.; Jensen, M.P.; Katz, N.P.; Kerns, R.D.; Stucki, G.; Allen, R.R.; Bellamy, N.; et al. Core outcome measures for chronic pain clinical trials: IMMPACT recommendations. *Pain* **2005**, *113*, 9–19. [CrossRef]
40. Haas, E.; Hill, R.D.; Lambert, M.J.; Morrell, B. Do early responders to psychotherapy maintain treatment gains? *J. Clin. Psychol.* **2002**, *58*, 1157–1172. [CrossRef]
41. Erekson, D.M.; Horner, J.; Lambert, M.J. Different lens or different picture? Comparing methods of defining dramatic change in psychotherapy. *Psychother. Res.* **2018**, *28*, 750–760. [CrossRef]
42. Stiles, W.B.; Leach, C.; Barkham, M.; Lucock, M.; Iveson, S.; Shapiro, D.A.; Iveson, M.; Hardy, G.E. Early sudden gains in psychotherapy under routine clinic conditions: Practice-based evidence. *J. Consult. Clin. Psychol.* **2003**, *71*, 14–21. [CrossRef]
43. Kleinstauber, M.; Lambert, M.J.; Hiller, W. Early response in cognitive-behavior therapy for syndromes of medically unexplained symptoms. *BMC Psychiatry* **2017**, *17*, 195. [CrossRef]
44. Hiller, W.; Schindler, A.C.; Lambert, M.J. Defining response and remission in psychotherapy research: A comparison of the RCI and the method of percent improvement. *Psychother. Res.* **2012**, *22*, 1–11. [CrossRef] [PubMed]

13

Mental Health Comorbidities in Pediatric Chronic Pain: A Narrative Review of Epidemiology, Models, Neurobiological Mechanisms and Treatment

Jillian Vinall [1], Maria Pavlova [2], Gordon J. G. Asmundson [3], Nivez Rasic [1] and Melanie Noel [2,4,*]

[1] Department of Anesthesia, University of Calgary, Calgary, AB T3B 6A8, Canada; jillian.vinall@ahs.ca (J.V.); nivez.rasic@ahs.ca (N.R.)
[2] Department of Psychology, University of Calgary, Calgary, AB T2N 1N4, Canada; mpavlova@ucalgary.ca
[3] Department of Psychology, University of Regina, Regina, SK S4S 0A2, Canada; Gordon.Asmundson@uregina.ca
[4] Division of Behaviour and the Developing Brain, Alberta Children's Hospital Research Institute, Calgary, AB T3B 6A8, Canada
* Correspondence: melanie.noel@ucalgary.ca

Academic Editor: Sari A. Acra

Abstract: Chronic pain during childhood and adolescence can lead to persistent pain problems and mental health disorders into adulthood. Posttraumatic stress disorders and depressive and anxiety disorders are mental health conditions that co-occur at high rates in both adolescent and adult samples, and are linked to heightened impairment and disability. Comorbid chronic pain and psychopathology has been explained by the presence of shared neurobiology and mutually maintaining cognitive-affective and behavioral factors that lead to the development and/or maintenance of both conditions. Particularly within the pediatric chronic pain population, these factors are embedded within the broader context of the parent–child relationship. In this review, we will explore the epidemiology of, and current working models explaining, these comorbidities. Particular emphasis will be made on shared neurobiological mechanisms, given that the majority of previous research to date has centered on cognitive, affective, and behavioral mechanisms. Parental contributions to co-occurring chronic pain and psychopathology in childhood and adolescence will be discussed. Moreover, we will review current treatment recommendations and future directions for both research and practice. We argue that the integration of biological and behavioral approaches will be critical to sufficiently address why these comorbidities exist and how they can best be targeted in treatment.

Keywords: chronic pain; posttraumatic stress disorder; anxiety; depression; neurobiology; stress; brain; comorbidity; parent; intervention

1. Introduction

Chronic pain, defined as pain occurring constantly or frequently for 3 months or more, is very prevalent in adolescence [1] and poses high costs to society ($11.8 billion/year) [2]. Poorly managed pain in childhood can lead to persistent pain problems and mental health disorders into adulthood [3,4]. In a longitudinal study, youth with chronic abdominal pain were found to be at greater risk of developing anxiety and depressive disorders as compared to youth without chronic pain [3,5]. Importantly, the risk of anxiety and depressive disorders were higher than controls regardless of whether or not chronic pain persisted into adulthood, suggesting that chronic pain in adolescence heightens the risk of developing mental health disorders, even when pain resolves [5]. Epidemiological research also suggests that youth with chronic pain have higher rates of anxiety disorders in adulthood [4]. This provides compelling evidence that youth with chronic pain are at risk for having and developing mental health conditions. Nevertheless, there remains limited understanding of the mechanisms associated with these comorbid mental health disorders that might impact children's response to pain and pain treatment.

The co-occurrence of chronic pain and mental health conditions (i.e., posttraumatic stress disorder (PTSD)), anxiety and depressive disorders) is high, and has been explained by the presence of shared neurobiology (e.g., genes, hormones, brain networks) and mutually maintaining cognitive (e.g., attention and memory biases) and behavioral (e.g., sleep disturbance) factors that lead to the development and/or maintenance of both conditions [6–8]. However, existing interventions generally fail to effectively target co-morbid mental health disorders and underlying mechanisms that maintain both conditions [9]. It is becoming increasingly clear that there is a need for treatments of pediatric chronic pain to move away from the "one-size-fits-all" approach, which may not sufficiently help a substantial portion of youth with mental health co-morbidities. Indeed, treatment effects for psychological therapies for pediatric chronic pain have generally been small [10], which could be due to heterogeneity within pediatric samples in terms of these underlying mental health conditions. It has been suggested that by increasing our understanding of the genetic and neurobiological mechanisms underlying these comorbidities, we may be able to better predict trajectories of pain and tailor interventional strategies [11]. Moreover, particularly in youth, one cannot underestimate the interaction and influence of the environment (e.g., the parents' influence) on children's pain and mental health conditions.

This review will explore the epidemiology of mental health disorders in pediatric chronic pain populations, and present current working models that have been put forth to explain this comorbidity. Given that the vast majority of work on this topic has emphasized cognitive, affective, and behavioral mechanisms, we will highlight recent research investigating the shared neurobiological mechanisms that may underlie these comorbidities. Parental contributions to comorbid chronic pain and psychopathology in childhood will also be discussed. Finally, we will discuss current treatment recommendations and future directions for both research and practice. Given the high prevalence [1], large economic burden [12], and sometimes debilitating nature of pediatric chronic pain on physical and mental health [13] that can persist into adulthood [4], identifying and modifying mechanisms underlying these conditions has powerful implications for preventing adult-onset chronic pain and mental health disorders.

2. Epidemiology of Internalizing Mental Health Disorders in Pediatric Chronic Pain Population

2.1. Longitudinal Studies of Pediatric Chronic Pain and Internalizing Mental Health Issues in Adulthood

Evidence demonstrating the comorbidity of chronic pain and mental health disorders is accumulating (Table 1). One of the seminal epidemiological studies examining the co-occurrence of pediatric chronic pain and psychiatric disorders was undertaken by Hotopf et al. [5]. The 1946 birth cohort, followed for over two decades examined the relationship between chronic abdominal pain in childhood and medically unexplained symptoms, and mental health disorders in adulthood. They found that while the presence of pediatric abdominal pain was not associated with physical symptoms in adulthood, the risk of developing a psychiatric disorder by the age of 36 years was higher in children who had recurrent abdominal pain versus those who did not [5]. A similar study reported recurrent headaches in childhood to be related to an increased risk of psychiatric morbidity and multiple physical symptoms at the age of 33 years [3]. Despite the reliance on maternal and self-report, and failure to use a conventional definition of chronic pain (e.g., that included pain frequency in addition to pain duration), these studies laid an important foundation for the field of pediatric pain. They provided evidence that while pediatric chronic pain may or may not persist into adulthood, it confers risk of developing mental health disorders in adulthood.

Table 1. Summary of epidemiological studies of internalizing mental health issues in youth with chronic pain.

Study	n	Design	Age (Year)	Assessment Time Points	Pain assessment	Internalizing Disorders/Symptoms Assessment	Findings
Longitudinal studies of pediatric chronic pain and internalizing mental health issues into adulthood							
Egger et al, 1998 [14]	1013	Longitudinal cohort study	5–15	Assessed annually over 3 years	CAPA somatization section	CAPA	40.8% of girls with depression reported headaches as compared to girls without depression (10.5%). 34.1% of girls with an anxiety disorder reported having headaches as compared with girls without an anxiety disorder (10%). 19.2% of boys with CD and 10% of boys with ODD reported having headaches as compared to boys without externalizing disorders (9.6%).
Egger et al, 1999 [15]	3733	Longitudinal cohort study	9–16	Assessed annually over 3 years	CAPA somatization section	CAPA	Girls with stomach aches (OR 7.2, CI 2.8–18.5) and musculoskeletal pain (OR 3.4, CI 1.5–8.0) were more likely to have anxiety as compared to pain-free girls. Boys with stomach aches were likely to have ODD (OR 3.6, CI 1.6–8.1) and ADHD (OR 3.5, CI 1.8–7.1) as compared to boys without stomach aches. Both girls (OR 12.9, CI 4.5–37.0) and boys (OR 10.5, CI 2.3–48.0) with musculoskeletal pain were more likely to report depression compared to children without musculoskeletal pain.
Hotopf et al, 1998 [5]	3637	Longitudinal cohort study	7–36	7, 11, 15 years old	Parent report of abdominal pain at ages 7, 11 and 15 years	N/A	Youth who had abdominal pain were more likely to develop a psychiatric disorder by Time 2 (OR 2.72, CI 1.65–4.49). Pain in childhood was not associated with heightened risk of physical symptoms in adulthood (OR 1.39, CI 0.83–2.36).
				36 years old	Self-report of physical symptoms (back pain, headache, abdominal pain, chest pain, dizziness, and rheumatism)	Semi–structured psychiatric interview (Present State Examination)	
Fearon et al, 2001 [3]	11,407	Longitudinal cohort study	7–33	7, 11, 16, 23 years old	Parent report of headache at ages 7 and 11 (binary variable)	Bristol Social Adjustment Guide	Youth suffering from frequent headaches were more likely to have recurrent headaches in adulthood (OR 2.22, CI 1.62–3.06), physical symptoms (OR 1.75, CI 1.46–2.10), and psychiatric disorders (OR 1.41, CI 1.20–1.66).
				33 years old	Self-report of physical symptoms (back pain, headache, twitches, rheumatism, indigestion, heart racing, worries about health)	Presence of four or more symptoms on a psychiatric morbidity self-report scale	
Walker et al, 2012 [16]	843	Longitudinal cohort study	12–21	12 years old	API, CSI	N/A	At 21 years, participants with High Pain Dysfunctional profile were at a higher risk of having a pain-related FGID (OR 3.45, CI 1.95–6.11), FGID and non-abdominal chronic pain (OR 2.6, CI 1.45–4.66), FGID and anxiety or depressive disorder (OR 2.84, CI 1.35–6.00) as compared with Low Pain Adaptive profile participants.
				21 years old	Rome III, PPQ	ADIS	

Table 1. *Cont.*

Study	*n*	Design	Age (Year)	Assessment Time Points	Pain assessment	Internalizing Disorders/Symptoms Assessment	Findings
Longitudinal studies of pediatric chronic pain and internalizing mental health issues into adulthood							
Shelby et al, 2013 [4]	491	Longitudinal cohort study	8–21	8–17 years old	Vanderbilt Pediatric Gastroenterology Service evaluation of FAP	N/A	At follow-up, participants with FAP were more likely to meet criteria for lifetime (OR 4.9, CI 2.83–7.43) and current (OR 3.57, CI 2.00–6.36) anxiety disorder and lifetime depressive disorder (OR 2.62, CI 1.56–4.40) as compared to controls. Participants with FAP, who developed FGID by follow-up, were more likely to meet criteria for any lifetime (OR 7.31, CI 4.17–12.81) or current (OR 5.09, CI 2.70–9.59) anxiety disorder and any lifetime depressive disorder (OR 4.14, CI 2.31–7.40) as compared to controls. Participants with FAP, who have not met criteria for FGID by follow-up, were still more likely to have any lifetime (OR 3.36, CI 2.01–5.63) or current (OR 2.68, CI 1.44–4.99) anxiety disorder as compared to controls.
				4 years after initial assessment	Rome III	ADIS	
Shanahan et al, 2015 [17]	1420	Longitudinal cohort study	9–26	9–16 years old, assessed 4–7 times	Self- and parent-report of recurrent (at least one one-hour episode at least once a week in the past three months) pain (headache, abdominal or muscle pain)	CAPA	34.4% of children reported somatic complaints. Participants with somatic complaints were more likely to have depressive (OR 6.90, CI 3.57–13.34) or anxiety (OR2.75, CI 1.55–4.89) disorders in childhood versus pain-free peers. Children with somatic complaints in childhood were more likely to develop depressive (OR 3.21, CI 1.54–6.70) or any anxiety disorders (CI 2.32, CI 1.30–4.14) by young adulthood as compared to pain-free participants. Sex differences in the likelihood of developing psychiatric disorders in adulthood following somatic complaints in childhood were not revealed.
				19, 21, 24–26	Recurrent headache binomial variable within the YAPA	YAPA	
Noel et al, 2016 [18]	14,790	Longitudinal cohort study	12–32	Wave I and II: 12–18	Self-report general health survey—frequency of headache, stomach ache, muscle/joints pain. Chronic pain was defined as pain at wave I and/or wave II	N/A	21.9% of participants reported having chronic pain during adolescence. Youth with chronic pain reported higher rates of lifetime depressive (24.5%) and anxiety (21.1%) disorders versus youth without chronic pain. Chronic pain in youth was associated with a greater likelihood of having lifetime anxiety (OR 1.33, CI 1.09–1.63) and depressive (OR 1.38, CI 1.16–1.64) disorders.
				Wave IV: ages 24–32	N/A	Diagnosis of PTSD, anxiety, and/or depression by a health care provider	

Table 1. *Cont.*

Study	n	Design	Age (Year)	Assessment Time Points	Pain assessment	Internalizing Disorders/Symptoms Assessment	Findings
Studies of co-occurring pediatric chronic pain and internalizing mental health issues							
Balottin et al, 2013 [19]	1124	Meta-analysis	Mean ages: 11.6 (migraine), 12.3 (tension-type headache), 11.75 controls	N/A	ICHD I or II	CBCL	Having tension-type headaches was associated with higher internalizing symptoms (Hedge's $g = 2.344$).
Blaauw et al, 2014 [20]	4872	Cross-sectional study	12–17	N/A	Headache interview assessing frequency of migraine, tension-type headache or unclassifiable headache over the last year	SCL-5	Recurrent headache of any type (migraine, tension-type) was associated with anxiety and depression symptoms (at the age of 12–14 years, OR 2.50, CI 1.61–2.61; at the age of 15–17 years, OR 1.64, CI 1.39–1.93).
Coffelt et al, 2013 [21]	3752	Retrospective cohort study	Mean age 13.54	N/A	Hospital record of chronic pain diagnoses (e.g., psychogenic pain not otherwise specified, chronic pain syndrome, complex regional pain syndrome)	Hospital record of a psychiatric diagnosis.	44% of youth with chronic pain have been diagnosed with a psychiatric condition, specifically, an affective (28%), anxiety (18%), somatization (6%) disorder or PTSD (2.4%).
Noel et al, 2016 [22]	195	Cross-sectional study	10–17	N/A	Self-report of pain characteristics (i.e., pain intensity, frequency, location, unpleasantness, and duration over the previous seven days); pain interference sub-scale of the PROMIS-25 Pediatric Profile	CPSS-5	32% of youth with chronic pain reported clinically significant PTSD symptoms as compared to 8% of pain-free peers. Parents of youth with chronic pain had higher levels of clinically significant PTSD symptoms (8%) as compared with parents' of youth without chronic pain (1%). Among the chronic pain group, PTSD symptoms were significantly associated with pain intensity, unpleasantness, interference, and quality of life.
Simons et al, 2012 [23]	655	Retrospective chart review	8–17	N/A	11-point NRS	RCMAS	11% of youth with chronic pain reported clinically significant levels of anxiety, 31% underreported their anxiety levels.
Tegethoff et al, 2015 [24]	6483	Cross-sectional study	13–18 years	N/A	Self-report chronic pain conditions checklist	CIDI; parent-report SAQ	25.93% of youth reported having chronic pain and mental health disorder in their lifetime. Any type or chronic pain increased the risk of developing eating (OR 2.63, CI 1.63–4.24), anxiety (OR 2.42, CI 2.03–2.88), affective (OR 2.32, CI 1.85–2.91), or any mental (OR 2.51, CI 2.12–2.98) disorder. The onset of any mental health disorder preceded any chronic pain (OR 1.64, CI 1.44–1.86).

ADHD: attention-deficit/hyperactivity disorder; ADIS: Anxiety Disorders Interview Schedule-IV, Adult Lifetime and Child and Parent Versions; API: Abdominal pain index; CAPA: Child and Adolescent Psychiatric Assessment; CBCL: Child Behavior Checklist; CD: conduct disorder; CI: confidence interval; CIDI: Composite International Diagnostic interview; CPSS-5: Child PTSD Symptom Scale; CSI: Children's Somatization Inventory; FAP: functional abdominal pain; FGID: functional gastrointestinal disorders; ICHD: International Classification of Headache Disorders; NRS: Numerical Rating Scale; ODD: oppositional defiant disorder; OR: odds ratio; PPQ: Persistent Pain Questionnaire; PROMIS-25: Patient-Reported Outcomes Measurement Information System; PTSD: posttraumatic stress disorder; Rome III: diagnostic questionnaire for functional gastrointestinal disorders; RCMAS: Revised Children's Manifest Anxiety Scale; SAQ: self-administered questionnaire; SCL-5: Symptom Checklist; YAPA: Young Adult Psychiatric Assessment.

Building upon these previous epidemiological studies, Walker et al. [16] conducted a longitudinal study of youth diagnosed with chronic abdominal pain followed into adulthood, at which time their pain and mental health status was assessed. The authors used cluster analysis to categorize youth with persistent abdominal pain into three groups based on pain ratings, gastrointestinal and non-gastrointestinal symptoms, beliefs about pain threat, pain coping efficacy, pain catastrophizing, negative affect and functional disability assessed in adolescence (i.e., Low Pain Adaptive, High Pain Adaptive, and High Pain Dysfunctional) [16]. Follow-up clinical interviews at the mean age of 21 years revealed that high pain ratings in conjunction with poorer coping skills and psychological functioning (i.e., characteristic of the High Pain Dysfunctional group) were associated with higher risk of developing functional gastrointestinal disorder (FGID) and non-abdominal chronic pain in adulthood [16]. The odds of having an anxiety or depressive disorder comorbid with FGID in adulthood were significantly higher only in the High Pain Dysfunctional group [16]. These findings provided further evidence of reciprocal relationships between pediatric chronic pain and mental health disorders. This study demonstrated for the first time that it is not pain per se but, rather, the combination of pain and psychological functioning that predicts the co-occurrence of pain and mental health disorders into adulthood. In a second investigation, Shelby et al. [4] examined the same cohort of youth with functional abdominal pain (FAP), as well as a pain-free controls whose mental health was assessed in adulthood. Fifty-one percent of youth with a childhood history of FAP developed an anxiety disorder over their lifetime, and 30% of youth had a current anxiety disorder at follow-up [4]. Depressive symptoms followed a different pattern; lifetime, but not current, risk of developing a depressive disorder was higher for individuals with chronic abdominal pain in childhood [4]. Risk of developing anxiety or depressive disorders was heightened for youth with chronic pain (versus controls) even when their pain resolved by adulthood. Temporal associations (based on retrospective recall) between mental health status and chronic pain suggested that anxiety disorders preceded the onset of chronic pain, whereas a depressive disorder followed it [4].

Recent data from a cohort study found that in a sample of 1420 youth, somatic complaints during childhood predicted generalized anxiety and depressive disorders at the age of 19–26 years [17]. Findings of the most recent epidemiological study by Noel et al. [18] revealed a consistent pattern. The study conducted a secondary data analysis of a sample of 14,790 individuals from the National Longitudinal Study of Adolescent to Adult Health to examine the co-occurrence of adolescent chronic pain and lifetime rates of mental health disorders [18]. In contrast to previous research, a broader range of chronic pain conditions (i.e., headache, abdominal and musculoskeletal pain) were assessed in adolescence, and lifetime history of mental health disorders (i.e., depressive and anxiety disorders) were subsequently assessed in adulthood. Individuals with, versus without, chronic pain in adolescence subsequently reported significantly higher lifetime rates of anxiety (21.1%) and depressive (24.5%) disorders [18]. After controlling for established confounding factors (e.g., age, sex, insufficient sleep, general health), chronic pain in adolescence was associated with a greater likelihood of having anxiety (odds ratio (OR) 1.33) and depressive (OR 1.38) disorders over the lifetime [18].

2.2. Co-Occurrence of Pediatric Chronic Pain and Internalizing Mental Health Issues

Other studies have focused on establishing concurrent rates of mental health disorders and chronic pain status in youth. Coffelt et al. [21] analyzed retrospective data from 3752 youth admitted with a primary diagnosis of chronic pain. Forty-four percent of adolescents had a comorbid mental health condition [21]. The diagnoses included mood disorders (28%), anxiety disorders (18%), conversion and somatization disorders (6%), and PTSD (2.4%) [21]. Simons et al. [23] also investigated the prevalence of anxiety symptoms in a large sample of youth with chronic pain. While only 11% of the participants reported clinically significant levels of total anxiety, 31% may have underreported their anxiety symptoms given their heightened scores on a social desirability scale [23]. Children with diffuse pain reported significantly higher levels of anxiety as compared to youth with musculoskeletal, abdominal or neuropathic pain [23]. Recently, Noel et al. [25] compared prevalence of PTSD symptoms in a sample of youth with chronic pain and their parents to pain-free peers. Findings revealed significantly higher levels of PTSD symptoms (including clinically significant symptoms) in youth with chronic pain and their parents [25].

Similar patterns of co-occurring pain and mental health disorders were found among youth with chronic headaches. In a large sample of youth, recurrent headaches were positively related to higher levels of anxiety and depressive symptoms across two broad age groups (12–14 years, OR 2.05; 15–17 years, OR 1.64) [20]. These results are consistent with those of a meta-analysis of mental health conditions in pediatric headache populations, which revealed higher levels of psychopathology symptoms in children and adolescents with headache as compared to healthy controls [19]. Tension-type headaches were associated with higher internalizing symptoms, which included anxiety and depressive symptoms, withdrawal and somatic complaints [19]. A meta-analysis of FAP revealed that levels of concurrent anxiety, depression and psychological distress were significantly higher in youth with FAP as compared to pain-free youth [26].

The co-occurrence of pediatric chronic pain and mental health disorders has been shown to differ by child sex [14,27]. In a representative sample of 3733 youth, abdominal pain and headaches were associated with co-occurring anxiety disorders in girls, but not boys [27]. Musculoskeletal pain exhibited a similar pattern, showing a strong association with anxiety disorders in girls, but not boys [27]. Conversely, boys were more likely than girls to develop externalizing mental health disorders comorbid with recurrent abdominal pain [14,27]. Both girls and boys were at risk for developing depression in the presence of musculoskeletal pains [27].

In addition to establishing prevalence rates of pediatric chronic pain and mental disorders, Tegethoff et al. [24] sought to determine the temporal primacy of each condition using structured clinical interviews assessing mental health disorders, parental reports of youth mental health disorders and adolescent self-reports of chronic pain in a sample of 6000 youth. More than a quarter of youth reported having both a mental health disorder and chronic pain in their lifetime [24]. Most youth who experienced any type of chronic pain (i.e., back/neck pain, headache, or other chronic pain) reported having an anxiety disorder (17.4%) and an affective disorder (10.06%) [24]. Having experienced any type of chronic pain increased the risk of developing anxiety (OR 2.42), eating (OR 2.63) and depressive (OR 2.32) disorders [24]. Temporal associations (albeit assessed via retrospective report) were reported between the onset of mental health disorders in childhood and the subsequent onset of chronic pain. There were no significant temporal associations between the preceding onset of chronic pain and the subsequent onset of psychological disorders later in life.

Taken together, the available literature demonstrates high levels of co-occurrence of pediatric chronic pain and mental health disorders and symptoms. A major limitation of much of the epidemiological work to date has been the suboptimal assessment of pain. Indeed, chronic or recurrent pain status has often been limited to a single binary question that fails to capture crucial aspects of chronic pain assessment, such as pain frequency, distress due to pain, and pain interference or disability. Moreover, over-reliance on retrospective self-report of symptoms has precluded reliable conclusions about risk and temporal relationships between the onset of chronic pain and mental health issues. The few studies examining temporality suggest that anxiety issues may indeed precede the development of chronic pain; however, rigorous prospective research is needed. Arguably the most striking finding from this body of research is that, irrespective of whether or not pediatric chronic pain resolves by adulthood, the long-term risk for developing mental health disorders remains. This has important clinical implications and suggests that treatments for chronic pain that only target pain, may not be sufficient for interrupting a trajectory of illness into adulthood.

3. Models of Chronic Pain and Comorbid Anxiety, Depression and PTSD

Several models have been proposed to understand the mechanisms underlying comorbidities between various mental health disorders and chronic pain in adults. Sharp and Harvey's mutual maintenance model accounted for seven mechanisms through which PTSD and chronic pain might mutually maintain each other [8]. They proposed that cognitive (e.g., attentional biases), affective (e.g., depression) and behavioral (e.g., reduced activity levels) factors, characteristic of chronic pain, serve to exacerbate PTSD symptoms. Similarly, physiological (e.g., heightened alarm response to trauma reminder), affective (e.g., negative alterations on mood and cognitions) and behavioral (e.g., avoidance) aspects of PTSD contribute to the exacerbation of chronic pain [8]. The model, however, does not account for potential causal connections between those factors.

Liedl et al. [28] subsequently proposed the Perpetual Avoidance Model (PAM). The authors posited that trauma catalyzes dysfunctional cognitions and sensations of intrusion which lead to heightened arousal [28]. The role of hyperarousal is thought to be two-fold: it promotes avoidance behaviors that feed into PTSD-related dysfunctional cognitions and it amplifies pain sensations [28]. Intensified pain sensations further drive pain-related cognitions (e.g., catastrophizing, fear-avoidance beliefs), in turn, promoting avoidance of pain-inducing activities [28]. Avoidance (an element shared with PTSD) further intensifies pain sensations [28]. Hence, individuals get trapped in a cycle of perpetual avoidance that serves to maintain both PTSD and chronic pain. The PAM assumes no direct relationship between an inciting traumatic event and chronic pain. The pain model by Norman et al. [29] postulates that pain drives PTSD onset, whereas PTSD does not contribute to pain maintenance. Brown et al. [30] used structural equation modelling to test three theoretical models with a pediatric population (i.e., the PAM, mutual maintenance model, and the pain model). The authors used diagnostic interviews to assess PTSD and self-report to assess physical pain in a clinical sample of youth with traumatic brain injuries (TBIs) 3, 6 and 18 months after their injuries [30]. Sharp and Harvey's model fit the acquired data significantly better as compared to the Norman et al. pain model. The PAM did not differ significantly in terms of fit as compared to Sharp and Harvey's model, suggesting equally good fit [30]. The authors concluded that PTSD drives the presence of physical pain in this particular pediatric population.

Sharp and Harvey's mutual maintenance model was later expanded to distinguish between mutual maintaining versus shared vulnerability factors, the latter of which serve to precipitate both conditions [7]. The shared vulnerability model postulates that certain psychological symptom clusters (e.g., anxiety sensitivity) and physiological factors (e.g., lower alarm threshold) can precipitate the emergence of both chronic pain and PTSD and be causally related to cognitive and behavioral mechanisms [6,7]. Moreover, the model posits that the conditions only develop when an individual with such a diathesis is exposed to a traumatic life event [7]. Trauma initiates a diathesis-amplified psychological response that includes maladaptive levels of fear and anxiety, and results in an array of detrimental behavioral (e.g., avoidance), cognitive (e.g., hypervigilance) and physiological (e.g., autonomic nervous system responsivity) consequences [7]. These consequences, which are thought to be bi-directionally related, account for the development of PTSD, chronic pain and/or both comorbidities [7]. The shared vulnerability model is the first model to include anxiety disorders, in addition to PTSD. Just as symptoms of mental health disorders (e.g., physiological arousal in anxiety, lack of positive emotions in anxiety or anhedonia in depression) may intensify pain symptoms [7], pain-related cognitive biases, physiological responses and maladaptive behaviors may serve to aggravate symptoms of mental health disorders [7]. It is, therefore, likely that mental health conditions and chronic pain share certain predisposing factors that form a common diathesis.

Until only recently, existing models of co-occurring mental health disorders and chronic pain were specific to adults. In a recent topical review, Holley et al. [31] proposed a new pediatric model of PTSD and chronic pain comorbidity in youth. Central to this model are shared vulnerability and mutually maintaining factors that are thought to influence PTSD, chronic pain and the disorders' comorbidity in bi-directional ways. While many of the proposed factors are similar to those covered in the previous models (e.g., anxiety sensitivity, avoidance, hyperarousal), the authors drew evidence from pediatric research, confirming the important roles that these factors play in pain and mental health trajectories in childhood and adolescence [31]. Unique to this model is the integration of individual (e.g., trauma and pain-related variables), interpersonal (e.g., parent traumatic stress, peer victimization) and neurobiological (e.g., PTSD and pain influences on the developing brain) factors, all couched within a developmental context [31]. At all levels, PTSD and pain symptomatology are thought to reciprocally influence one another. For instance, catastrophic thoughts about pain in youth may lead to behavioral avoidance, and similar cognitions in parents may serve to exacerbate these cognitions and behaviors in their child [31]. Likewise, depressive symptoms characteristic of chronic pain and PTSD might be aggravated or even induced by peer difficulties and social isolation that are also commonly found in both conditions [31]. Overall, the proposed model fills a gap in the literature by being the first to integrate evidence from the pediatric PTSD and pain literatures, and positing developmentally relevant mechanisms that might underlie and serve to maintain both conditions in youth.

4. Potential Neurobiological Mechanisms Underlying Comorbid Chronic Pain and Anxiety, Depression or PTSD

As outlined in some of the models previously described (e.g., [6,7,31]), shared neurobiology of chronic pain and mental health conditions may in part explain the high co-occurrence of these disorders. Nevertheless, biological underpinnings of comorbidity have largely been overlooked relative to cognitive, affective and behavioral factors. There is accumulating evidence to suggest that genes, hormones and neural networks contribute to both the predisposition and maintenance of, chronic pain, PTSD, anxiety and depressive disorders. The following will provide a brief overview of some of the neurobiological factors that may underlie chronic pain and these associated mental health conditions. Presently, there are a limited number of studies that have examined mechanisms contributing to the development and maintenance of pediatric chronic pain and comorbid internalizing mental health issues. Therefore, in this particular section of the review, where there is an absence of child research, we draw from adult and animal literatures. We acknowledge that work in this area is preliminary. It is important that future research further investigate these factors and their developmental specificity to children and adolescents, so that interventions can be developed to effectively target the underlying mechanisms that maintain these conditions during the pediatric period.

4.1. The Hypothalamic–Pituitary–Adrenal Axis

Both stress and pain incite a cascade of neurobiological events, leading to the activation of the hypothalamic–pituitary–adrenal (HPA) axis and production of stress hormones (glucocorticoids (cortisol in humans)), which regulate the transcription of genes [32]. The process through which cortisol is secreted begins with the activation of the hypothalamus. This leads to the co-release of hormones [33–36] that stimulate the synthesis and release of adrenocorticotropin (ACTH) from the anterior pituitary gland. ACTH secretion influences the release of glucocorticoids from the adrenal cortex into general circulation [33–36]. Cortisol binds with glucocorticoid receptors in the hypothalamus, hippocampus and other brain regions to inhibit further production of cortisol (negative feedback) [33,34]. However, early and/or prolonged exposure to stress and/or pain can disrupt this cortisol feedback loop. Individuals with chronic pain often demonstrate HPA dysfunction [37,38], including altered glucocorticoid negative feedback [39,40] and abnormal cortisol levels [41–44]. Similarly, co-occurring stress-related mental health conditions (PTSD, anxiety and depressive disorders) are also associated with disruptions to the HPA axis [45–47].

Priming of the HPA axis begins in utero. Prenatal exposure to stress hormones leads to greater stress responses in adults, by reducing glucocorticoid receptors in the hippocampus [48,49]. Fewer glucocorticoid receptors in the hippocampus, leads to poorer negative feedback, and greater anxiety-related behavior during adulthood [48,49]. The postnatal environment also has considerable influence on the programming of the HPA axis. Natural variations in maternal behavior, such as the amount a rat licks and grooms their pups in the first week of life [50], incites a cascade of serotonin-mediated changes affecting hippocampal glucocorticoid receptor expression [51–57]. Adult offspring of low licking and grooming rat mothers showed reduced hippocampal glucocorticoid receptor expression, poorer glucocorticoid feedback sensitivity, and greater glucocorticoid production in comparison to pups reared by high licking and grooming mothers [52,53]. These changes in physiology are related to alterations in behavior as adults. Offspring of low licking and grooming mothers show greater anxiety-like behavior and alterations in cognitive functioning during adulthood [51,55,58–60], factors commonly associated with chronic pain [7]. Comparable disruption of cortisol reactivity in response to maternal behavior has been observed in humans. Early disruptions in the parent–child relationship have been associated with increased levels of cortisol in preschoolers [61]. Moreover, these heighted glucocorticoid responses were associated with increased behavioral and emotional problems both at school-age and adulthood [61,62]. Therefore, normal variations in early life experience and parent–child interactions can subsequently alter stress reactivity and behavior; this may contribute to the vulnerability and or mutual maintenance of psychopathology and chronic pain [7].

Cumulative life trauma also influences the development of chronic pain and psychopathology [63–65], which may, in part, be explained by dysregulation of the HPA axis. Youth with chronic pain report having a greater number of stressful life events compared to those without chronic pain, and cumulative trauma was associated with higher PTSD symptoms [25]. The timing and duration of traumatic events appears to largely influence glucocorticoid and behavioral responses to trauma. Both in humans and animals, prolonged pain and distress appears to be associated with a dampening of cortisol responses, in contrast to acute stressors that are associated with hyper-secretion of cortisol [52,53,66–70]. For example, among rhesus monkeys during the first month of life, when abuse is most prevalent, abused infants had elevated plasma cortisol levels as compared to non-abused infants [71]. However, by 6 months of age, the monkeys exhibited lower basal cortisol levels and attenuated ACTH to corticotropin-releasing factor (CRF) compared to control monkeys [71]. In humans, children who experienced abuse in their home environments, showed enhanced ACTH responses and normal cortisol levels [72]. However, adult survivors of childhood abuse or those with PTSD demonstrate lower ACTH responses following CRF injections [73]. Moreover, in a sample of youth exposed to interpersonal violence, if the trauma occurred in the last year of assessment, higher levels of salivary cortisol were positively associated with PTSD [74]. Conversely, in individuals with traumas exceeding a year prior to assessment, PTSD symptoms were associated lower levels of cortisol [74]. Ultimately, previous and/or prolonged physiological arousal associated with stress initiated by exposure to the threat of or actual death, serious injury, or violence can have detrimental effects on activation of neural and hormonal processes, and may contribute to the development of chronic pain and mental health disorders. This research also suggests that timing of exposure to traumatic/stressful events as well as assessment can influence the patterns of activation found.

Therefore, prolonged activation of the HPA axis may lead to stress-related conditions as chronic pain, PTSD, anxiety and depressive disorders. At this time, the mechanisms underlying the relationships between chronic pain and mental health conditions have not been well characterized. However, given the widespread actions of cortisol on multiple neurobiological systems, prolonged exposure to glucocorticoids may lead to changes in gene expression, the immune system and to the developing brain, thereby increasing the vulnerability and maintenance of these conditions.

4.2. Serotonin

Serotonin (5-hydroxytryptamine (5-HT)) is a widely distributed neurotransmitter that is a key modulator of stress responses (i.e., HPA axis) [75,76]. It is also an important molecule for pain processing, and is centrally involved in chronic pain states [77,78]. Previous studies have shown that individuals with chronic pain have decreased levels of 5-HT in their serum and cerebrospinal fluid [79,80]. This led to an investigation as to whether variants of 5-HT genes were associated with increased risk of developing chronic pain. One of the major 5HT receptor subtypes is the serotonin 2A receptor (5-HT2AR). It was found that following nerve injury, 5-HT2AR promotes spinal hyper-excitation and impairs spinal μ-opioid mechanisms, thereby contributing to the development of mechanical allodynia [81]. Using 2 population-based cohorts, Nicholl et al. [82] were able to demonstrate for the first time that single-nucleotide polymorphisms (SNP) of the 5-HT2AR gene were associated with musculoskeletal pain in adult males, even after adjustment for symptoms of depressive disorders. Therefore, 5-HT availability appears to have a role in the development of chronic pain conditions. Central to the reuptake of 5-HT is the transporter protein (5-HTT). Genetic variants of the transporter promoter region (5-HTTLPR) play a critical role in determining intra-synaptic 5-HT signaling [83]. In humans it has been found that the short (S) allele of 5-HTTLPR results in ~50% reduction in 5-HT reuptake compared to the long (L) allele [84]. The S allele has been found to increase the risk of chronic pain [85,86]. Chronic pain patients with the S allele also demonstrated higher levels of anxiety and depressive disorders [85]. It has been theorized that the inability for rapid 5-HT clearance from the synaptic cleft may result in serotonin 1A receptor (5-HT1A) subtype negative feedback, causing an overall decreased in 5-HT neurotransmission for individuals with the S allele [85]. Converging evidence from both human and nonhuman primates suggests that S allele carriers may also have greater vulnerability for anxiety and depressive disorders [87]. Indeed, a recent meta-analysis found a significant association between 5-HTTLPR genotype and HPA-axis reactivity to acute psychosocial stress, with homozygous carriers of the S allele displaying increased stress hormone reactivity compared with individuals with the S/L and L/L genotype [88]. The 5-HTTLPR genotype also modulates brain activation during emotional processing tasks [89,90]. Human adult functional magnetic resonance imaging (fMRI) studies have found consistent associations between the short allele and greater amygdala reactivity to aversive versus neutral stimuli [91,92]. This is important given that the amygdala plays a key role in activating the HPA axis. Altogether, it would appear that 5-HT availability modifies brain responses and predisposes individuals to developing chronic pain and/or mental health conditions.

4.3. *Brain-Derived Neurotrophic Factor*

Serotonin interacts closely with brain-derived neurotrophic factor (BDNF), a neurotrophin that is widely expressed in stress-related brain regions (e.g., prefrontal cortex and hippocampus) and is intrinsic to neurogenesis and synaptogenesis [93]. Both human and animal studies have demonstrated that stress hormones modify BDNF expression, such that there is decreased BDNF expression in the hippocampus and increased expression in the amygdala [94–96]. This finding is consistent with recent neuroimaging studies, which have reported significant loss in hippocampal neuroconnectivity with the medial prefrontal cortex [97], and exaggerated amygdalar connectivity with the central executive network (dorsolateral prefrontal cortex and posterior parietal cortex) in individuals with chronic pain compared to healthy controls [98]. Therefore, genetically determined BDNF availability may modify brain connections contributing to the development and maintenance of chronic pain conditions. To that effect, it has been shown that induced chronic inflammatory pain dampens hippocampal *BDNF* gene expression in rats [99]. Deletion of *BDNF* also produces chronic pain and depressive-like behavior in mice [100], and stimulators of BDNF synthesis have been shown to have an analgesic effect and reduce depression-like behavior in rats with chronic pain [101]. Similar to 5-HT, there are variants of *BDNF*, which are important determinants of intracellular processing and secretion [102]. Unlike Val66Met (rs6265), the 66Met allele results in lower BDNF availability, and is associated with alterations of human hippocampal function [103]. Both human and mouse 66Met allele carriers have been shown to have smaller bilateral hippocampi, in addition to lower gray mater volumes (e.g., prefrontal cortex), and reduced white matter tract integrity when compared to 66Val homozygote controls [104–110]. Furthermore, adult human and rat studies have shown that 66Met carriers may be at higher risk for developing chronic pain, PTSD, anxiety and depressive disorders [111–119]. Therefore, stress-regulated *BDNF* may be another mechanism through which genes may increase susceptibility to chronic pain and comorbid mental health conditions.

4.4. Inflammation

Another important factor to consider in the co-occurrence of chronic pain and mental health disorders is the effect that chronic pain and stress can have on immune function. Injury leads to the activation of microglia in the dorsal horn of the spinal cord, which results in the release of cytokines and growth factors that excite nociceptive dorsal horn neurons, contributing to the development of central sensitization and hyperalgesia [120] as well as the pathogenesis of chronic pain [121,122]. It is important to note that chronic inflammatory processes are not specific to pain (e.g., autoimmune diseases, aging) [123,124] and may arise from acute immune challenges [125]. Therefore, other conditions that incite neuro-inflammatory responses may also lead to chronic pain and comorbid conditions. Post-mortem immunohistochemical studies of the spinal cord in patients with complex regional pain syndrome [126] and human immunodeficiency virus-related neuropathic pain [127], and cerebral spinal fluid sampling of patients with fibromyalgia and chronic low back pain [128,129], have provided support for the involvement of glia in the pathogenesis of chronic pain. A recent study using positron emission tomography–magnetic resonance imaging showed for the first time, in vivo, that the occurrence of glial activation, as measured by an increase in [^{11}C]PBR28 binding, was greater in the thalamus of patients with chronic pain as compared to controls [130]. Preclinical research involving nerve injury models have shown that chronic pain evokes anatomically specific neuroinflammation in brain regions that is causally linked to anxiety and depressive-like symptoms [131]. Specifically, nerve injury elicits the production of pro-inflammatory cytokines both in the periphery and centrally, which can cause a reduction in BDNF (neurogenesis) and glucocorticoid receptor expression and function, and an increase in excitoxicity in brain regions that are critical for behavior regulation (i.e., hippocampus, hypothalamus, amygdala, prefrontal cortex) [131–135]. Altering the connectivity of these regions can lead to alterations in function and behavioral disturbances. In humans, the production capacity of several cytokines has been positively associated with severity of depressive and anxiety symptoms, even while taking lifestyle and health factors into account [136]. Furthermore, it has been shown that among chronic pain patients, higher levels of tumor necrosis factor-α (TNF-α) and interleukin-6 (IL-6) were associated with less improvement in pain intensity, greater psychological inflexibility and lower mental health-related quality of life following a pain intervention, compared to patients with lower levels of these cytokines [137]. Therefore, inflammation may not only act as a precipitating factor for pain and mental health conditions, but also may be a perpetuating factor that deters patient recovery.

To date, very little research has been completed examining inflammatory factors and its contribution to the chronicity of pediatric pain and comorbid mental health disorders. Therefore, this represents an important, cutting-edge area for future research. We know that early life pain and/or stress also appears to dysregulate the developing immune system. Rat pups surgically incised on postnatal day 3 show priming of the central neuroimmune response, such that upon re-injury during adulthood, they demonstrate an enhanced degree and duration of microglial reactivity [138]. This is one of the first studies to demonstrate how early tissue injury can modify the neuroimmune profile to shape nociceptive processing throughout life, and may yield valuable insights into the potential link between pediatric and adult chronic pain conditions [138]. To the best of our knowledge, this has not yet been demonstrated in humans. However, Mitchell and Goldstein [139] reviewed 67 studies including nearly 4000 youth with mental health conditions and found preliminary evidence for elevated markers of inflammation in this population. In particular, associations with depressive disorders and PTSD converge with the extant adult literature demonstrating associations with inflammatory markers [139]. Early-life stress leads to a suppression of inflammatory markers during development, but causes a shift towards a pro-inflammatory state in later life [140]. For children born extremely preterm, this change in inflammatory responses may coincide with the dampening of HPA activity over time [69,70]. Prolonged stress appears to have a similar effect on inflammatory responses, such that in adult patients with comorbid PTSD and major depressive disorder demonstrated higher IL-6 activity concurrent with reduced sensitivity to glucocorticoids as compared to PTSD patients alone [141]. Furthermore, another study found that combat veterans with PTSD demonstrated abnormally elevated neuroinflammatory responses to deep pain stimuli relative to combat veterans without PTSD [142]. Taken together, inflammatory responses appear to play an important role in the development and maintenance of comorbid chronic pain and mental health disorders. Currently, many new pharmacological agents that target cytokines are being synthesized for different clinical indicators [143], which may result in better control of chronic inflammation, as well as improved treatment outcomes for patients with chronic pain and PTSD, anxiety and depressive disorder comorbidities.

4.5. Neuroimaging Chronic Pain and Psychopathology

In recent years, several neuroimaging studies have attempted to characterize nociceptive systems, their central nervous system targets (e.g., primary and secondary somatosensory cortices, insula, anterior cingulate cortex, and thalamus) [144–148], and correlate these regions with the modality and intensity of noxious input [144,149–151]. For example, in a recent fMRI study involving 114 healthy adult participants, Wager et al. [151] found a highly sensitive and specific neurologic signature of physical pain. It included both medial (e.g., affective; anterior cingulate cortex) and lateral (e.g., sensory; somatosensory cortices) pain systems that were consistent across individuals [151]. However, in the transition from an acute and adaptive pain state to a chronic, maladaptive neuropathic disease state, there is extensive functional and metabolic reorganization in pain-related brain circuitry. A recent study by Hubbard et al. [152] examined functional brain changes over time in response to acetone application to the left hindpaw in rats that either received a spared nerve injury (SNI) or sham surgery. The SNI rats demonstrated early hyperactivity of sensory areas (ventroposterior lateral nucleus of the thalamus, primary somatosensory cortex) and later hyperactivity of affective areas (anterior cingulate cortex, prelimbic cortex), and early and sustained hypoactivity of the medial thalamus and periaqueductal gray matter [152]. Moreover, for the SNI rats, these functional brain changes were associated with early and sustained increases in behavioral measures of mechanical and cold sensitivity [152]. Therefore, it would appear that as an individual transitions from an acute to chronic pain state, activations within the brain move from primarily somatosensory regions to limbic regions, indicating a shift from primarily physical to emotional neural processing. These findings were recently corroborated by Jensen et al. [153]. Using an activation likelihood estimate to analyze 138 independent data sets, they demonstrated that chronic pain patients were less likely to activate key nociceptive regions compared to healthy controls [153]. In low back pain patients followed longitudinally, Mutso et al. [97] showed that over the course of 1 year, patients acquired significant losses in hippocampal connectivity with the medial prefrontal cortex. This cellular loss between the hippocampus and cortex seemed to contribute to the transition from subacute to chronic pain and was thought to be a factor in the known aversive learning and heightened anxiety associated with chronic pain. Baliki et al. [154] also noted over the same time course that gray matter brain density decreased in patients with low back pain relative to healthy controls. However, adult chronic low back pain patients also tended to have exaggerated amygdalar connectivity with the central executive network (dorsolateral prefrontal cortex and posterior parietal cortex) as compared to healthy controls [98]. Moreover, this greater connectivity has been associated with increased tendencies to engage in catastrophic thinking about pain [98]. In support of this finding, in adolescents with irritable bowel syndrome, disease duration is associated with cortical thickness in bilateral dorsolateral prefrontal cortex and left supramarginal gyri [155]. Additionally, higher levels of pain intensity were associated with significant cortical thickening in the bilateral orbitofrontal cortex [155]. Thus, similar to the animal research described above, in humans, the transition from acute to chronic pain is characterized by reorganization within the limbic structures, thereby altering cognitive and emotional processes. This also supports the potential role of cognitive (e.g., memory and attentional biases) and affective (e.g., depressive symptoms) factors as potential mechanisms that may maintain the comorbidity between chronic pain and mental health conditions.

To date, very few neuroimaging studies have been conducted in pediatric chronic pain populations. However, among the few pediatric studies, similar findings to studies in adults have been reported. Youth with complex regional pain syndrome have been shown to have greater connectivity of the left and right amygdala to several cortical and subcortical areas as compared to healthy controls [156]. However, despite this greater connectivity, Simons et al. [157] found decreased evoked responses to fearful stimuli in patients with complex regional pain syndrome compared to healthy sex- and age-matched controls in prefrontal and limbic regions, particularly within the striatum, amygdala, insula and dorsolateral prefrontal cortex. Furthermore, blunted responses to fearful expressions in the caudate, putamen, centromedial amygdala, and anterior insula were associated with pain-related fear levels. Simons et al. [157] postulated that these results corroborate accumulating research demonstrating alterations in cognitive-affective brain regions in the chronic pain state [158] and may reflect either allostatic over-load [159,160] or pain avoidance, a maladaptive behavior often used in an effort to manage chronic pain [157].

Although the majority of neuroimaging studies of pediatric chronic pain have focused on the amygdala and its functional connections, pain is a multidimensional experience, with sensory, cognitive, and evaluative aspects. Therefore, other networks may be simultaneously activated during the transmission of pain signals in the brain. Differences in intrinsic brain networks were observed in pediatric complex regional pain syndrome patients as compared to controls, with the most prominent differences in the central executive, default mode, sensorimotor, and salience (anterior insula, mid-cingulate cortex, temperoparietal junction, and dorsolateral prefrontal cortex) networks [161]. Given the extent of neural networks that are affected by chronic pain, it is not surprising that comorbidities (i.e., PTSD, anxiety and depressive disorders) exist among individuals with chronic pain. Indeed, these same networks have also been shown to be altered in individuals with PTSD, anxiety and depressive disorders [162–165]. The majority of neuroimaging studies to date have only examined one to two of these disorders in conjunction with pain and their effects on the brain. Therefore, the specificity of the overlap within the brain between each of these disorders requires further investigation. However, it is becoming increasingly clear that chronic pain, anxiety, depression and/or PTSD, are not completely independent and the predisposing factors and neurobiological mechanisms, which lead to the presence and/or comorbidity of these disorders, are intrinsically related.

5. Parental Mental Health Disorders in Pediatric Chronic Pain Population

As previously mentioned, the neurobiology of pediatric chronic pain is deeply embedded in the broader social context of the family and parent–child relationship. It is, therefore, essential to examine parental factors that co-occur with pediatric pain or that might contribute to the development of chronic pain and comorbid mental health conditions. Several studies and reviews have confirmed a strong relationship between familial history of chronic pain with pediatric chronic pain [166,167]. Hoftun et al. [168] used a large community sample of Norwegian youth and at least one of their parents to examine the relationship between parental chronic pain history and pediatric chronic pain. The youth were more likely to have chronic pain if their mother or father reported recurrent pain issues; the risk was much higher if both parents were suffering from chronic pain [168].

There is evidence to suggest that genes, in combination with early environments, contribute to the risk of developing chronic pain and comorbid mental health conditions. Parents with the *5-HTTLPR* S allele exhibit significantly less observed positive parenting than those with the L genotype [169]. The S allele results in ~50% reduction in 5-HT reuptake compared to the long (L) allele [84], which is thought to cause an overall decrease of 5-HT neurotransmission in individuals with the short *5-HTTLPR* allele [85]. Lower 5-HT availability, leads to reduced glucocorticoid receptor expression, and greater circulating cortisol [51–57]. As previously described, children of mothers that have increased stress hormones during pregnancy are more likely to have greater stress responses as adults [48,49]. However, the postnatal environment is also important for HPA axis programming, such that parent behaviors can either reduce or increase cortisol activity, thereby modifying gene expression [52,53,170,171]. Glucocorticoid dysfunction is associated with chronic pain and mental health conditions (PTSD, anxiety and depressive disorders) [45–47]. Therefore, parent factors contribute to their child's risk of subsequently developing chronic pain and comorbid mental health conditions.

Other studies have also reported associations between parental mental health and chronic pain in children. Garber et al. [167] examined children with recurrent abdominal pain (RAP) with and without known "organic cause", children with psychiatric issues and a healthy control group. Parental self-reports of psychiatric symptoms were significantly different between the groups. Mothers (but not fathers) of children with RAP were more anxious than mothers of children who had pain with a known "organic" origin and mothers in the control group [167]. Mothers of children who had RAP without a known "organic cause" reported more depressive and somatization symptoms than mothers of healthy controls. Walker et al. [172] reported similar findings: mothers of children with RAP reported higher levels of depressive, anxiety, and somatization symptoms as compared to mothers of healthy children. Parental reports did not differ significantly between the groups. Campo et al. [173] examined a clinical sample of children with FAP and their mothers, finding the latter were significantly more likely to report a lifetime incidence of anxiety or depressive disorders as compared to mothers of children without recurrent pain. The UK child development cohort study mirrored those findings: high levels of maternal neuroticism was a risk factor for pediatric abdominal pain [5], and family history of mental health issues were linked to recurrent headaches in childhood [3,21]. Williamson et al. [174] examined a small clinical sample of youth with chronic pain and their mothers. In addition to child ratings of pain, another significant predictor of child-reported depression was maternal depression. Similarly, Wolff et al. [175] assessed anxiety and depressive symptoms in pregnant women as a part of a population-based cohort study (the Generation R). Among other factors (e.g., maternal stress and child temperament), higher anxiety symptoms in mothers increased the risk of somatic complaints in their 18 month old children [175]. While the number of studies in this area is rather limited, a pattern of high co-occurrence between pediatric chronic pain and parental mental health disorders and symptoms is evident.

Moreover, as reported in a recent meta-analysis, children of parents who have versus who do not have chronic pain are more likely to develop a host of physical and mental health problems from early in life [176]. Starting as early as perinatal period, children of mothers with chronic pain were at higher risk for preterm delivery, C-section, and adverse birth outcomes (e.g., low birth weight, congenital abnormalities) [176]. In addition to increased pain problems, offspring of parents with chronic pain were at higher risk for poorer mental health outcomes [176]. Limited evidence was found for higher rates of externalizing problems [176]; however, consistent patterns were found for internalizing problems. Levels of both parent- and youth-reported internalizing problems (including symptoms of depression, anxiety and obsessive–compulsive disorder) in youth whose parents had chronic pain were higher as compared to controls (i.e., children of pain-free parents) [176]. Other research has examined parent–child transmission of gastrointestinal illness (GI) behaviors and psychosocial mechanisms underlying this transmission [177,178]. In a study of parents with and without irritable bowel syndrome and their children, a stronger relationship between maternal and child psychological distress was found among the clinical group [178].

Stone and Wilson [179] recently developed an integrative conceptual model addressing the apparent clustering of chronic pain within families. The model outlines possible mechanisms (e.g., pain-specific social learning, general parenting style) and child vulnerabilities (e.g., altered pain processing, pain-related cognitions, pain coping behaviors, physical health, emotion regulation) that contribute to intergenerational transmission of chronic pain risk and may lead to adverse pain-related child outcomes (chronic pain, poor psychological functioning, disability) [179]. The authors also identified potential moderators that exacerbate the risk of transmitting chronic pain to offspring. Thus, chronic pain status of the second parent increases the risk of child developing chronic pain, whereas a pain-free second parent may buffer this risk [179]. Earlier and longer exposure to parental chronic pain, that is, in the same location as child pain is more detrimental as it increases the chances of child learning and adopting pain-related behaviors and beliefs [179]. Girls, African American youth and youth exposed to parental chronic pain at earlier ages may be at higher risk for developing chronic pain as compared to boys, non-Hispanic White youth, and youth who were exposed to parental chronic pain during late adolescence [179]. Importantly, it was proposed that positive affectivity in the child might buffer against the negative influence of parental chronic pain on children, whereas negative affectivity and attention control (i.e., effortful control) in the child may have the opposite effect [179].

Many of the same mechanisms that have been proposed to underlie parental and child chronic pain may also underlie the familial transmission of chronic pain and internalizing mental health symptoms between parents and youth. These proposed mechanisms include: (1) genetic contributions; (2) modeling of behavior (i.e., mothers with higher levels of anxiety model associated patterns of behavior to their children) and pain-specific learning; (3) changes in parenting style, behavior, and interactions with the child (e.g., withdrawal associated with depression, excessive attention to child's pain in cases of heightened anxiety); (4) early neurobiological changes; (5) general familial health; and (6) exposure to stressful environment [167,179]. However, it remains unclear whether parental mental health is a risk factor for development of pediatric pain or a result of having a child with a pain problem. Certainly, parenting a child with chronic pain is associated with high emotional burden to the parent and the broader family system, and recent efforts have been made to directly target parental distress in pediatric chronic pain for this very reason [180]. Twenty percent of parents of youth with chronic pain (versus 1% of parents of pain free peers) have been found to experience clinically significant levels of PTSD [25], however, their PTSD symptoms were not related to those of their child [25].

Any temporal and/or causal connections between pediatric chronic pain and parental psychological health are premature and require further longitudinal and epidemiological investigations. It will also be important to consider that parental mental health might be comorbid and have a bi-directional influence on youth's psychological functioning in chronic pain populations. Palermo et al. [181] developed a conceptual three-level model that elucidates factors at play in pediatric chronic pain. Parental level variables (mental health and emotions, behaviors, physical health status) connect to the other two levels including family variables and developmental factors, by the means of bi-directional relationships. Clearly there is a necessity to further investigate parental factors to gain a more comprehensive understanding of their role in the onset and trajectories of pediatric chronic pain and mental health.

6. Treatments for Comorbid Chronic Pain in Youth

Despite growing recognition of the high co-occurrence of mental health disorders in children and adolescents with chronic pain, treatment approaches to address this growing problem have lagged behind. Currently, psychological treatments for chronic pain have taken a "one-size-fits-all" approach and predominantly focus on changing pain-related cognitions and behaviors without adequately addressing elevations in anxiety and depressive symptoms that often accompany the pain. This could, in part, explain the small and non-significant treatment effects that have been found for face-to-face psychological interventions in reducing pain and disability among headache and non-headache pain populations, respectively. While it may also account for a lack of lasting reductions found in anxiety and depressive symptoms following treatment, this could also reflect the small number of trials that have analyzed mental health conditions as outcomes [10]. Similarly, in a recent meta-analysis of remotely delivered psychological interventions (e.g., via the internet, computers, smartphone applications or telephone), there were no beneficial effects found in reducing depressive symptoms and only small effects in reducing headache pain in the short-term [182]. However, it should be noted that there were only a small number of (small) trials conducted, and, like the face-to-face trials, many did not assess both anxiety and depressive symptoms as primary outcomes. Taken together, the evidence to date suggests that our existing interventions for chronic pain emphasize changing pain cognitions and behaviors without adequate emphasis on co-occurring mental health conditions. Although more trials assessing pain and mental health disorders as primary outcomes are needed, it is possible that existing treatments may not be sufficient for interrupting a trajectory of pain and comorbid mental health conditions from persisting long-term.

Recent research suggests that mental health comorbidities and symptoms can impede recovery among youth with chronic pain. Cunningham et al. [183] examined 175 children seen in a pediatric pain management center, 40 of who completed cognitive–behavioral therapy for chronic pain. Findings revealed that children who had clinically significant symptoms of anxiety at the time of initial evaluation (albeit similar levels of pain and functioning) showed greater initiation in and completion of the pain intervention but poorer treatment response (i.e., less reductions in pain intensity and functional disability) as compared to youth with subclinical anxiety symptoms. Research also suggests that modifying anxiety is important for reducing pain and improving functioning during intensive interdisciplinary rehabilitation pain programs. Specifically, Benore et al. [184] found that over and above the effect of age, sex and pain at admission and 1-month post-discharge, reductions in general anxiety, pain-specific anxiety and pain catastrophizing predicted improved physical quality of life, as well as pain intensity, but, not the number of missed school days. Taken together, this evidence demonstrates that mental health (anxiety) symptom elevations impede recovery in psychological pain treatments and should be reduced in order to see improvements in pain and functional outcomes. This suggests that youth with chronic pain are not a homogenous group and treatment approaches that are tailored to addressing co-morbid anxiety symptoms are likely necessary for subgroups of youth who exhibit clinically significant anxiety symptoms. Moreover, youth who appear to be most engaged in treatment (i.e., those with clinically significant anxiety symptoms) might be the very ones who are least likely to recover. Research on treatment response among youth with other mental health conditions (e.g., depression, PTSD) is needed.

Like Cunningham et al. [183], recent authors have argued for the use of mental health screening tools to identify mental health disorder co-morbidities [31,185,186] in order to predict outcomes and inform clinician-use of treatment approaches. Some authors have also provided treatment recommendations [31,185], albeit largely based on adult research. Adult guidelines recommend treating overlapping pain and PTSD symptoms (e.g., fears and avoidance behaviors) concurrently [9,187]. Dually targeted interventions have been developed for adults that combine PTSD behavioral activation, pain education and emphasis on exercise [9,188]. Similarly, other programs developed for adult veterans have combined cognitive processing therapy for PTSD with CBT for chronic pain [9,189]. Pediatric researchers have stressed the importance of understanding comorbid PTSD and chronic pain within a developmental context [31] and cautioned against simply downwardly extending adult recommendations to pediatric populations. Attempts have been made to apply a unified, transdiagnostic treatment for adolescents with chronic pain and comorbid anxiety and depressive disorders (Unified Protocol for the Treatment of Emotions in Youth With Pain (UP-YP)) [190]. The UP-YP is a modular-based individual treatment protocol [190]. Treatment is offered between 8 to 21 50-min sessions over a front-loaded 6-month period [190]. The UP-YP modules include: (a) psychoeducation about emotions and pain; (b) awareness of emotions and pain; (c) flexibility in thinking; (d) modifying emotion-driven behaviors through exposures; and (e) treatment review and relapse prevention [190]. Several optional modules are available as well (e.g., parenting the emotional adolescent with pain) [190]. Although similar in its application to traditional CBT therapy, the UP-YP aims to modify both pain and emotions [190]. Using two case studies, Allen et al. [190] provided initial evidence that the UP-YP can be used to broaden the scope of treatment to include both emotion regulation skills and cognitive–behavioral treatment strategies to assist individuals with complex medical and psychological conditions. After completing the training modules, case 1 was back at school nearly full-time, engaging in social activities, and showed significant improvement in his anxiety and disability, although his pain levels remained more or less the same. Case 2, was somewhat less successful as her pain symptoms were initially being addressed by the program, but her physical illness towards the end of treatment precluded her from the continued benefits of UP-YP. As an alternative to this method of intervention, clinicians may choose to stagger treatment delivery by treating the condition that causes the most distress first and then addressing remaining symptoms of the other condition; however, treatment algorithms based on evidence are needed. Clearly, knowing when and how to integrate versus stagger treatment is a critical area for future research in this area.

Another reason why existing interventions may not help a substantial portion of youth may be due to the fact that they do not effectively target the underlying mechanisms that maintain these conditions. Genetic screening for alleles associated with these conditions may help to identify patients at risk for developing chronic pain and a comorbid mental health condition, allowing clinicians to intervene prior to significant neural remodeling. A better understanding of the neural "signature(s)" associated with chronic pain, PTSD, anxiety and depressive disorders will also help to evaluate the effectiveness of clinical interventions for altering this neural circuitry. New therapies, which directly target the underlying mechanisms of these conditions, may also be a promising new direction for clinical intervention. For example, transcranial magnetic stimulation (rTMS) involves using a magnetic field generator to stimulate small regions of the affected brain region. Thus far, rTMS has been shown to be an effective treatment for burning mouth syndrome [191], complex regional pain syndrome [192], fibromyalgia [193,194], neuropathic pain [195–197], depressive disorders [198] and to a lesser degree PTSD and other anxiety disorders [199,200]. It has been proposed to prevent or revert the ongoing maladaptive plasticity within the pain matrix [201], and modify opioidergic, glutamatergic, gamma-aminobutyric acidergic, and serotoninergic neurotransmissions [202]. The application of screening, implementation of early interventions at the individual and familial level (e.g., teaching coping mechanisms, parent sensitivity training), refining current intervention strategies, and the innovation of new, targeted therapies, holds promise for addressing and reducing these comorbidities.

7. Discussion

High levels of comorbid chronic pain and mental health conditions have been reported in pediatric populations, and persistent pain reportedly increases the risk of PTSD, anxiety and depressive disorders later in adulthood [3–5,16,17]. Chronic pain and mental health disorders (as well as their subclinical symptoms) reciprocally influence each other, significantly decrease youth quality of life and impose a large health care and economic burden in childhood and adulthood [2,7,18,31]. While studies have attempted to identify mechanisms underlying these relationships, they often focus on one to two factors, which cannot account for the complex interplay between genetic, epigenetic, chemical, neuronal and environmental factors that may interact synergistically to influence the development and maintenance of chronic pain and mental health conditions. This review highlights some of the ways in which pre-determined and concurrent neurobiology and genetics interact with parental influences to influence chronic pain and mental health conditions in youth (Figure 1). It extends previous pediatric and adult work on mental health conditions/symptoms and chronic pain, which have focused primarily on cognitive, affective, and behavioral mechanisms. We suggest that an integrative approach combining biological and behavioral factors is needed to push forward this important line of inquiry, and ultimately inform how to interrupt this trajectory, to prevent issues from persisting into adulthood. However, systematic review methodology is warranted as more evidence accumulates on this topic.

Theoretical work is critical for synthesizing existing (and often disparate) bodies of evidence and guiding future scientific inquiry. Existing models that address comorbidity of mental health disorders and chronic pain are scarce. Moreover, they focus primarily on the relationship between PTSD and chronic pain, and are primarily based on adult populations [7,8,28]. While mutual maintenance [8] and shared vulnerability [6] models account for the relationship between PTSD and persistent pain in adults, they do not account for an array of dynamic changes that occur during childhood and adolescence and the unique influence of parents. The new developmentally informed model of Holley et al. [31] begins to fill this gap by placing shared PTSD and chronic pain factors within interpersonal (e.g., parent context) and neurobiological (e.g., impact of pain and PTSD on the developing brain) developmental contexts. A more generalized model addressing the comorbidity between several mental health disorders/symptoms (depression, anxiety and PTSD) and chronic pain in youth would help guide future research and inform clinical practice in this area.

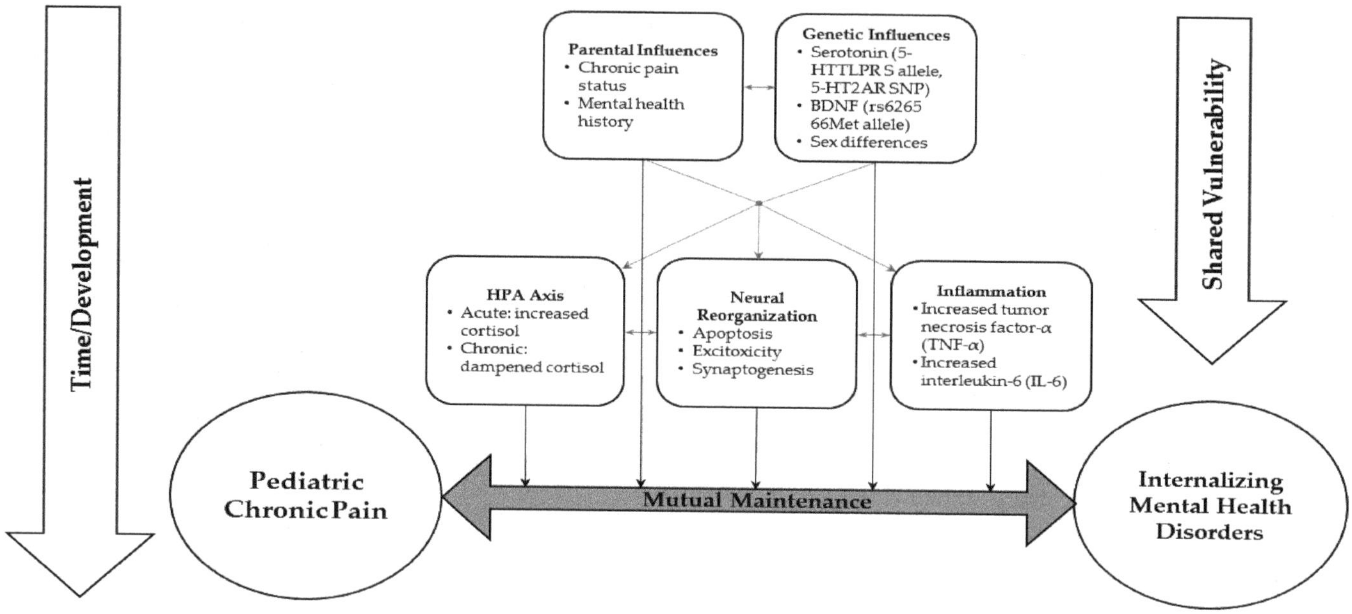

Figure 1. Possible mechanisms underlying the shared vulnerability and mutual maintenance of pediatric chronic pain and internalizing mental health disorders. 5-HTTLPR: Serotonin-transporter-linked polymorphic region; BDNF: Brain-derived neurotrophic factor; HPA: hypothalamic–pituitary–adrenal; S allele: Short allele.

There has been extensive literature examining the contribution of specific genes and neurobiological pathways underlying chronic pain, anxiety, depression and PTSD in adults and animals. However, these studies are often conducted in isolation of one another and focus specifically on the neurobiological influence on one or two outcomes in particular. We have demonstrated in this review that many of the same genes (e.g., 5-HT, *BDNF*), hormones (e.g., cortisol), neurotransmitters (e.g., 5-HT), cytokines (e.g., TNF-α, IL-6) have been implicated in each of these conditions and are inextricably related to one another, either directly or indirectly through the HPA axis. For example, individuals with the short (S) allele of 5-HTTLPR have ~50% reduction in 5-HT reuptake compared to the long (L) allele [84], which may result in decreased 5-HT neurotransmission [85]. Reduced 5-HT availability leads to lower glucocorticoid receptor expression, which results in poorer negative feedback and greater cortisol secretion [51–57]. Stress hormones modify BDNF expression, such that there is decreased BDNF expression in the hippocampus and increased expression in the amygdala [94–96]. BDNF is intrinsic to neurogenesis and synaptogenesis [93], therefore, BDNF availability may contribute to the patterns of neuroconnectivity that develop as pain becomes comorbid and chronic [97,98]. Prolonged exposure to pain leads to a dampening of cortisol responses [52,53,66–70]. Inhibition of the HPA axis leads to heightened inflammatory/immune responses [203,204]. Therefore, following exposure to pain, large inflammatory responses in both the periphery and central systems may cause a reduction in neurogenesis and an increase in excitoxicity leading to both the chronification of pain and its comorbidities. Furthermore, glucocorticoids are involved in normal brain maturation and cell survival [205–207], and both an excess of or too low levels of cortisol can have deleterious effects on the brain, leading to long-term changes in behavior. HPA activity is programmed at birth [48,49], modified by the environment (e.g., parent behavior) [51–57,72], has significant effects in the developing brain [52,53], and influences responses to pain and behavior [63–65]. Pain, anxiety, depression and PTSD are all stress-related conditions influenced by either hyper- or hypo-glucocorticoid activity [63–65]. Evidence suggests that the combination of predisposing factors, along with the timing and duration of environmental influences, modifies HPA activity, which has widespread effects on the neurobiological (e.g., brain organization/function), physiological (e.g., arousal), and psychological systems (e.g., stress, anxiety sensitivity), and may lead to the maintenance of these conditions.

Precedence of mental health disorders onset prior to chronic pain have been reported [24,30]; however, the studies examining temporal relationships between the conditions are scarce, conflicting [208], and come with methodological limitations (e.g., reliance on retrospective report). Clinician-administered interviews (as opposed to self- and parental report) to prospectively assess mental and physical health in childhood, adolescence and early to middle adulthood would be a methodological advance that would help determine temporal relationships between chronic pain and psychiatric disorders.

When examining mental health and chronic pain in youth, it is crucial to take into account the parent–child relational context and the influential role of parental factors. Indeed, parents of youth with chronic pain report more anxiety, depression, and somatization symptoms than pain-free peers [167,173]. Moreover, maternal anxiety and depressive disorders were associated with depressive and somatic symptoms of children with chronic pain [167,172]. Therefore, it is possible that parents with mental health disorders through interactions with their genes and environment influence the comorbidity of chronic pain and mental health conditions in the child. It is necessary to further investigate the role of parental factors in the development and maintenance of pediatric chronic pain and comorbid mental health disorders and symptoms. Additionally, there is a paucity of research examining mental health in fathers of youth with chronic pain. Given the profound influence that pediatric chronic pain has on the entire family, it will be important to address paternal factors in addition to, and in combination with, maternal contributions to pediatric chronic pain and mental health conditions.

While psychological treatments for chronic pain have led to some changes in pain and disability, there is currently no evidence to suggest that it leads to lasting reductions in mental health symptoms. Moreover, many randomized controlled trials of psychological interventions for pediatric chronic pain have not included (or reported on) measures of PTSD, anxiety and depressive disorders over the course of treatment. These mental health conditions are often comorbid with one another, and many of the proposed mechanisms (e.g., avoidance, cognitive biases, sleep disturbances) underlying them are similar. Research in this area has tended to focus on these conditions and symptoms in isolation. Future research examining all of these mental health symptoms in the context of pediatric chronic pain is needed. Moreover, despite increasing evidence demonstrating that these comorbidities are common and debilitating, there is currently minimal empirically based guidance for how to treat children and adolescents who present with comorbid chronic pain and mental health conditions, and clinicians often rely on adult recommendations and/or clinical intuition. Clearly, treatment development and research on comorbid mental health conditions and chronic pain in youth is critically needed at this time. New therapies, which directly target the underlying neural mechanisms (e.g., rTMS; targeted anti-inflammatories) may also be a promising new direction for clinical intervention. However, whether or not these new treatments will be effective for treating chronic pain together with comorbid mental health disorders will need to be determined. Given potential intergenerational transmission of chronic pain and high levels of mental health symptoms among parents, research is needed to determine how to best address parents' emotional burden. Novel parenting interventions to reduce parent distress in the context of pediatric chronic pain have been developed and tested and show promising evidence for improving parent and child emotional outcomes [180]. Addressing parent mental health conditions is likely a necessary first step before they can engage in behavior change that is often required in psychological treatments for their child's chronic pain.

Sex differences in 5-HT signaling systems, stress responses, and neuroimmune interactions are being increasingly recognized [209,210]. Estrogens are often regarded as a central nervous system stimulant, and androgen receptor-mediated actions are often related to inhibition, which may underlie the lower incidence of many forms of chronic pain in males [211]. However, given the scope of this narrative review, in which we examined developmental trajectories of potentially shared neurobiological mechanisms underlying pain, PTSD, anxiety and depressive disorders, we were not able to describe the influence of sex hormones on each of these conditions, and how this changes across development. This is an important area for future research.

Given the debilitating impact of comorbid chronic pain and mental health disorders on youth there is an increasing need for prospective, interdisciplinary studies to identify the primary mechanisms underlying this co-occurrence in youth. This will inform the development and refinement of evidence-based interventions that can interrupt or possibly prevent the maintenance of these chronic conditions. Developmentally sensitive research integrating biological, behavioral, and social perspectives will be critical in driving forward this field of inquiry and addressing this growing epidemic.

Acknowledgments: Jillian Vinall is supported by a Fellowship in Pediatric Pain Research from the Louise and Allan Edward Foundation, and received a Postdoctoral Scholarship from the Alberta Children's Hospital Research Institute/Cumming School of Medicine at the University of Calgary. Jillian Vinall is also a member of the Pain in Child Health research training initiative. Gordon J.G. Asmundson is supported by the University of Regina President's Chair for Academic Excellence in Adult Mental Health Research. Melanie Noel's research is supported by the Alberta Children's Hospital Research Institute, Canadian Institutes of Health Research, and American Pain Society.

Author Contributions: M.N. and G.J.G.A. conceptualized the manuscript. J.V. M.P. and M.N. drafted the manuscript for review. All authors provided critical review of the manuscript for publication.

References

1. King, S.; Chambers, C.T.; Huguet, A.; MacNevin, R.C.; McGrath, P.J.; Parker, L.; MacDonald, A.J. The epidemiology of chronic pain in children and adolescents revisited: A systematic review. *Pain* **2011**, *152*, 2729–2738. [CrossRef] [PubMed]
2. Groenewald, C.B.; Essner, B.S.; Wright, D.; Fesinmeyer, M.D.; Palermo, T.M. The economic costs of chronic pain among a cohort of treatment-seeking adolescents in the united states. *J. Pain* **2014**, *15*, 925–933. [CrossRef] [PubMed]
3. Fearon, P.; Hotopf, M. Relation between headache in childhood and physical and psychiatric symptoms in adulthood: National birth cohort study. *BMJ* **2001**, *322*, 1145. [CrossRef] [PubMed]
4. Shelby, G.D.; Shirkey, K.C.; Sherman, A.L.; Beck, J.E.; Haman, K.; Shears, A.R.; Horst, S.N.; Smith, C.A.; Garber, J.; Walker, L.S. Functional abdominal pain in childhood and long-term vulnerability to anxiety disorders. *Pediatrics* **2013**, *132*, 475–482. [CrossRef] [PubMed]
5. Hotopf, M.; Carr, S.; Mayou, R.; Wadsworth, M.; Wessely, S. Why do children have chronic abdominal pain, and what happens to them when they grow up? Population based cohort study. *BMJ* **1998**, *316*, 1196–1200. [CrossRef] [PubMed]
6. Asmundson, G.J.; Coons, M.J.; Taylor, S.; Katz, J. Ptsd and the experience of pain: Research and clinical implications of shared vulnerability and mutual maintenance models. *Can. J. Psychiatry* **2002**, *47*, 930–937. [PubMed]
7. Asmundson, G.J.; Katz, J. Understanding the co-occurrence of anxiety disorders and chronic pain: State-of-the-art. *Depress. Anxiety* **2009**, *26*, 888–901. [CrossRef] [PubMed]
8. Sharp, T.J.; Harvey, A.G. Chronic pain and posttraumatic stress disorder: Mutual maintenance? *Clin. Psychol. Rev.* **2001**, *21*, 857–877. [CrossRef]
9. Asmundson, G.J. The emotional and physical pains of trauma: Contemporary and innovative approaches for treating co-occurring ptsd and chronic pain. *Depress. Anxiety* **2014**, *31*, 717–720. [CrossRef] [PubMed]
10. Eccleston, C. Systematic review and meta-analysis of psychological therapies for children with chronic pain. *Clin. Pract. Pediatr. Psychol.* **2014**, *39*, 763–782.
11. Shipton, E.A. The transition from acute to chronic post surgical pain. *Anaesth. Intensive Care* **2011**, *39*, 824–836. [PubMed]

12. Groenewald, C.B.; Wright, D.R.; Palermo, T.M. Health care expenditures associated with pediatric pain-related conditions in the united states. *Pain* **2015**, *156*, 951–957. [CrossRef] [PubMed]
13. Palermo, T.M. Impact of recurrent and chronic pain on child and family daily functioning: A critical review of the literature. *J. Dev. Behav. Pediatr.* **2000**, *21*, 58–69. [CrossRef] [PubMed]
14. Egger, H.L.; Angold, A.; Costello, E.J. Headaches and psychopathology in children and adolescents. *J. Am. Acad. Child Adolesc. Psychiatry* **1998**, *37*, 951–958. [CrossRef] [PubMed]
15. Egger, H.L.; Costello, E.J.; Erkanli, A.; Angold, A. Somatic complaints and psychopathology in children and adolescents: Stomach aches, musculoskeletal pains, and headaches. *J. Am. Acad. Child Adolesc. Psychiatry* **1999**, *38*, 852–860.
16. Walker, L.S.; Sherman, A.L.; Bruehl, S.; Garber, J.; Smith, C.A. Functional abdominal pain patient subtypes in childhood predict functional gastrointestinal disorders with chronic pain and psychiatric comorbidities in adolescence and adulthood. *Pain* **2012**, *153*, 1798–1806. [CrossRef] [PubMed]
17. Shanahan, L.; Zucker, N.; Copeland, W.E.; Bondy, C.L.; Egger, H.L.; Costello, E.J. Childhood somatic complaints predict generalized anxiety and depressive disorders during young adulthood in a community sample. *Psychol. Med.* **2015**, *45*, 1721–1730. [CrossRef] [PubMed]
18. Noel, M.; Groenewald, C.B.; Beals-Erickson, S.E.; Gebert, J.T.; Palermo, T.M. Chronic pain in adolescence and internalizing mental health disorders: A nationally representative study. *Pain* **2016**, *157*, 1333–1338. [CrossRef] [PubMed]
19. Balottin, U.; Fusar Poli, P.; Termine, C.; Molteni, S.; Galli, F. Psychopathological symptoms in child and adolescent migraine and tension-type headache: A meta-analysis. *Cephalalgia* **2013**, *33*, 112–122. [CrossRef] [PubMed]
20. Blaauw, B.A.; Dyb, G.; Hagen, K.; Holmen, T.L.; Linde, M.; Wentzel-Larsen, T.; Zwart, J.A. Anxiety, depression and behavioral problems among adolescents with recurrent headache: The young-hunt study. *J. Headache Pain* **2014**, *15*, 38. [CrossRef] [PubMed]
21. Coffelt, T.A.; Bauer, B.D.; Carroll, A.E. Inpatient characteristics of the child admitted with chronic pain. *Pediatrics* **2013**, *132*, e422–e429. [CrossRef] [PubMed]
22. Noel, M.; Beals-Erickson, S.E.; Law, E.F.; Alberts, N.; Palermo, T.M. Characterizing the pain narratives of parents of youth with chronic pain. *Clin. J. Pain* **2016**, *32*, 849–858. [CrossRef] [PubMed]
23. Simons, L.E.; Sieberg, C.B.; Claar, R.L. Anxiety and functional disability in a large sample of children and adolescents with chronic pain. *Pain Res. Manag.* **2012**, *17*, 93–97. [CrossRef] [PubMed]
24. Tegethoff, M.; Belardi, A.; Stalujanis, E.; Meinlschmidt, G. Comorbidity of mental disorders and chronic pain: Chronology of onset in adolescents of a national representative cohort. *J. Pain* **2015**, *16*, 1054–1064. [CrossRef] [PubMed]
25. Noel, M.; Wilson, A.C.; Holley, A.L.; Durkin, L.; Patton, M.; Palermo, T.M. Posttraumatic stress disorder symptoms in youth with versus without chronic pain. *Pain* **2016**, *157*, 2277–2284. [CrossRef] [PubMed]
26. Korterink, J.J.; Diederen, K.; Benninga, M.A.; Tabbers, M.M. Epidemiology of pediatric functional abdominal pain disorders: A meta-analysis. *PLoS ONE* **2015**, *10*, e0126982. [CrossRef] [PubMed]
27. Egger, H.L.; Costello, E.J.; Erkanli, A.; Angold, A. Somatic complaints and psychopathology in children and adolescents: Stomach aches, musculoskeletal pains, and headaches. *J. Am. Acad. Child Adolesc. Psychiatry* **1999**, *38*, 852–860. [CrossRef] [PubMed]
28. Liedl, A.; Knaevelsrud, C. Chronic pain and PTSD: The perpetual avoidance model and its treatment implications. *Torture* **2008**, *18*, 69–76. [PubMed]
29. Norman, S.B.; Stein, M.B.; Dimsdale, J.E.; Hoyt, D.B. Pain in the aftermath of trauma is a risk factor for post-traumatic stress disorder. *Psychol. Med.* **2008**, *38*, 533–542. [CrossRef] [PubMed]
30. Brown, E.A.; Kenardy, J.A.; Dow, B.L. Ptsd perpetuates pain in children with traumatic brain injury. *J. Pediatr. Psychol.* **2014**, *39*, 512–520. [CrossRef] [PubMed]
31. Holley, A.L.; Wilson, A.C.; Noel, M.; Palermo, T.M. Post-traumatic stress symptoms in children and adolescents with chronic pain: A topical review of the literature and a proposed framework for future research. *Eur. J. Pain* **2016**, *20*, 1371–1383. [CrossRef] [PubMed]
32. Chrousos, G.P. Stress and disorders of the stress system. *Nat. Rev. Endocrinol.* **2009**, *5*, 374–381. [CrossRef] [PubMed]
33. Francis, D.D.; Champagne, F.A.; Liu, D.; Meaney, M.J. Maternal care, gene expression, and the development of individual differences in stress reactivity. *Ann. N. Y. Acad. Sci.* **1999**, *896*, 66–84. [CrossRef] [PubMed]

34. Gunnar, M.; Quevedo, K. The neurobiology of stress and development. *Annu. Rev. Psychol.* **2007**, *58*, 145–173. [CrossRef] [PubMed]
35. Heim, C.; Nemeroff, C.B. The role of childhood trauma in the neurobiology of mood and anxiety disorders: Preclinical and clinical studies. *Biol. Psychiatry* **2001**, *49*, 1023–1039. [CrossRef]
36. Peters, K.L. Neonatal stress reactivity and cortisol. *J. Perinat. Neonatal Nurs.* **1998**, *11*, 45–59. [CrossRef] [PubMed]
37. Shanks, N.; Harbuz, M.S.; Jessop, D.S.; Perks, P.; Moore, P.M.; Lightman, S.L. Inflammatory disease as chronic stress. *Ann. N. Y. Acad. Sci.* **1998**, *840*, 599–607. [CrossRef] [PubMed]
38. Lentjes, E.G.; Griep, E.N.; Boersma, J.W.; Romijn, F.P.; de Kloet, E.R. Glucocorticoid receptors, fibromyalgia and low back pain. *Psychoneuroendocrinology* **1997**, *22*, 603–614. [CrossRef]
39. Heim, C.; Ehlert, U.; Hanker, J.P.; Hellhammer, D.H. Abuse-related posttraumatic stress disorder and alterations of the hypothalamic-pituitary-adrenal axis in women with chronic pelvic pain. *Psychosom. Med.* **1998**, *60*, 309–318. [CrossRef] [PubMed]
40. Blumer, D.; Zorick, F.; Heilbronn, M.; Roth, T. Biological markers for depression in chronic pain. *J. Nerv. Ment. Dis.* **1982**, *170*, 425–428. [CrossRef] [PubMed]
41. Tennant, F.; Hermann, L. Normalization of serum cortisol concentration with opioid treatment of severe chronic pain. *Pain Med.* **2002**, *3*, 132–134. [CrossRef] [PubMed]
42. Geiss, A.; Varadi, E.; Steinbach, K.; Bauer, H.W.; Anton, F. Psychoneuroimmunological correlates of persisting sciatic pain in patients who underwent discectomy. *Neurosci. Lett.* **1997**, *237*, 65–68. [CrossRef]
43. Griep, E.N.; Boersma, J.W.; Lentjes, E.G.; Prins, A.P.; van der Korst, J.K.; de Kloet, E.R. Function of the hypothalamic-pituitary-adrenal axis in patients with fibromyalgia and low back pain. *J. Rheumatol.* **1998**, *25*, 1374–1381. [PubMed]
44. Korszun, A.; Young, E.A.; Singer, K.; Carlson, N.E.; Brown, M.B.; Crofford, L. Basal circadian cortisol secretion in women with temporomandibular disorders. *J. Dent. Res.* **2002**, *81*, 279–283. [CrossRef] [PubMed]
45. Blackburn-Munro, G.; Blackburn-Munro, R.E. Chronic pain, chronic stress and depression: Coincidence or consequence? *J. Neuroendocrinol.* **2001**, *13*, 1009–1023. [CrossRef] [PubMed]
46. Yehuda, R. Biology of posttraumatic stress disorder. *J. Clin. Psychiatry* **2001**, *62* (Suppl. 17), 41–46. [PubMed]
47. Boyer, P. Do anxiety and depression have a common pathophysiological mechanism? *Acta Psychiatr. Scand. Suppl.* **2000**, 24–29. [CrossRef]
48. Levitt, N.S.; Lindsay, R.S.; Holmes, M.C.; Seckl, J.R. Dexamethasone in the last week of pregnancy attenuates hippocampal glucocorticoid receptor gene expression and elevates blood pressure in the adult offspring in the rat. *Neuroendocrinology* **1996**, *64*, 412–418. [CrossRef] [PubMed]
49. Harris, A.; Seckl, J. Glucocorticoids, prenatal stress and the programming of disease. *Horm. Behav.* **2011**, *59*, 279–289. [CrossRef] [PubMed]
50. Champagne, F.A.; Francis, D.D.; Mar, A.; Meaney, M.J. Variations in maternal care in the rat as a mediating influence for the effects of environment on development. *Physiol. Behav.* **2003**, *79*, 359–371. [CrossRef]
51. Caldji, C.; Tannenbaum, B.; Sharma, S.; Francis, D.; Plotsky, P.M.; Meaney, M.J. Maternal care during infancy regulates the development of neural systems mediating the expression of fearfulness in the rat. *Proc. Natl. Acad. Sci. USA* **1998**, *95*, 5335–5340. [CrossRef] [PubMed]
52. Francis, D.; Diorio, J.; Liu, D.; Meaney, M.J. Nongenomic transmission across generations of maternal behavior and stress responses in the rat. *Science* **1999**, *286*, 1155–1158. [CrossRef] [PubMed]
53. Liu, D.; Diorio, J.; Tannenbaum, B.; Caldji, C.; Francis, D.; Freedman, A.; Sharma, S.; Pearson, D.; Plotsky, P.M.; Meaney, M.J. Maternal care, hippocampal glucocorticoid receptors, and hypothalamic-pituitary-adrenal responses to stress. *Science* **1997**, *277*, 1659–1662. [CrossRef] [PubMed]
54. Menard, J.L.; Champagne, D.L.; Meaney, M.J. Variations of maternal care differentially influence 'fear' reactivity and regional patterns of cfos immunoreactivity in response to the shock-probe burying test. *Neuroscience* **2004**, *129*, 297–308. [CrossRef] [PubMed]
55. van Hasselt, F.N.; Cornelisse, S.; Zhang, T.Y.; Meaney, M.J.; Velzing, E.H.; Krugers, H.J.; Joels, M. Adult hippocampal glucocorticoid receptor expression and dentate synaptic plasticity correlate with maternal care received by individuals early in life. *Hippocampus* **2012**, *22*, 255–266. [CrossRef] [PubMed]
56. Weaver, I.C.; Cervoni, N.; Champagne, F.A.; D'Alessio, A.C.; Sharma, S.; Seckl, J.R.; Dymov, S.; Szyf, M.; Meaney, M.J. Epigenetic programming by maternal behavior. *Nat. Neurosci.* **2004**, *7*, 847–854. [CrossRef] [PubMed]

57. Zhang, T.Y.; Bagot, R.; Parent, C.; Nesbitt, C.; Bredy, T.W.; Caldji, C.; Fish, E.; Anisman, H.; Szyf, M.; Meaney, M.J. Maternal programming of defensive responses through sustained effects on gene expression. *Biol. Psychol.* **2006**, *73*, 72–89. [CrossRef] [PubMed]
58. Liu, D.; Diorio, J.; Day, J.C.; Francis, D.D.; Meaney, M.J. Maternal care, hippocampal synaptogenesis and cognitive development in rats. *Nat. Neurosci.* **2000**, *3*, 799–806. [PubMed]
59. Pena, C.J.; Neugut, Y.D.; Calarco, C.A.; Champagne, F.A. Effects of maternal care on the development of midbrain dopamine pathways and reward-directed behavior in female offspring. *Eur. J. Neurosci.* **2014**, *39*, 946–956. [CrossRef] [PubMed]
60. Starr-Phillips, E.J.; Beery, A.K. Natural variation in maternal care shapes adult social behavior in rats. *Dev. Psychobiol.* **2014**, *56*, 1017–1026. [CrossRef] [PubMed]
61. Essex, M.J.; Klein, M.H.; Cho, E.; Kalin, N.H. Maternal stress beginning in infancy may sensitize children to later stress exposure: Effects on cortisol and behavior. *Biol. Psychiatry* **2002**, *52*, 776–784. [CrossRef]
62. Barry, T.J.; Murray, L.; Fearon, R.M.; Moutsiana, C.; Cooper, P.; Goodyer, I.M.; Herbert, J.; Halligan, S.L. Maternal postnatal depression predicts altered offspring biological stress reactivity in adulthood. *Psychoneuroendocrinology* **2015**, *52*, 251–260. [CrossRef] [PubMed]
63. McCauley, J.; Kern, D.E.; Kolodner, K.; Dill, L.; Schroeder, A.F.; DeChant, H.K.; Ryden, J.; Derogatis, L.R.; Bass, E.B. Clinical characteristics of women with a history of childhood abuse: Unhealed wounds. *JAMA* **1997**, *277*, 1362–1368. [CrossRef] [PubMed]
64. Yaari, A.; Eisenberg, E.; Adler, R.; Birkhan, J. Chronic pain in holocaust survivors. *J. Pain Symptom Manag.* **1999**, *17*, 181–187. [CrossRef]
65. Young Casey, C.; Greenberg, M.A.; Nicassio, P.M.; Harpin, R.E.; Hubbard, D. Transition from acute to chronic pain and disability: A model including cognitive, affective, and trauma factors. *Pain* **2008**, *134*, 69–79. [CrossRef] [PubMed]
66. Young, E.A.; Haskett, R.F.; Murphy-Weinberg, V.; Watson, S.J.; Akil, H. Loss of glucocorticoid fast feedback in depression. *Arch. Gen. Psychiatry* **1991**, *48*, 693–699. [CrossRef] [PubMed]
67. Yehuda, R. Biology of posttraumatic stress disorder. *J Clin Psychiatry* **2000**, *61* (Suppl. 7), 14–21. [PubMed]
68. Muhtz, C.; Rodriguez-Raecke, R.; Hinkelmann, K.; Moeller-Bertram, T.; Kiefer, F.; Wiedemann, K.; May, A.; Otte, C. Cortisol response to experimental pain in patients with chronic low back pain and patients with major depression. *Pain Med.* **2013**, *14*, 498–503. [CrossRef] [PubMed]
69. Grunau, R.E.; Cepeda, I.L.; Chau, C.M.; Brummelte, S.; Weinberg, J.; Lavoie, P.M.; Ladd, M.; Hirschfeld, A.F.; Russell, E.; Koren, G.; et al. Neonatal pain-related stress and nfkbia genotype are associated with altered cortisol levels in preterm boys at school age. *PLoS ONE* **2013**, *8*, e73926. [CrossRef] [PubMed]
70. Brummelte, S.; Chau, C.M.; Cepeda, I.L.; Degenhardt, A.; Weinberg, J.; Synnes, A.R.; Grunau, R.E. Cortisol levels in former preterm children at school age are predicted by neonatal procedural pain-related stress. *Psychoneuroendocrinology* **2015**, *51*, 151–163. [CrossRef] [PubMed]
71. McCormack, K.; Sanchez, M.M.; Bardi, M.; Maestripieri, D. Maternal care patterns and behavioral development of rhesus macaque abused infants in the first 6 months of life. *Dev. Psychobiol.* **2006**, *48*, 537–550. [CrossRef] [PubMed]
72. Kaufman, J.; Birmaher, B.; Perel, J.; Dahl, R.E.; Moreci, P.; Nelson, B.; Wells, W.; Ryan, N.D. The corticotropin-releasing hormone challenge in depressed abused, depressed nonabused, and normal control children. *Biol. Psychiatry* **1997**, *42*, 669–679. [CrossRef]
73. De Bellis, M.D.; Chrousos, G.P.; Dorn, L.D.; Burke, L.; Helmers, K.; Kling, M.A.; Trickett, P.K.; Putnam, F.W. Hypothalamic-pituitary-adrenal axis dysregulation in sexually abused girls. *J. Clin. Endocrinol. Metab.* **1994**, *78*, 249–255. [PubMed]
74. Weems, C.F.; Carrion, V.G. The association between ptsd symptoms and salivary cortisol in youth: The role of time since the trauma. *J. Trauma. Stress* **2007**, *20*, 903–907. [CrossRef] [PubMed]
75. Laplante, P.; Diorio, J.; Meaney, M.J. Serotonin regulates hippocampal glucocorticoid receptor expression via a 5-ht7 receptor. *Brain Res. Dev. Brain Res.* **2002**, *139*, 199–203. [CrossRef]
76. Charnay, Y.; Leger, L. Brain serotonergic circuitries. *Dialogues Clin. Neurosci.* **2010**, *12*, 471–487. [PubMed]
77. Suzuki, R.; Rygh, L.J.; Dickenson, A.H. Bad news from the brain: Descending 5-ht pathways that control spinal pain processing. *Trends Pharmacol. Sci.* **2004**, *25*, 613–617. [CrossRef] [PubMed]
78. Sommer, C. Is serotonin hyperalgesic or analgesic? *Curr. Pain Headache Rep.* **2006**, *10*, 101–106. [CrossRef] [PubMed]

79. Wolfe, F.; Russell, I.J.; Vipraio, G.; Ross, K.; Anderson, J. Serotonin levels, pain threshold, and fibromyalgia symptoms in the general population. *J. Rheumatol.* **1997**, *24*, 555–559. [PubMed]
80. Russell, I.J.; Vaeroy, H.; Javors, M.; Nyberg, F. Cerebrospinal fluid biogenic amine metabolites in fibromyalgia/fibrositis syndrome and rheumatoid arthritis. *Arthritis Rheumatol.* **1992**, *35*, 550–556. [CrossRef] [PubMed]
81. Aira, Z.; Buesa, I.; Salgueiro, M.; Bilbao, J.; Aguilera, L.; Zimmermann, M.; Azkue, J.J. Subtype-specific changes in 5-ht receptor-mediated modulation of c fibre-evoked spinal field potentials are triggered by peripheral nerve injury. *Neuroscience* **2010**, *168*, 831–841. [CrossRef] [PubMed]
82. Nicholl, B.I.; Holliday, K.L.; Macfarlane, G.J.; Thomson, W.; Davies, K.A.; O'Neill, T.W.; Bartfai, G.; Boonen, S.; Casanueva, F.F.; Finn, J.D.; et al. Association of htr2a polymorphisms with chronic widespread pain and the extent of musculoskeletal pain: Results from two population-based cohorts. *Arthritis Rheumatol.* **2011**, *63*, 810–818. [CrossRef] [PubMed]
83. Hanley, G.E.; Oberlander, T.F. Neurodevelopmental outcomes following prenatal exposure to serotonin reuptake inhibitor antidepressants: A "social teratogen" or moderator of developmental risk? *Birth Defects Res. A Clin. Mol. Teratol.* **2012**, *94*, 651–659. [CrossRef] [PubMed]
84. Heils, A.; Teufel, A.; Petri, S.; Stober, G.; Riederer, P.; Bengel, D.; Lesch, K.P. Allelic variation of human serotonin transporter gene expression. *J. Neurochem.* **1996**, *66*, 2621–2624. [CrossRef] [PubMed]
85. Offenbaecher, M.; Bondy, B.; de Jonge, S.; Glatzeder, K.; Kruger, M.; Schoeps, P.; Ackenheil, M. Possible association of fibromyalgia with a polymorphism in the serotonin transporter gene regulatory region. *Arthritis Rheumatol.* **1999**, *42*, 2482–2488. [CrossRef]
86. Cohen, H.; Buskila, D.; Neumann, L.; Ebstein, R.P. Confirmation of an association between fibromyalgia and serotonin transporter promoter region (5- httlpr) polymorphism, and relationship to anxiety-related personality traits. *Arthritis Rheumatol.* **2002**, *46*, 845–847. [CrossRef] [PubMed]
87. Homberg, J.R.; Lesch, K.P. Looking on the bright side of serotonin transporter gene variation. *Biol. Psychiatry* **2011**, *69*, 513–519. [CrossRef] [PubMed]
88. Miller, R.; Wankerl, M.; Stalder, T.; Kirschbaum, C.; Alexander, N. The serotonin transporter gene-linked polymorphic region (5-httlpr) and cortisol stress reactivity: A meta-analysis. *Mol. Psychiatry* **2013**, *18*, 1018–1024. [CrossRef] [PubMed]
89. Hariri, A.R.; Mattay, V.S.; Tessitore, A.; Kolachana, B.; Fera, F.; Goldman, D.; Egan, M.F.; Weinberger, D.R. Serotonin transporter genetic variation and the response of the human amygdala. *Science* **2002**, *297*, 400–403. [CrossRef] [PubMed]
90. Heinz, A.; Braus, D.F.; Smolka, M.N.; Wrase, J.; Puls, I.; Hermann, D.; Klein, S.; Grusser, S.M.; Flor, H.; Schumann, G.; et al. Amygdala-prefrontal coupling depends on a genetic variation of the serotonin transporter. *Nat. Neurosci.* **2005**, *8*, 20–21. [CrossRef] [PubMed]
91. Hariri, A.R.; Holmes, A. Genetics of emotional regulation: The role of the serotonin transporter in neural function. *Trends Cogn. Sci.* **2006**, *10*, 182–191. [CrossRef] [PubMed]
92. Canli, T.; Lesch, K.P. Long story short: The serotonin transporter in emotion regulation and social cognition. *Nat. Neurosci.* **2007**, *10*, 1103–1109. [CrossRef] [PubMed]
93. Huang, E.J.; Reichardt, L.F. Neurotrophins: Roles in neuronal development and function. *Annu. Rev. Neurosci.* **2001**, *24*, 677–736. [CrossRef] [PubMed]
94. Rasmusson, A.M.; Shi, L.; Duman, R. Downregulation of bdnf mrna in the hippocampal dentate gyrus after re-exposure to cues previously associated with footshock. *Neuropsychopharmacology* **2002**, *27*, 133–142. [CrossRef]
95. Govindarajan, A.; Rao, B.S.; Nair, D.; Trinh, M.; Mawjee, N.; Tonegawa, S.; Chattarji, S. Transgenic brain-derived neurotrophic factor expression causes both anxiogenic and antidepressant effects. *Proc. Natl. Acad. Sci. USA* **2006**, *103*, 13208–13213. [CrossRef] [PubMed]
96. Lakshminarasimhan, H.; Chattarji, S. Stress leads to contrasting effects on the levels of brain derived neurotrophic factor in the hippocampus and amygdala. *PLoS ONE* **2012**, *7*, e30481. [CrossRef] [PubMed]
97. Mutso, A.A.; Petre, B.; Huang, L.; Baliki, M.N.; Torbey, S.; Herrmann, K.M.; Schnitzer, T.J.; Apkarian, A.V. Reorganization of hippocampal functional connectivity with transition to chronic back pain. *J. Neurophysiol.* **2014**, *111*, 1065–1076. [CrossRef] [PubMed]

98. Jiang, Y.; Oathes, D.; Hush, J.; Darnall, B.; Charvat, M.; Mackey, S.; Etkin, A. Perturbed connectivity of the amygdala and its subregions with the central executive and default mode networks in chronic pain. *Pain* **2016**, *157*, 1970–1978. [CrossRef] [PubMed]
99. Duric, V.; McCarson, K.E. Effects of analgesic or antidepressant drugs on pain- or stress-evoked hippocampal and spinal neurokinin-1 receptor and brain-derived neurotrophic factor gene expression in the rat. *J. Pharmacol. Exp. Ther.* **2006**, *319*, 1235–1243. [CrossRef] [PubMed]
100. Heldt, S.A.; Stanek, L.; Chhatwal, J.P.; Ressler, K.J. Hippocampus-specific deletion of bdnf in adult mice impairs spatial memory and extinction of aversive memories. *Mol. Psychiatry* **2007**, *12*, 656–670. [CrossRef] [PubMed]
101. Fukuhara, K.; Ishikawa, K.; Yasuda, S.; Kishishita, Y.; Kim, H.K.; Kakeda, T.; Yamamoto, M.; Norii, T.; Ishikawa, T. Intracerebroventricular 4-methylcatechol (4-mc) ameliorates chronic pain associated with depression-like behavior via induction of brain-derived neurotrophic factor (bdnf). *Cell. Mol. Neurobiol.* **2012**, *32*, 971–977. [CrossRef] [PubMed]
102. Egan, M.F.; Goldberg, T.E.; Kolachana, B.S.; Callicott, J.H.; Mazzanti, C.M.; Straub, R.E.; Goldman, D.; Weinberger, D.R. Effect of comt val108/158 met genotype on frontal lobe function and risk for schizophrenia. *Proc. Natl. Acad. Sci. USA* **2001**, *98*, 6917–6922. [CrossRef] [PubMed]
103. Egan, M.F.; Kojima, M.; Callicott, J.H.; Goldberg, T.E.; Kolachana, B.S.; Bertolino, A.; Zaitsev, E.; Gold, B.; Goldman, D.; Dean, M.; et al. The bdnf val66met polymorphism affects activity-dependent secretion of bdnf and human memory and hippocampal function. *Cell* **2003**, *112*, 257–269. [CrossRef]
104. Pezawas, L.; Verchinski, B.A.; Mattay, V.S.; Callicott, J.H.; Kolachana, B.S.; Straub, R.E.; Egan, M.F.; Meyer-Lindenberg, A.; Weinberger, D.R. The brain-derived neurotrophic factor val66met polymorphism and variation in human cortical morphology. *J. Neurosci.* **2004**, *24*, 10099–10102. [CrossRef] [PubMed]
105. Kennedy, K.M.; Rodrigue, K.M.; Land, S.J.; Raz, N. Bdnf val66met polymorphism influences age differences in microstructure of the corpus callosum. *Front. Hum. Neurosci.* **2009**, *3*, 19. [CrossRef] [PubMed]
106. Montag, C.; Weber, B.; Fliessbach, K.; Elger, C.; Reuter, M. The bdnf val66met polymorphism impacts parahippocampal and amygdala volume in healthy humans: Incremental support for a genetic risk factor for depression. *Psychol. Med.* **2009**, *39*, 1831–1839. [CrossRef] [PubMed]
107. Soliman, F.; Glatt, C.E.; Bath, K.G.; Levita, L.; Jones, R.M.; Pattwell, S.S.; Jing, D.; Tottenham, N.; Amso, D.; Somerville, L.H.; et al. A genetic variant bdnf polymorphism alters extinction learning in both mouse and human. *Science* **2010**, *327*, 863–866. [CrossRef] [PubMed]
108. Hajek, T.; Kopecek, M.; Hoschl, C. Reduced hippocampal volumes in healthy carriers of brain-derived neurotrophic factor val66met polymorphism: Meta-analysis. *World J. Biol. Psychiatry* **2012**, *13*, 178–187. [CrossRef] [PubMed]
109. Molendijk, M.L.; Bus, B.A.; Spinhoven, P.; Kaimatzoglou, A.; Oude Voshaar, R.C.; Penninx, B.W.; van, I.M.H.; Elzinga, B.M. A systematic review and meta-analysis on the association between bdnf val(66)met and hippocampal volume–a genuine effect or a winners curse? *Am. J. Med. Genet. B Neuropsychiatr. Genet.* **2012**, *159B*, 731–740. [CrossRef] [PubMed]
110. Kim, S.N.; Kang, D.H.; Yun, J.Y.; Lee, T.Y.; Jung, W.H.; Jang, J.H.; Kwon, J.S. Impact of the bdnf val66met polymorphism on regional brain gray matter volumes: Relevance to the stress response. *Psychiatry Investig.* **2013**, *10*, 173–179. [CrossRef] [PubMed]
111. Xu, H.; Qing, H.; Lu, W.; Keegan, D.; Richardson, J.S.; Chlan-Fourney, J.; Li, X.M. Quetiapine attenuates the immobilization stress-induced decrease of brain-derived neurotrophic factor expression in rat hippocampus. *Neurosci. Lett.* **2002**, *321*, 65–68. [CrossRef]
112. Chen, Z.Y.; Jing, D.; Bath, K.G.; Ieraci, A.; Khan, T.; Siao, C.J.; Herrera, D.G.; Toth, M.; Yang, C.; McEwen, B.S.; et al. Genetic variant bdnf (val66met) polymorphism alters anxiety-related behavior. *Science* **2006**, *314*, 140–143. [CrossRef] [PubMed]
113. Garcia, L.S.; Comim, C.M.; Valvassori, S.S.; Reus, G.Z.; Barbosa, L.M.; Andreazza, A.C.; Stertz, L.; Fries, G.R.; Gavioli, E.C.; Kapczinski, F.; et al. Acute administration of ketamine induces antidepressant-like effects in the forced swimming test and increases bdnf levels in the rat hippocampus. *Prog. Neuropsychopharmacol. Biol. Psychiatry* **2008**, *32*, 140–144. [CrossRef] [PubMed]
114. Pivac, N.; Kozaric-Kovacic, D.; Grubisic-Ilic, M.; Nedic, G.; Rakos, I.; Nikolac, M.; Blazev, M.; Muck-Seler, D. The association between brain-derived neurotrophic factor val66met variants and psychotic symptoms in posttraumatic stress disorder. *World J. Biol. Psychiatry* **2012**, *13*, 306–311. [CrossRef] [PubMed]

115. Gao, S.; Cui, Y.L.; Yu, C.Q.; Wang, Q.S.; Zhang, Y. Tetrandrine exerts antidepressant-like effects in animal models: Role of brain-derived neurotrophic factor. *Behav. Brain Res.* **2013**, *238*, 79–85. [CrossRef] [PubMed]
116. Lee, L.C.; Tu, C.H.; Chen, L.F.; Shen, H.D.; Chao, H.T.; Lin, M.W.; Hsieh, J.C. Association of brain-derived neurotrophic factor gene val66met polymorphism with primary dysmenorrhea. *PLoS ONE* **2014**, *9*, e112766. [CrossRef] [PubMed]
117. Reddy, S.Y.; Rasmussen, N.A.; Fourie, N.H.; Berger, R.S.; Martino, A.C.; Gill, J.; Longchamps, R.; Wang, X.M.; Heitkemper, M.M.; Henderson, W.A. Sleep quality, bdnf genotype and gene expression in individuals with chronic abdominal pain. *BMC Med. Genom.* **2014**, *7*, 61. [CrossRef] [PubMed]
118. Zhang, L.; Benedek, D.M.; Fullerton, C.S.; Forsten, R.D.; Naifeh, J.A.; Li, X.X.; Hu, X.Z.; Li, H.; Jia, M.; Xing, G.Q.; et al. Ptsd risk is associated with bdnf val66met and bdnf overexpression. *Mol. Psychiatry* **2014**, *19*, 8–10. [CrossRef] [PubMed]
119. Generaal, E.; Milaneschi, Y.; Jansen, R.; Elzinga, B.M.; Dekker, J.; Penninx, B.W. The brain-derived neurotrophic factor pathway, life stress, and chronic multi-site musculoskeletal pain. *Mol. Pain* **2016**, *12*. [CrossRef] [PubMed]
120. Trang, T.; Beggs, S.; Salter, M.W. Brain-derived neurotrophic factor from microglia: A molecular substrate for neuropathic pain. *Neuron. Glia Biol.* **2011**, *7*, 99–108. [CrossRef] [PubMed]
121. Watkins, L.R.; Hutchinson, M.R.; Ledeboer, A.; Wieseler-Frank, J.; Milligan, E.D.; Maier, S.F. Norman cousins lecture. Glia as the "bad guys": Implications for improving clinical pain control and the clinical utility of opioids. *Brain Behav. Immun.* **2007**, *21*, 131–146. [CrossRef] [PubMed]
122. Uceyler, N.; Sommer, C. Cytokine-related and histological biomarkers for neuropathic pain assessment. *Pain Manag.* **2012**, *2*, 391–398. [CrossRef] [PubMed]
123. Ransohoff, R.M. How neuroinflammation contributes to neurodegeneration. *Science* **2016**, *353*, 777–783. [CrossRef] [PubMed]
124. Pankratz, S.; Bittner, S.; Kehrel, B.E.; Langer, H.F.; Kleinschnitz, C.; Meuth, S.G.; Gobel, K. The inflammatory role of platelets: Translational insights from experimental studies of autoimmune disorders. *Int. J. Mol. Sci.* **2016**, *17*. [CrossRef] [PubMed]
125. Benson, S.; Engler, H.; Schedlowski, M.; Elsenbruch, S. Experimental endotoxemia as a model to study neuroimmune mechanisms in human visceral pain. *Ann. N. Y. Acad. Sci.* **2012**, *1262*, 108–117. [CrossRef] [PubMed]
126. Del Valle, L.; Schwartzman, R.J.; Alexander, G. Spinal cord histopathological alterations in a patient with longstanding complex regional pain syndrome. *Brain Behav. Immun.* **2009**, *23*, 85–91. [CrossRef] [PubMed]
127. Shi, Y.; Gelman, B.B.; Lisinicchia, J.G.; Tang, S.J. Chronic-pain-associated astrocytic reaction in the spinal cord dorsal horn of human immunodeficiency virus-infected patients. *J. Neurosci.* **2012**, *32*, 10833–10840. [CrossRef] [PubMed]
128. Brisby, H.; Olmarker, K.; Rosengren, L.; Cederlund, C.G.; Rydevik, B. Markers of nerve tissue injury in the cerebrospinal fluid in patients with lumbar disc herniation and sciatica. *Spine* **1999**, *24*, 742–746. [CrossRef]
129. Kadetoff, D.; Lampa, J.; Westman, M.; Andersson, M.; Kosek, E. Evidence of central inflammation in fibromyalgia-increased cerebrospinal fluid interleukin-8 levels. *J. Neuroimmunol.* **2012**, *242*, 33–38. [CrossRef] [PubMed]
130. Loggia, M.L.; Chonde, D.B.; Akeju, O.; Arabasz, G.; Catana, C.; Edwards, R.R.; Hill, E.; Hsu, S.; Izquierdo-Garcia, D.; Ji, R.R.; et al. Evidence for brain glial activation in chronic pain patients. *Brain* **2015**, *138*, 604–615. [CrossRef] [PubMed]
131. Fiore, N.T.; Austin, P.J. Are the emergence of affective disturbances in neuropathic pain states contingent on supraspinal neuroinflammation? *Brain Behav. Immun.* **2016**, *56*, 397–411. [CrossRef] [PubMed]
132. Goshen, I.; Kreisel, T.; Ben-Menachem-Zidon, O.; Licht, T.; Weidenfeld, J.; Ben-Hur, T.; Yirmiya, R. Brain interleukin-1 mediates chronic stress-induced depression in mice via adrenocortical activation and hippocampal neurogenesis suppression. *Mol. Psychiatry* **2008**, *13*, 717–728. [CrossRef] [PubMed]
133. Goshen, I.; Kreisel, T.; Ounallah-Saad, H.; Renbaum, P.; Zalzstein, Y.; Ben-Hur, T.; Levy-Lahad, E.; Yirmiya, R. A dual role for interleukin-1 in hippocampal-dependent memory processes. *Psychoneuroendocrinology* **2007**, *32*, 1106–1115. [CrossRef] [PubMed]
134. Besedovsky, H.O.; del Rey, A. Immune-neuro-endocrine interactions: Facts and hypotheses. *Endocr. Rev.* **1996**, *17*, 64–102. [CrossRef] [PubMed]

135. Pace, T.W.; Hu, F.; Miller, A.H. Cytokine-effects on glucocorticoid receptor function: Relevance to glucocorticoid resistance and the pathophysiology and treatment of major depression. *Brain Behav. Immun.* **2007**, *21*, 9–19. [CrossRef] [PubMed]
136. Vogelzangs, N.; de Jonge, P.; Smit, J.H.; Bahn, S.; Penninx, B.W. Cytokine production capacity in depression and anxiety. *Transl. Psychiatry* **2016**, *6*, e825. [CrossRef] [PubMed]
137. Lasselin, J.; Kemani, M.K.; Kanstrup, M.; Olsson, G.L.; Axelsson, J.; Andreasson, A.; Lekander, M.; Wicksell, R.K. Low-grade inflammation may moderate the effect of behavioral treatment for chronic pain in adults. *J. Behav. Med.* **2016**. [CrossRef] [PubMed]
138. Beggs, S.; Currie, G.; Salter, M.W.; Fitzgerald, M.; Walker, S.M. Priming of adult pain responses by neonatal pain experience: Maintenance by central neuroimmune activity. *Brain* **2012**, *135*, 404–417. [CrossRef] [PubMed]
139. Mitchell, R.H.; Goldstein, B.I. Inflammation in children and adolescents with neuropsychiatric disorders: A systematic review. *J. Am. Acad. Child Adolesc. Psychiatry* **2014**, *53*, 274–296. [CrossRef] [PubMed]
140. Ganguly, P.; Brenhouse, H.C. Broken or maladaptive? Altered trajectories in neuroinflammation and behavior after early life adversity. *Dev. Cogn. Neurosci.* **2015**, *11*, 18–30. [CrossRef] [PubMed]
141. Gill, J.; Luckenbaugh, D.; Charney, D.; Vythilingam, M. Sustained elevation of serum interleukin-6 and relative insensitivity to hydrocortisone differentiates posttraumatic stress disorder with and without depression. *Biol. Psychiatry* **2010**, *68*, 999–1006. [CrossRef] [PubMed]
142. Lerman, I.; Davis, B.A.; Bertram, T.M.; Proudfoot, J.; Hauger, R.L.; Coe, C.L.; Patel, P.M.; Baker, D.G. Posttraumatic stress disorder influences the nociceptive and intrathecal cytokine response to a painful stimulus in combat veterans. *Psychoneuroendocrinology* **2016**, *73*, 99–108. [CrossRef] [PubMed]
143. Kopf, M.; Bachmann, M.F.; Marsland, B.J. Averting inflammation by targeting the cytokine environment. *Nat. Rev. Drug Discov.* **2010**, *9*, 703–718. [CrossRef] [PubMed]
144. Apkarian, A.V.; Bushnell, M.C.; Treede, R.D.; Zubieta, J.K. Human brain mechanisms of pain perception and regulation in health and disease. *Eur. J. Pain* **2005**, *9*, 463–484. [CrossRef] [PubMed]
145. Bushnell, M.C.; Ceko, M.; Low, L.A. Cognitive and emotional control of pain and its disruption in chronic pain. *Nat. Rev. Neurosci.* **2013**, *14*, 502–511. [CrossRef] [PubMed]
146. Duerden, E.G.; Albanese, M.C. Localization of pain-related brain activation: A meta-analysis of neuroimaging data. *Hum. Brain Mapp.* **2013**, *34*, 109–149. [CrossRef] [PubMed]
147. Iadarola, M.J.; Coghill, R.C. Imaging of pain: Recent developments. *Curr. Opin. Anaesthesiol.* **1999**, *12*, 583–589. [CrossRef] [PubMed]
148. Willis, W.D.; Westlund, K.N. Neuroanatomy of the pain system and of the pathways that modulate pain. *J. Clin. Neurophysiol.* **1997**, *14*, 2–31. [CrossRef] [PubMed]
149. Atlas, L.Y.; Lindquist, M.A.; Bolger, N.; Wager, T.D. Brain mediators of the effects of noxious heat on pain. *Pain* **2014**, *155*, 1632–1648. [CrossRef] [PubMed]
150. Coghill, R.C.; Sang, C.N.; Maisog, J.M.; Iadarola, M.J. Pain intensity processing within the human brain: A bilateral, distributed mechanism. *J. Neurophysiol.* **1999**, *82*, 1934–1943. [PubMed]
151. Wager, T.D.; Atlas, L.Y.; Lindquist, M.A.; Roy, M.; Woo, C.W.; Kross, E. An fmri-based neurologic signature of physical pain. *N. Engl. J. Med.* **2013**, *368*, 1388–1397. [CrossRef] [PubMed]
152. Hubbard, C.S.; Khan, S.A.; Xu, S.; Cha, M.; Masri, R.; Seminowicz, D.A. Behavioral, metabolic and functional brain changes in a rat model of chronic neuropathic pain: A longitudinal mri study. *Neuroimage* **2015**, *107*, 333–344. [CrossRef] [PubMed]
153. Jensen, K.B.; Regenbogen, C.; Ohse, M.C.; Frasnelli, J.; Freiherr, J.; Lundstrom, J.N. Brain activations during pain: A neuroimaging meta-analysis of patients with pain and healthy controls. *Pain* **2016**, *157*, 1279–1286. [CrossRef] [PubMed]
154. Baliki, M.N.; Petre, B.; Torbey, S.; Herrmann, K.M.; Huang, L.; Schnitzer, T.J.; Fields, H.L.; Apkarian, A.V. Corticostriatal functional connectivity predicts transition to chronic back pain. *Nat. Neurosci.* **2012**, *15*, 1117–1119. [CrossRef] [PubMed]
155. Hubbard, C.S.; Becerra, L.; Heinz, N.; Ludwick, A.; Rasooly, T.; Wu, R.; Johnson, A.; Schechter, N.L.; Borsook, D.; Nurko, S. Abdominal pain, the adolescent and altered brain structure and function. *PLoS ONE* **2016**, *11*, e0156545. [CrossRef] [PubMed]

156. Simons, L.E.; Pielech, M.; Erpelding, N.; Linnman, C.; Moulton, E.; Sava, S.; Lebel, A.; Serrano, P.; Sethna, N.; Berde, C.; et al. The responsive amygdala: Treatment-induced alterations in functional connectivity in pediatric complex regional pain syndrome. *Pain* **2014**, *155*, 1727–1742. [CrossRef] [PubMed]
157. Simons, L.E.; Erpelding, N.; Hernandez, J.; Serrano, P.; Zhang, K.; Lebel, A.; Sethna, N.; Berde, C.; Prabhu, S.; Becerra, L.; et al. Fear and reward circuit alterations in pediatric crps. *Front. Hum. Neurosci.* **2016**, *9*, 1–13. [CrossRef] [PubMed]
158. Lebel, A.; Becerra, L.; Wallin, D.; Moulton, E.A.; Morris, S.; Pendse, G.; Jasciewicz, J.; Stein, M.; Aiello-Lammens, M.; Grant, E.; et al. Fmri reveals distinct cns processing during symptomatic and recovered complex regional pain syndrome in children. *Brain* **2008**, *131*, 1854–1879. [CrossRef] [PubMed]
159. McEwen, B.S.; Kalia, M. The role of corticosteroids and stress in chronic pain conditions. *Metabolism* **2010**, *59* (Suppl. 1), S9–S15. [CrossRef] [PubMed]
160. Karatsoreos, I.N.; McEwen, B.S. Psychobiological allostasis: Resistance, resilience and vulnerability. *Trends Cogn. Sci.* **2011**, *15*, 576–584. [CrossRef] [PubMed]
161. Becerra, L.; Sava, S.; Simons, L.E.; Drosos, A.M.; Sethna, N.; Berde, C.; Lebel, A.A.; Borsook, D. Intrinsic brain networks normalize with treatment in pediatric complex regional pain syndrome. *Neuroimage Clin.* **2014**, *6*, 347–369. [CrossRef] [PubMed]
162. Coutinho, J.F.; Fernandesl, S.V.; Soares, J.M.; Maia, L.; Goncalves, O.F.; Sampaio, A. Default mode network dissociation in depressive and anxiety states. *Brain Imaging Behav.* **2016**, *10*, 147–157. [CrossRef] [PubMed]
163. Geng, H.; Li, X.; Chen, J.; Li, X.; Gu, R. Decreased intra- and inter-salience network functional connectivity is related to trait anxiety in adolescents. *Front. Behav. Neurosci.* **2015**, *9*, 350. [CrossRef] [PubMed]
164. Lei, D.; Li, L.; Li, L.; Suo, X.; Huang, X.; Lui, S.; Li, J.; Bi, F.; Kemp, G.J.; Gong, Q. Microstructural abnormalities in children with post-traumatic stress disorder: A diffusion tensor imaging study at 3.0t. *Sci. Rep.* **2015**, *5*, 8933. [CrossRef] [PubMed]
165. Pannekoek, J.N.; van der Werff, S.J.; Meens, P.H.; van den Bulk, B.G.; Jolles, D.D.; Veer, I.M.; van Lang, N.D.; Rombouts, S.A.; van der Wee, N.J.; Vermeiren, R.R. Aberrant resting-state functional connectivity in limbic and salience networks in treatment–naive clinically depressed adolescents. *J. Child Psychol. Psychiatry* **2014**, *55*, 1317–1327. [CrossRef] [PubMed]
166. Schanberg, L.E.; Anthony, K.K.; Gil, K.M.; Lefebvre, J.C.; Kredich, D.W.; Macharoni, L.M. Family pain history predicts child health status in children with chronic rheumatic disease. *Pediatrics* **2001**, *108*, E47. [CrossRef] [PubMed]
167. Garber, J.; Zeman, J.; Walker, L.S. Recurrent abdominal pain in children: Psychiatric diagnoses and parental psychopathology. *J. Am. Acad. Child Adolesc. Psychiatry* **1990**, *29*, 648–656. [CrossRef] [PubMed]
168. Hoftun, G.B.; Romundstad, P.R.; Rygg, M. Factors associated with adolescent chronic non-specific pain, chronic multisite pain, and chronic pain with high disability: The young-hunt study 2008. *J. Pain* **2012**. [CrossRef] [PubMed]
169. Morgan, J.E.; Hammen, C.; Lee, S.S. Parental serotonin transporter polymorphism (5-httlpr) moderates associations of stress and child behavior with parenting behavior. *J. Clin. Child Adolesc. Psychol.* **2016**, 1–12. [CrossRef] [PubMed]
170. Roth, T.L.; Lubin, F.D.; Funk, A.J.; Sweatt, J.D. Lasting epigenetic influence of early-life adversity on the bdnf gene. *Biol. Psychiatry* **2009**, *65*, 760–769. [CrossRef] [PubMed]
171. van der Doelen, R.H.; Arnoldussen, I.A.; Ghareh, H.; van Och, L.; Homberg, J.R.; Kozicz, T. Early life adversity and serotonin transporter gene variation interact to affect DNA methylation of the corticotropin-releasing factor gene promoter region in the adult rat brain. *Dev. Psychopathol.* **2015**, *27*, 123–135. [CrossRef] [PubMed]
172. Walker, L.S.; Greene, J.W. Children with recurrent abdominal pain and their parents: More somatic complaints, anxiety, and depression than other patient families? *J. Pediatr. Psychol.* **1989**, *14*, 231–243. [CrossRef] [PubMed]
173. Campo, J.V.; Bridge, J.; Lucas, A.; Savorelli, S.; Walker, L.; Di Lorenzo, C.; Iyengar, S.; Brent, D.A. Physical and emotional health of mothers of youth with functional abdominal pain. *Arch. Pediatr. Adolesc. Med.* **2007**, *161*, 131–137. [CrossRef] [PubMed]
174. Williamson, G.M.; Walters, A.S.; Shaffer, D.R. Caregiver models of self and others, coping, and depression: Predictors of depression in children with chronic pain. *Health Psychol.* **2002**, *21*, 405–410. [CrossRef] [PubMed]

175. Wolff, N.; Darlington, A.S.; Hunfeld, J.; Verhulst, F.; Jaddoe, V.; Hofman, A.; Passchier, J.; Tiemeier, H. Determinants of somatic complaints in 18-month-old children: The generation r study. *J. Pediatr. Psychol.* **2010**, *35*, 306–316. [CrossRef] [PubMed]
176. Higgins, K.S.; Birnie, K.A.; Chambers, C.T.; Wilson, A.C.; Caes, L.; Clark, A.J.; Lynch, M.; Stinson, J.; Campbell-Yeo, M. Offspring of parents with chronic pain: A systematic review and meta-analysis of pain, health, psychological, and family outcomes. *Pain* **2015**, *156*, 2256–2266. [CrossRef] [PubMed]
177. Levy, R.L.; Whitehead, W.E.; Von Korff, M.R.; Feld, A.D. Intergenerational transmission of gastrointestinal illness behavior. *Am. J. Gastroenterol.* **2000**, *95*, 451–456. [CrossRef] [PubMed]
178. van Tilburg, M.A.; Levy, R.L.; Walker, L.S.; Von Korff, M.; Feld, L.D.; Garner, M.; Feld, A.D.; Whitehead, W.E. Psychosocial mechanisms for the transmission of somatic symptoms from parents to children. *World J. Gastroenterol.* **2015**, *21*, 5532–5541. [CrossRef] [PubMed]
179. Stone, A.L.; Wilson, A.C. Transmission of risk from parents with chronic pain to offspring: An integrative conceptual model. *Pain* **2016**. [CrossRef] [PubMed]
180. Palermo, T.M.; Law, E.F.; Fales, J.; Bromberg, M.H.; Jessen-Fiddick, T.; Tai, G. Internet-delivered cognitive-behavioral treatment for adolescents with chronic pain and their parents: A randomized controlled multicenter trial. *Pain* **2016**, *157*, 174–185. [CrossRef] [PubMed]
181. Palermo, T.M.; Valrie, C.R.; Karlson, C.W. Family and parent influences on pediatric chronic pain: A developmental perspective. *Am. Psychol.* **2014**, *69*, 142–152. [CrossRef] [PubMed]
182. Fisher, E.; Law, E.; Palermo, T.M.; Eccleston, C. Psychological therapies (remotely delivered) for the management of chronic and recurrent pain in children and adolescents. *Cochrane Database Syst. Rev.* **2014**, *2014*.
183. Cunningham, N.R.; Jagpal, A.; Tran, S.T.; Kashikar-Zuck, S.; Goldschneider, K.R.; Coghill, R.C.; Lynch-Jordan, A.M. Anxiety adversely impacts response to cognitive behavioral therapy in children with chronic pain. *J. Pediatr.* **2016**, *171*, 227–233. [CrossRef] [PubMed]
184. Benore, E.; D'Auria, A.; Banez, G.A.; Worley, S.; Tang, A. The influence of anxiety reduction on clinical response to pediatric chronic pain rehabilitation. *Clin. J. Pain* **2015**, *31*, 375–383. [CrossRef] [PubMed]
185. Sullivan, A.; Goodison-Farnsworth, E.; Jaaniste, T. Posttraumatic stress disorder in children with chronic pain. *Pediatr. Pain Lett.* **2015**, *17*, 35–39.
186. Nelson, S.M.; Cunningham, N.R.; Kashikar-Zuck, S. A conceptual framework for understanding the role of adverse childhood experiences in pediatric chronic pain. *Clin. J. Pain* **2016**. [CrossRef] [PubMed]
187. Bosco, M.A.; Gallinati, J.L.; Clark, M.E. Conceptualizing and treating comorbid chronic pain and ptsd. *Pain Res. Treat.* **2013**, *2013*, 174728. [CrossRef] [PubMed]
188. Plagge, J.M.; Lu, M.W.; Lovejoy, T.I.; Karl, A.I.; Dobscha, S.K. Treatment of comorbid pain and ptsd in returning veterans: A collaborative approach utilizing behavioral activation. *Pain Med.* **2013**, *14*, 1164–1172. [CrossRef] [PubMed]
189. Otis, J.D.; Keane, T.M.; Kerns, R.D.; Monson, C.; Scioli, E. The development of an integrated treatment for veterans with comorbid chronic pain and posttraumatic stress disorder. *Pain Med.* **2009**, *10*, 1300–1311. [CrossRef] [PubMed]
190. Allen, L.B.; Tsao, J.C.I.; Seidman, L.C.; Ehrenreich-May, J.; Zeltzer, L.K. A unified, transdiagnositc treatment for adolescents with chronic pain and comorbid anxiety and depression. *Cogn. Behav. Pract.* **2012**, *19*, 56–67. [CrossRef]
191. Umezaki, Y.; Badran, B.W.; DeVries, W.H.; Moss, J.; Gonzales, T.; George, M.S. The efficacy of daily prefrontal repetitive transcranial magnetic stimulation (rtms) for burning mouth syndrome (bms): A randomized controlled single-blind study. *Brain Stimul.* **2016**, *9*, 234–242. [CrossRef] [PubMed]
192. Picarelli, H.; Teixeira, M.J.; de Andrade, D.C.; Myczkowski, M.L.; Luvisotto, T.B.; Yeng, L.T.; Fonoff, E.T.; Pridmore, S.; Marcolin, M.A. Repetitive transcranial magnetic stimulation is efficacious as an add-on to pharmacological therapy in complex regional pain syndrome (crps) type i. *J. Pain* **2010**, *11*, 1203–1210. [CrossRef] [PubMed]
193. Mendonca, M.E.; Simis, M.; Grecco, L.C.; Battistella, L.R.; Baptista, A.F.; Fregni, F. Transcranial direct current stimulation combined with aerobic exercise to optimize analgesic responses in fibromyalgia: A randomized placebo-controlled clinical trial. *Front. Hum. Neurosci.* **2016**, *10*, 68. [CrossRef] [PubMed]
194. Short, E.B.; Borckardt, J.J.; Anderson, B.S.; Frohman, H.; Beam, W.; Reeves, S.T.; George, M.S. Ten sessions of adjunctive left prefrontal rtms significantly reduces fibromyalgia pain: A randomized, controlled pilot study. *Pain* **2011**, *152*, 2477–2484. [CrossRef] [PubMed]

195. Lefaucheur, J.P.; Ayache, S.S.; Sorel, M.; Farhat, W.H.; Zouari, H.G.; Ciampi de Andrade, D.; Ahdab, R.; Menard-Lefaucheur, I.; Brugieres, P.; Goujon, C. Analgesic effects of repetitive transcranial magnetic stimulation of the motor cortex in neuropathic pain: Influence of theta burst stimulation priming. *Eur. J. Pain* **2012**, *16*, 1403–1413. [CrossRef] [PubMed]
196. Fregni, F.; Boggio, P.S.; Lima, M.C.; Ferreira, M.J.; Wagner, T.; Rigonatti, S.P.; Castro, A.W.; Souza, D.R.; Riberto, M.; Freedman, S.D.; et al. A sham-controlled, phase ii trial of transcranial direct current stimulation for the treatment of central pain in traumatic spinal cord injury. *Pain* **2006**, *122*, 197–209. [CrossRef] [PubMed]
197. Defrin, R.; Grunhaus, L.; Zamir, D.; Zeilig, G. The effect of a series of repetitive transcranial magnetic stimulations of the motor cortex on central pain after spinal cord injury. *Arch. Phys. Med. Rehabil.* **2007**, *88*, 1574–1580. [CrossRef] [PubMed]
198. Perera, T.; George, M.S.; Grammer, G.; Janicak, P.G.; Pascual-Leone, A.; Wirecki, T.S. The clinical tms society consensus review and treatment recommendations for tms therapy for major depressive disorder. *Brain Stimul.* **2016**, *9*, 336–346. [CrossRef] [PubMed]
199. Canadian Agency for Drugs and Technologies in Health. Cadth rapid response reports. In *Transcranial Magnetic Stimulation for the Treatment of Adults with Ptsd, Gad, or Depression: A Review of Clinical Effectiveness and Guidelines*; Canadian Agency for Drugs and Technologies in Health: Ottawa, ON, Canada, 2014.
200. Paes, F.; Machado, S.; Arias-Carrion, O.; Velasques, B.; Teixeira, S.; Budde, H.; Cagy, M.; Piedade, R.; Ribeiro, P.; Huston, J.P.; et al. The value of repetitive transcranial magnetic stimulation (rtms) for the treatment of anxiety disorders: An integrative review. *CNS Neurol. Disord. Drug Targets* **2011**, *10*, 610–620. [CrossRef] [PubMed]
201. Naro, A.; Milardi, D.; Russo, M.; Terranova, C.; Rizzo, V.; Cacciola, A.; Marino, S.; Calabro, R.S.; Quartarone, A. Non-invasive brain stimulation, a tool to revert maladaptive plasticity in neuropathic pain. *Front. Hum. Neurosci.* **2016**, *10*, 376. [CrossRef] [PubMed]
202. DosSantos, M.F.; Ferreira, N.; Toback, R.L.; Carvalho, A.C.; DaSilva, A.F. Potential mechanisms supporting the value of motor cortex stimulation to treat chronic pain syndromes. *Front. Neurosci.* **2016**, *10*. [CrossRef] [PubMed]
203. Chrousos, G.P. The hypothalamic-pituitary-adrenal axis and immune-mediated inflammation. *N. Engl. J. Med.* **1995**, *332*, 1351–1362. [PubMed]
204. Elenkov, I.J.; Webster, E.L.; Torpy, D.J.; Chrousos, G.P. Stress, corticotropin-releasing hormone, glucocorticoids, and the immune/inflammatory response: Acute and chronic effects. *Ann. N. Y. Acad. Sci.* **1999**, *876*, 1–11; discussion 11-13. [CrossRef] [PubMed]
205. Meyer, J.S. Early adrenalectomy stimulates subsequent growth and development of the rat brain. *Exp. Neurol.* **1983**, *82*, 432–446. [CrossRef]
206. Meaney, M.J.; Diorio, J.; Francis, D.; Widdowson, J.; LaPlante, P.; Caldji, C.; Sharma, S.; Seckl, J.R.; Plotsky, P.M. Early environmental regulation of forebrain glucocorticoid receptor gene expression: Implications for adrenocortical responses to stress. *Dev. Neurosci.* **1996**, *18*, 49–72. [CrossRef] [PubMed]
207. Korte, S.M. Corticosteroids in relation to fear, anxiety and psychopathology. *Neurosci. Biobehav. Rev.* **2001**, *25*, 117–142. [CrossRef]
208. Knook, L.M.; Lijmer, J.G.; Konijnenberg, A.Y.; Taminiau, B.; van Engeland, H. The course of chronic pain with and without psychiatric disorders: A 6-year follow-up study from childhood to adolescence and young adulthood. *J. Clin. Psychiatry* **2012**, *73*, e134–e139. [CrossRef] [PubMed]
209. Mulak, A.; Tache, Y.; Larauche, M. Sex hormones in the modulation of irritable bowel syndrome. *World J. Gastroenterol.* **2014**, *20*, 2433–2448. [CrossRef] [PubMed]
210. Karshikoff, B.; Lekander, M.; Soop, A.; Lindstedt, F.; Ingvar, M.; Kosek, E.; Olgart Hoglund, C.; Axelsson, J. Modality and sex differences in pain sensitivity during human endotoxemia. *Brain Behav. Immun.* **2015**, *46*, 35–43. [CrossRef] [PubMed]
211. Aloisi, A.M.; Bachiocco, V.; Costantino, A.; Stefani, R.; Ceccarelli, I.; Bertaccini, A.; Meriggiola, M.C. Cross-sex hormone administration changes pain in transsexual women and men. *Pain* **2007**, *132* (Suppl. 1), S60–S67. [CrossRef] [PubMed]

14

A Systematic Review of the Effects of Exercise and Physical Activity on Non-Specific Chronic Low Back Pain

Rebecca Gordon * and Saul Bloxham

Department of Sport and Health Sciences, University of St Mark and St John, Plymouth PL6 8BH, UK; sbloxham@marjon.ac.uk

* Correspondence: rgordon@marjon.ac.uk

Academic Editor: Robert J. Gatchel

Abstract: Back pain is a major health issue in Western countries and 60%–80% of adults are likely to experience low back pain. This paper explores the impact of back pain on society and the role of physical activity for treatment of non-specific low back pain. A review of the literature was carried out using the databases SPORTDiscuss, Medline and Google Scholar. A general exercise programme that combines muscular strength, flexibility and aerobic fitness is beneficial for rehabilitation of non-specific chronic low back pain. Increasing core muscular strength can assist in supporting the lumbar spine. Improving the flexibility of the muscle-tendons and ligaments in the back increases the range of motion and assists with the patient's functional movement. Aerobic exercise increases the blood flow and nutrients to the soft tissues in the back, improving the healing process and reducing stiffness that can result in back pain.

Keywords: aerobic fitness; non-specific chronic low back pain; pedometer; physical activity

---

1. An Introduction to the Impact of Back Pain on Society and the Importance of Physical Activity

Back pain is a major health issue in Western countries and is associated with increasing medical expenditure, work absence [1,2] and is the most common musculoskeletal condition [3–5]. Sixty to eighty percent of adults will at some point in their lives experience low back pain [6–8], and 16% of adults in the United Kingdom (UK) consult their general practitioner every year [9]. Back pain costs the National Health Service (NHS) £1.3 million every day [10] and results in 12.5% of all work absence in the UK [11]. However, the most appropriate intervention to treat non-specific chronic low back pain (NSCLBP) remains elusive [12].

It is recommended for patients with NSCLBP to remain physically active, as long periods of inactivity will adversely affect recovery [13,14]. A variety of different types of exercise have been explored to treat CLBP, including low-to-moderate intensity aerobic exercise [15,16], high intensity aerobic exercise [17,18], core stabilization and muscular strength exercises [19–24] and flexibility programmes [25–27]. However, the most effective form of exercise as a method of rehabilitation for NSCLBP is unknown [6,28] reflecting its complexity [17] and more research is required [29].

Physical activity (PA) to increase aerobic capacity and muscular strength, especially of the lumbar extensor muscles, is important for patients with CLBP in assisting them to complete activities of daily living [30]. However, different exercises have been found to result in varying levels of effectiveness in reducing lower back pain [31]. In addition, too much or too little PA can be associated with low back pain [32], suggesting that PA as an intervention for low back pain is complex.

Eight-five percent of back pain cases have an unknown cause [33], normally diagnosed after undergoing tests such as X-ray, MRI scan and blood tests [34]. Understanding the cause of back pain is important in order to remove it from the patient's life and not to replicate the movement during therapy [35]. However, when the cause of the back pain is unknown, prescribing targeted therapy can prove difficult, and general exercise is often recommended [36]. Typically intervention programmes have adopted a monodisciplinary approach to rehabilitate NSCLBP [15,21,25]. Although promising findings were reported following a multicomponent exercise programme [37]. Thirty-seven patients with NSCLBP were allocated into control, (who just maintained their current rehabilitation programme), or training groups, which combined an additional functional training programme of aerobic exercise, muscular strength and flexibility. Back pain was found to significantly decrease by 52.5% in the training group compared to no significant change in the control group. In addition, disability significantly decreased by 27.3% in the training group according to the Oswestry Disability Index, compared to no significant change in the control group. The aim of this article is to review the effects of PA and exercise interventions involving aerobic exercise, muscular strength and stabilisation exercises and/or flexibility training on NSCLBP to identify effective strategies for treatment.

2. Method

A systematic review was carried out between 2014 and 2015 using the databases SPORTDiscuss, Medline and Google Scholar. The first author selected intervention programmes published between 2005 and 2015 which investigated the effect of PA or exercise interventions for NSCLBP patients involving aerobic exercise, muscular strength and stabilisation exercises and/or flexibility training on NSCLBP. The first author read and reviewed the articles. Chronic pain was defined as pain remaining for longer than three months and further inclusion criteria was that the participants involved in the studies should be ⩾18 years old. The intervention programmes were identified using the search terms "non-specific chronic low back pain and exercise" which returned 141 results. Other search terms included "chronic low back pain and aerobic exercise" (187 results), "chronic low back pain and muscular strength" (120 results) and "non-specific chronic low back pain" (173 results). A total of 14 studies were included within the final review. The review summarised the effect on NSCLBP within the included intervention programmes.

2.1. *Eligibility Criteria*

Studies were included within the final review based on the following: population, intervention and the outcome.

2.2. *Inclusion Criteria*

Population: NSCLBP patients aged 18 years or older.

Intervention: Aerobic exercise, muscular strength or stabilisation exercises and/or flexibility training intervention programmes. There was no restriction on the inclusion of a follow up in the included studies.

Outcome: Investigate effect of the intervention on NSCLBP which was not limited to one specific measure for pain.

2.3. *Exclusion Criteria*

Literature reviews and any article which did not involve a delivery of an intervention programme to NSCLBP patients.

3. Defining Back Pain and the Impact of Physical Activity and Exercise

Back pain is defined as chronic when the pain remains for longer than three months [38]. CLBP can have a debilitating effect on patients' lives, resulting in disability and reducing their ability to carry out activities of daily living [29]. Acute back pain is pain that remains for less than 6 weeks [39,40] and sub-acute back pain is back pain for between 6 weeks and 3 months. Forty percent of patients with acute low back pain are at an elevated risk of developing CLBP [41].

Back pain is then further categorised into specific or non-specific back pain. Non-specific back pain is diagnosed when the cause of the back pain is unknown [42,43], and specific back pain refers to a specific cause for the pain, for example an infection or a fracture [44]. Non-specific low back pain is the most common type of back pain to occur [45,46], and accounts for 85% of all back pain cases [39,47].

PA increases the blood flow to the back which is important for the healing process of the soft tissues in the back [48]. Being physically active, through activities of daily living, has been highlighted as important in assisting the recovery of acute and NSCLBP [49]. However, following a review of 39 trials into the effects of exercise on non-specific acute low back pain [2], it was suggested there is strong evidence that an exercise programme was not more effective for recovery of non-specific acute low back pain, compared to inactivity. Thus, patients with acute low back pain should not start an exercise programme for rehabilitation [50].

The difference between PA and exercise is that exercise is planned and structured which involves disrupting homeostasis by concentric, eccentric and isometric muscular activity and involves repetitive movements [51]. PA is not structured, and includes any movement that involves contraction of skeletal muscles requiring energy expenditure [52] typified by activities of daily living such as walking and housework [53].

Most people with non-specific acute low back pain recover in 4–6 weeks with or without a treatment [5]. Therefore if acute low back pain patients recover without a treatment in a similar timescale to patients with a treatment, there is no added benefit in completing an exercise programme such as muscle strengthening exercises. Muscle strengthening exercises could potentially cause extra damage to acute back pain due to the additional strain on the ligaments and muscles in the back, which may have swelling [48]. It is important to stop exercise in order to reduce the swelling of the affected area and therefore reduce the back pain [39], suggesting it is a case of waiting for acute low back pain to recover.

Furthermore, a review of six randomised controlled trials researched the effect of exercise programmes on patients with non-specific sub-acute low back pain [54]. The review suggested that there was moderate evidence that a graded-activity exercise programme is effective for improving absenteeism from work for patients with non-specific sub-acute low back pain, however it was unclear if other types of exercise programmes are effective.

4. Results

4.1. Aerobic Exercise

Aerobic exercise can benefit CLBP as it increases the blood flow and nutrients to the soft tissues in the back, improving the healing process and reducing stiffness that results in back pain [55]. In addition 30–40 min of aerobic exercise increases the body's production of endorphins [55], a brain chemical that bind to the opiate receptors in the pain control system in the brain and spinal cord to decrease the perception of pain [56]. Endorphins act in a similar way to pain reducing drugs such as morphine and codeine [57]. However increasing the body's endorphin production is a natural alternative for pain relief for the body [58], and can reduce CLBP [59]. Rehabilitation involving aerobic exercise can be used as a conservative method for reducing CLBP, and could prevent patients relying on medication for pain reduction.

A low aerobic fitness level is associated with CLBP [60,61], and maximum oxygen consumption (VO_{2max}) was significantly lower by 10 mL/kg in men with CLBP compared to men without [62]. VO_{2max} was also significantly lower by 5.6 mL/kg in women with CLBP compared to healthy counterparts.

Aerobic exercise for 20 min on a cycle ergometer at 70% peak oxygen uptake reduced the pain perception for more than 30 min for patients with CLBP [63]. Aerobic exercise also provides additional benefits such as improving functional status [64], and reducing the fear of movement [65]. Fear of movement is a predictor for functional limitations [66] and is associated with disability in patients with CLBP [67]. Aerobic exercise can reduce disability and improve the functional status of patients with CLBP by increasing fitness levels, helping patients conduct activities of daily living.

4.1.1. Impact of Aerobic Exercise Interventions on Chronic Low Back Pain

A 6-week moderate intensity aerobic exercise programme (walking on a treadmill at 50% heart rate reserve) for 52 sedentary NSCLBP patients was compared to a 6-week programme involving specific strengthening exercises for the trunk and upper and lower limbs [16]. CLBP significantly reduced by 20% in the aerobic exercise group and 15% in the muscle strengthening group, although there was no significant difference between the two groups. This suggests that patients could be provided with a choice of which type of exercise programme they would most enjoy. This is important as enjoyment of exercise is an important factor in exercise adherence [68]. However this study involved a 6-week intervention, and an 8-week intervention programme is important to significantly improve aerobic fitness [69], by allowing greater physiological adaptions to occur [15].

An 8-week moderate intensity aerobic exercise intervention at 40%–60% of heart rate reserve combined with conventional physiotherapy, significantly reduced NSCLBP by 47% [15]. This was compared to a significant reduction of 42% in NSCLBP in the control group, involving only conventional physiotherapy. However there was no significant difference between the two groups, suggesting the combination of moderate intensity aerobic exercise and conventional physiotherapy does not provide any additional benefits to CLBP.

The 8-week intervention programme was also found to increase aerobic fitness by 3.3% as measured by VO_{2max}. This increase was not significant, and also suggests that additional factors excluding aerobic fitness levels must have had an influence on reducing CLBP. This was in contrast to previous research which suggested aerobic fitness levels to be associated with CLBP [60,61]. The conventional physiotherapy involved activities such as back mobilisation exercises, core stabilisation exercise and education on back care, suggesting a general programme involving a range of activities may be optimal.

A 12-week high intensity aerobic exercise programme involving running on a treadmill at 85% of heart rate reserve and was compared to passive treatment (ultrasound and did not include any form of PA) [17]. The 12-week high intensity exercise programme significantly reduced NSCLBP by 41% compared to no improvement in the passive treatment group.

The effect of high intensity aerobic exercise on CLBP was further supported by a 12-week high intensity aerobic exercise programme (running on a treadmill at 85% heart rate reserve) which significantly reduced NSCLBP by 30% [18]. This study involved a larger sample size of 64 patients, compared to the previous study [17].

However the study [18] excluded patients with NSCLBP who were obese, classified by a body mass index of 30 or over [70,71]. The researcher stated this was due to possible cardiovascular problems and the risk of injury to the patients, as the study involved high intensity exercise. Therefore the results from this study cannot be generalised to obese NSCLBP patients, despite obesity being associated with NSCLBP [72].

Walking is known to be a safe form of exercise for CLBP patients as it is associated with a low injury rate [73] and does not involve twisting or vigorous forward flexion [74]. Although, exercising at a low intensity at 40% VO_{2max} does not significantly increase cortisol levels [75], and low cortisol levels are associated with CLBP [76].

These studies indicate that although similar outcomes can be achieved despite differences in aerobic exercise intensity. Thus moderate exercise should be promoted over high or low intensity programmes given the reduced risks, enhanced compliance, optimal benefits and reduced impact [55].

Exercising at a comfortable intensity for the patient is important in reducing fear avoidance [77], which is important for increasing PA levels [78] as CLBP patients who are more fear avoidant report higher levels of disability [79]. Patients should be encouraged to increase their levels of PA at an intensity that is comfortable for them, and that can be integrated into activities of daily living [53]. Such an approach is more sustainable long term [80]. See Table 1 for a summary of each of the discussed aerobic exercise intervention programmes.

Table 1. Aerobic exercise intervention programmes for NSCLBP patients.

Reference Number	Type of Population	Length of Intervention	Effect on Back Pain	Significance Levels
(Hoffman *et al.*, 2005) [63]	8 individuals with NSCLBP (4 male, 4 female)	25 min of cycle ergometry. 5 min at 50% peak oxygen uptake, then 20 min at 70% peak oxygen uptake	Pressure pain test. Pain significantly decreased by 28% at 2 min and 22% at 32 min post exercise compared to pre-exercise values. No gender/age differences in results	$p < 0.05$
(Shnayderman & Katz-Leurer, 2013) [16]	52 sedentary NSCLBP patients aged 18-65 years	Experimental group (walking on treadmill at 50% heart rate reserve). Control group: specific low back strengthening exercises. Both twice a week for 6 weeks	Low Back Pain Functional Scale: Significantly improved by 20% in experimental group and 15% in control group. No gender/age differences in results	$p < 0.05$
(Chan *et al.*, 2011) [15]	46 NSCLBP patients (10 male, 36 female)	8-week intervention. Both intervention and control groups received conventional physiotherapy. Intervention group only also prescribed aerobic exercise (40%–60% heart rate reserve)	Visual Analogue Scale (VAS): Intervention group: 47% significant reduction post intervention. Control: 42% significant reduction post intervention. No gender/age differences in results	$p < 0.001$
(Chatzitheodorou *et al.*, 2007) [17]	20 NSCLBP patients (11 male, 9 female). Excludes patients with BMI > 30	12-week intervention. Exercise group: high intensity aerobic exercise (running on treadmill at 85% of heart rate reserve). Control group: Passive treatment (ultrasound and did not include any form of PA)	McGill Pain Questionnaire. Exercise group: 41% significant reduction post intervention. Control: no significant change. No gender/age differences in results	$p < 0.001$
(Chatzitheodorou *et al.*, 2008) [18]	64 NSCLBP patients (26 male, 38 female) Excludes patients with BMI > 30	Patients randomly allocated into positive or negative dexamethasone suppression test. Both groups completed 12-week aerobic exercise programme (running on treadmill at 85% heart rate reserve)	McGill Pain Questionnaire. Positive suppression group: 30% significant reduction post intervention. Negative suppression group: 8% significant reduction post intervention. No gender/age differences in results	$p < 0.001$

4.1.2. Summary

Moderate intensity aerobic exercise (40%–60% heart rate reserve) should be promoted for NSCLBP rehabilitation. Aerobic fitness, behavioural treatment and multi-disciplinary treatment programmes are important for reducing CLBP and improving disability [81].

4.2. Muscle Strength and Stabilisation Training

A reduction in core strength can lead to lumbar instability [82], and lumbar instability also reduces the flexibility of the lumbar spine [83]. CLBP patients restrict their trunk movement to reduce the pain in the lumbosacral area, however this only further reduces core strength and increases lumbar instability, resulting in low back pain [84]. Exercises to activate the deep abdominal muscles including the superficial muscles, transversus abdominis muscle and the multifidus are important for CLBP patients [85]. The deep abdominal muscles are essential for supporting the lumbar spine and strengthening these muscles can reduce back pain [86].

A high volume of stress placed on the vertebral column muscles can lead to back pain [87], and poor muscle recruitment of the deep abdominal muscles has been shown in NSCLBP patients [19]. The transversus abdominis is important in muscular stabilisation of the spine which assists in supporting posture [88] and a delayed muscle contraction during movement is often prevalent in patients [89]. Spinal stabilisation exercises aim to increase the strength and endurance of these muscles [90], improving spine stability [91].

Stabilisation exercises have been shown to be effective in reducing NSCLBP [19,21,24], but not acute low back pain [92]. It is important to identify the specific exercises which are most effective for a specific population, as opposed to a generic group [93]. Lumbar stabilisation programmes increase the stability of the spine by training the muscular motor patterns in order to reduce low back pain [94].

Strengthening exercises are considered the most effective treatment for functional gain including walking speed [16]. This is because the deep trunk muscles are active when walking [16], suggesting that strengthening these muscles can help with completing activities of daily living [95].

4.2.1. Muscular Strength and Stabilisation Intervention Programmes

Core stabilisation programmes [19,21,23,24] have been shown to significantly reduce CLBP by 39%–76.8%, and a muscular strength programme significantly reduced CLBP by 61.6% [20].

A 3-month intervention involving 30 NSCLBP patients compared core stabilisation exercises including slow curl ups, bird dog, the plank and sit ups (raising the head and shoulders off the ground with the hands under the head) to conventional spine exercises [19]. The conventional spine exercises included static stretching of muscles found to be tight, however the study does not state which form of assessment was used to identify tight muscles.

Core stabilisation exercises significantly reduced NSCLBP by 76.8% compared to a 62.8% significant reduction following the conventional exercises. These findings suggested both core stabilisation and conventional exercises to be significantly beneficial in reducing CLBP. However the core stabilisation group reported a significantly greater improvement compared to conventional exercises, highlighting the importance of core stability for CLBP patients.

An 8-week core stability intervention programme for 10 NSCLBP patients involved activating core stability responses using unstable standing surfaces and unexpected movements of the upper limbs [21]. CLBP significantly reduced by 39.5%. These results were lower in comparison to the other study [19] which reported a 76.8% significant decrease in CLBP. However this study involved a 3-month intervention [19] compared to the 8-week core stability intervention [21], suggesting the longer a stabilisation intervention programme is, the more positive impact upon CLBP there is.

Another study involved an 8-week stabilisation programme [24] involving 40 NSCLBP patients and investigated the effects of combining ankle dorsiflexion exercises with drawing in the abdominal wall (experimental group), to drawing in the abdominal wall exercises alone (control group). The ankle dorsiflexion exercises were completed at 30% of maximal voluntary isometric contraction of the tibialis anterior muscle, using a resistance band for 10 sets of 20s.

Ankle dorsiflexion exercises were included in the exercise programme because the proprioceptive neuromuscular facilitation irradiation technique, increases core muscular strength by stimulating stronger muscles from the lower body [96], which provides a resistance and stimulus to increase muscle fibres and muscle activity in abdominal muscles [97]. This suggests that to contract the deep target muscle the transversus abdominis, resistance should be applied to the stronger ankle dorsiflexors combined with drawing in the abdominal wall. The transversus abdominis and internal oblique muscles are important for core stability as they are attached to the thoracolumbar fascia, and increase the stiffness of the tissue which improves the core stability [98]. In addition an increase in the stiffness of the tissue in the core, can help to resist the stress placed on the spine and help to reduce back pain [99].

The study reported that the experimental group significantly reduced NSCLBP by 32.5% (according to the VAS), 23.2% (Pain Disability Index) and 21.5% (Pain Rating Scale). The control group significantly reduced CLBP by 16.8% (VAS), 12.4% (Pain Disability Index) and 8% (Pain Rating Scale).

This study [24] also included a follow up measurement after 2 months, in which time patients were instructed to continue the exercises of combining ankle dorsiflexion to drawing in the abdominal wall (experimental group), or only drawing in the abdominal wall (control group). The results identified CLBP had significantly reduced further to 46.8% (VAS), 39.2% (Pain Disability Index) and 30.7% (Pain Rating Scale) in the experimental group and 38.7% (VAS), 18.8% (Pain Disability Index) and 14.6% (Pain Rating Scale) in the control group. These results provide additional support for the benefits of a longer intervention programme and also for the inclusion of ankle dorsiflexion exercises in rehabilitation of NSCLBP.

Core stability measured by the active straight leg raise was also shown to improve by 56.1% in the experimental group, and 27.4% in the control group after 8 weeks. The results highlighted the importance of core stability in reducing CLBP, especially as core stability had improved by an additional 33.8% at the two month follow up compared to the 8-week measurement in the experimental group, and consequently CLBP had been shown to reduce further. Therefore the results suggested that the addition of ankle dorsiflexion exercises when combined with drawing in the abdominal wall to be an effective exercise in reducing CLBP.

The addition of ankle dorsiflexion exercises to drawing in the abdominal wall is a unique technique for improving core stability for NSCLBP patients, as this technique has only been previously researched in 40 healthy participants [100]. This study [100] reported that the combination of drawing in the abdominal wall and ankle dorsiflexion exercises, resulted in a significantly greater increase in the thickness of the transverse abdominal muscle measured using ultrasonography, compared to drawing in the abdominal wall alone. This is important for improving core strength [101].

The importance of core stability and muscular strength was emphasised by research which had reported that a slumped sitting posture involving lumbar flexion, resulted in a lower activation of the core muscles such as the lumbar multifidus, iliocostalis lumborum pars thoracis and the transverse fibers of internal oblique [102]. Consequently the muscles become weaker which negatively impacts upon the ability to maintain an upright posture [103]. This is because the intervertebral discs are composed of the annulus fibrosus, which connects the spinal vertebrae above and below the disk [104]. The annulus fibrosus requires a highly structured organisation involving aligned collagen fibres within the transverse axis of the spine, which forms an angle-ply laminate structure [105]. However, when the intervertebral disk degenerates the annulus fibrosus becomes unorganised, which can result in low back pain [106]. This is due to mechanical and structural problems such as tears and delamination [107], as the annulus fibrosus distributes force on the intervertebral discs to prevent the gelatinous material in the soft inner core of the intervertebral disc from leaking out [104].

Patients with low back pain adopt a sitting posture with significantly more lumbar flexion than those without low back pain [108,109]. Therefore this suggested a relationship between a poor sitting posture and low back pain, and highlighted the importance of improving core strength and stability [86] to support an upright sitting posture. In contrast no relationship was reported between low back pain and lumbar flexion when sitting in 170 female undergraduate nursing students, with either minor or significant low back pain or without lower back pain [110]. However this study involved only female participants, and males had been shown to be more associated with lumbar flexion when sitting, with an average of 12.2° more flexion than females [103].

A 12-month exercise programme focused on increasing control of the lumbar neutral zone [23] and involved 106 middle aged working men who had a reported episode of non-specific low back pain within the previous 3 months, but did not have severe disability. The participants exercised twice a week undergoing exercises which aimed to improve lumbar stability, such as abdominal curl up with slight rotation and squat exercises. This exercise programme was combined with educating the patients on back pain and providing training on correct techniques for lifting. Low back pain significantly decreased by 39%, suggesting exercises focusing on lumbar stability combined with education to be effective at reducing low back pain. However it was suggested that the participants may have reported a reduced lower back pain as they knew they were involved in the intervention group and therefore expected to experience less back pain [23].

A muscular strength 8-week intervention programme involving 47 women with NSCLBP [20] investigated the effect of different angles of inversion traction on muscular strength and NSCLBP. The study reported that the inversion −30° group and inversion −60° group was more effective at reducing NSCLBP, and improving core muscular strength than the supine group. NSCLBP significantly reduced by 61.6% in both the inversion −30° group and inversion −60° group, compared to 34.9% in the supine group. In addition extensor back muscle strength was also found to increase by 22.5% (inversion −30° group) and 47% (inversion −60° group), however muscular strength was found to reduce by 6% in the supine group. This suggested that another factor other than muscular strength influenced the decrease in back pain for the supine group.

Trunk extension flexibility was also shown to improve in all three groups. However the biggest increase of 22% was reported in the inversion −60° group compared to an increase of 13.3% in the inversion −30° group, and 4.8% in the supine group. This suggested that a range of factors are responsible for the decrease in NSCLBP, and indicates that a general intervention programme focusing on a range of different areas of fitness is important for NSCLBP rehabilitation.

A 4-week core muscular strength programme (control group) was compared to a core stability programme in addition to core muscular strength exercises (experimental group), in 160 patients with NSCLBP [22]. NSCLBP significantly reduced in the experimental group by 35% compared to 14% in the control group. The results suggested that an intervention programme for NSCLBP which incorporates both core stability and core muscular strength exercises, is more effective at reducing NSCLBP than muscular strength exercises alone.

Four variables exist which may determine the success of a stabilisation exercise programme for CLBP [94]. The four variables include age as participants under the age of 40 have been shown to have higher odds by 3.7 of the stabilisation treatment being a success, an active straight leg raise test higher than 91°, the presence of aberrant movement during lumbar range of motion and a positive prone instability test. Three or more of the four named variables being present is a predictor for the stabilisation exercise programme being successful in reducing CLBP. Therefore it is important to consider the four variables when designing an intervention programme involving stabilisation exercises for CLBP.

Finally, a 15-item questionnaire on clinical instability has been identified [111], which revealed whether patients with NSCLBP respond better to motor control exercises to increase the activation of muscles, including the transversus abdominis, multifidus, and pelvic-floor muscles, or graded activity involving submaximal exercises to increase exercise tolerance. This suggests the questionnaire can help to identify the most effective form of rehabilitation for NSCLBP patients. See Table 2 for a summary of each of the discussed muscular strength and stabilisation intervention programmes.

Table 2. Muscular strength and stabilisation intervention programmes for NSCLBP patients.

Reference Number	Type of Population	Length of Intervention	Effect on Back Pain	Significance Levels
(Inani & Selkar, 2013) [19]	30 NSCLBP patients (20 male, 10 female) aged 20–50 years	3-month intervention. Experimental group: Completed core stabilization exercises including slow curl ups, bird dog, the plank and sit ups (raising head and shoulders off the ground with hands under the head). Control group: Completed conventional spine exercises including static stretching of muscles found to be tight	Visual Analogue Scale. Experimental group: 76.8% significant reduction post intervention. Control group: 62.8% significant reduction post intervention. No gender/age differences in results	$p < 0.001$
(Šarabon, 2011) [21]	10 NSCLBP patients (3 male, 7 female)	8-week core stability intervention programme involving activating core stability responses using unstable standing surfaces and unexpected movements of the upper limbs	Visual Analogue Scale. 39.5% significant reduction post intervention. No gender/age differences in results	$p < 0.01$
(Suni *et al.*, 2006) [23]	106 middle aged working men who had a reported episode of non-specific low back pain within the previous 3 months, but did not have severe disability	12-month programme in which participants exercised twice a week undergoing exercises to improve lumbar stability e.g., abdominal curl up with slight rotation and squat exercises. This exercise programme was combined with educating the patients on back pain and providing training on correct techniques for lifting.	Visual Analogue Scale. Significant 39% reduction	$p < 0.01$
(You *et al.*, 2014) [24]	40 NSCLBP patients (19 male, 21 female)	8-week stabilisation programme and follow up measurement after 2 months. Patients continued exercises throughout 2-month follow up period. Experimental group: Combined ankle dorsiflexion exercises (completed at 30% of maximal voluntary isometric contraction using resistance band for 10 sets of 20 s) with drawing in the abdominal wall. Control group: Drawing in the abdominal wall exercises alone	Experimental group, post intervention: Significant reduction of 32.5% (VAS), 23.2% (Pain Disability Index) and 21.5% (Pain Rating Scale). Control group, post intervention: Significant reduction of 16.8% (VAS), 12.4% (Pain Disability Index) and 8% (Pain Rating Scale). Experimental group, follow up measurement: Significant reduction of 46.8% (VAS), 39.2% (Pain Disability Index) and 30.7% (Pain Rating Scale) compared to pre intervention. Control Group, follow up measurement: Significant reduction of 38.7% (VAS), 18.8% (Pain Disability Index) and 14.6% (Pain Rating Scale) compared to pre intervention. No gender/age differences in results	$p < 0.001$
(Kim *et al.*, 2013) [20]	47 women with NSCLBP	Muscular strength 8-week intervention programme which investigated different angles of inversion traction on NSCLBP. Patients randomly allocated into 3 groups: supine, inversion −30° and inversion −60°. Each group completed a 3 min x 3 set inversion traction protocol at 0°, inverted −30° or inverted −60° for 4 days a week during 8 weeks	Visual Analogue Scale. Significant reduction of 61.6% in both inversion −30° and inversion −60° groups. Significant reduction of 34.9% in the supine group	$p < 0.009$
(Stankovic *et al.*, 2012) [22]	160 NSCLBP patients (63 male, 97 female) 18–75 years	4-week core muscular strength programme (control group) was compared to a core stability programme in addition to core muscular strength exercises (experimental group)	Experimental group: Significantly reduced by 35% post intervention. Control group: Significantly reduced by 14% post intervention. No gender/age differences in results	$p < 0.001$

4.2.2. Summary

Increasing the strength of deep abdominal muscles and improving the stabilisation of the spine is effective at reducing NSCLBP. A core stabilisation programme combined with muscular strength should be considered for NSCLBP patients, as this was shown to be more effective than core muscular strength exercises alone [22]. This suggested a more general programme as opposed to focusing on one particular area of fitness to be more effective at reducing NSCLBP.

4.3. Flexibility Training

Stretching the soft tissues in the back, legs and buttock such as the hamstrings, erector muscles of the spine and hip flexor muscles, ligaments and tendons can help to mobilise the spine, and an increase in the range of motion of the spine can assist back pain [112]. This is because stretching can improve the flexibility of the muscle-tendons and ligaments in the back, which is important to increase the range of motion of the joints [113].Therefore an improved range of motion assists with patients' movement and ability to complete activities of daily living, as most everyday tasks such as lifting and bending require trunk flexion, which involves a complex movement combining lumbar and hip motion [114]. Also stretching exercises decrease the muscle stiffness as a result of changes in viscoelastic properties, due to the decreased actin-myosin cross-bridges and the reflex muscle inhibition [113].

According to the pelvic cross syndrome theory, muscle abnormalities in the postural muscles such as a decreased flexibility and shortening of the hip flexor and back extensor muscles, can result in additional mechanical stress to the joints and soft tissue of the lumbar spine, and can cause lumbar lordosis [87]. Lumbar lordosis is an excessive inward curving of the lumbar spine [115], as a weakening of the abdominal muscles can tilt the pelvis posteriorly, and can result in CLBP [116,117]. In addition the pelvic cross syndrome theory states that hamstring muscle shortening is also important in controlling lumbar lordosis [87]. Hamstring muscle shortening reduces the hip flexion range of motion due to being attached to the posterior leg and the ischial tuberosity, which can affect the lumbopelvic movement during forward bending and can cause low back pain [114].

Flexibility exercises are often used in exercise rehabilitation programmes as they have been shown to be effective at reducing the pain associated with CLBP [25,27]. However CLBP patients must be careful not to perform exercises that result in pain, especially when stretching the flexors and extensors of the trunk and hips [50].

4.3.1. Flexibility Programmes

A 4-week intervention programme involving 40 female NSCLBP patients between 45 and 65 years [27] included 10 exercises for the lumbo-pelvic spine to improve the lumbar flexibility and stability. The exercises were completed in positions which were non-weight bearing such as in a supine position, side lying and prone and were completed twice a week with 10 repetitions of each exercise.

The study reported a 54% significant increase for lumbar flexion and 98% for lumbar extension. Back pain also significantly improved by 58%. The results suggested that completing exercises to improve lumbar flexion and extension is important in reducing NSCLBP in women. This is because during the baseline measurements lumbar flexion was found to be correlated with back pain ($r = -0.581$). However these results cannot be generalised to men.

Lumbar extension exercises can reduce tension in the posterior annular fibers, and alter intradiscal pressure which allows anterior migration of the nucleus pulposus [115] which is important for the vertebral disc to withstand compression [118]. In addition lumbar flexion exercises stretch the hip flexors and lumbar extensors, and decrease the compressive forces on the posterior disc [115].

A further study researched the effect of a 6-week Pilates programme on hamstring and lower back flexibility and CLBP [25]. The study involved 34 NSCLBP patients aged 18–60 years, and were randomly assigned to either the Pilates group or the control group. The Pilates exercises were completed during a one hour class each week taught by a certified Pilates Institute Instructor, and two 30 min sessions each week at home without any supervision. The control group did not participate in the Pilates exercises and continued with their normal PA levels.

The study identified that flexibility significantly increased by 52.9% in the Pilates group, compared to a 7.8% increase in the control group which was not significantly different. Back pain also significantly decreased by 18.5% in the Pilates group, and there was no change in the back pain for the patients in the control group. The results suggested that Pilates exercises can significantly improve back pain and hamstring and lower back flexibility for NSCLBP patients.

The relationship between low back pain, lumbar flexion and hamstring flexibility was researched in a study involving 26 male University rowers who participated in rowing training six times a week [119]. Participants were assigned into groups according to whether they were currently suffering from low back pain (acute, sub-acute or chronic), had suffered from low back pain at some point in their lives or had never suffered from low back pain.

The study reported that the participants with current low back pain (11 participants) had a significantly reduced lumbar flexion compared to the participants without current low back pain (15 participants). However no significant difference was identified in hamstring flexibility between the two groups. In addition no significant difference was identified in lumbar flexion or hamstring flexibility between the participants who had experienced low back pain at some point in their lives (21 participants), or had not experienced low back pain (5 participants).

The results suggested that hamstring flexibility was not associated with low back pain occurrence, and therefore improving hamstring flexibility is not important for preventing low back pain or for an intervention programme for a patient with low back pain. Although, the results did highlight the importance of improving lumbar flexion for patients with current low back pain, and also suggested that a reduced lumbar flexion is an important factor for an occurrence of low back pain.

However the study [119] did not specifically focus on CLBP patients as the participants reported any experiences of low back pain, current or previous, and therefore could have included a range of acute, sub-acute or CLBP. In addition, the results from the study were in contrast to findings previously discussed [25], which suggested that improving hamstring flexibility is important for reducing NSCLBP.

A 3-month intervention programme for 86 NSCLBP patients [26] investigated the effects of progressive therapeutic exercise on spinal and muscle flexibility and back pain by dividing the patients into three groups: intensive training group, home exercise group and the control group. Follow up measurements at 6 and 12 months after baseline tests was also conducted. The intensive training group and home exercise group completed seven exercises for various parts of the body using either gym equipment, such as pulleys and bar bells (intensive training group) or without the use of extra equipment (home exercise group). The control group maintained their normal PA levels throughout the duration of the study and did not participate in an organised exercise programme. However no information was provided on which exercises were completed.

Back pain significantly decreased post intervention by 44% in the intensive training group, 32% in the home exercise group and 39% in the control group. The 6-month follow up identified that back pain had decreased further in the home exercise group to a 47% reduction which was significantly different to baseline. The intensive training group which increased compared to post intervention to a 32% reduction compared to baseline, although this was still significantly different. The control group also increased compared to post intervention to 28% and was not significantly different to baseline.

The flexibility of the hamstrings significantly increased at post intervention from 87°–90° in the intensive training group and 83°–87° in the home exercise group. However at the 12-month follow up hamstring flexibility had reduced to 83° in the intensive training group and 82° in the home exercise group. This suggests the importance of maintaining exercise which is aimed at improving flexibility, as both exercise groups lost the improved degree of hamstring flexibility. Although there was no correlation between back pain and flexibility which suggested the importance of other factors on back pain, such as an increase in core strength and aerobic fitness [16,19,23]. However the study [26] did not measure core strength or aerobic fitness. In addition the study [26] suggested improving flexibility could be important for preventing CLBP from occurring, as opposed to using exercises to improve flexibility as a rehabilitation from CLBP. See Table 3 for a summary of each of the discussed flexibility intervention programmes.

Table 3. Flexibility intervention programmes for NSCLBP patients.

Reference Number	Type of Population	Length of Intervention	Effect on Back Pain	Significance Levels
(Masharawi & Nadaf, 2013) [27]	40 female NSCLBP patients between 45 and 65 years	Study group: Activities of daily living guidance and a 45 min group exercise session aimed at improving lumbar flexibility and stability. Exercise session was completed twice a week for 4 weeks with 10 repetitions of each exercise. Control group: Activities of daily living guidance only	Visual Analogue Scale. Study group: 58% significant improvement following intervention. Control group: no significant change	$p < 0.001$
(Gladwell *et al.*, 2006) [25]	34 NSCLBP patients aged 18–60 years	Pilates group: Completed Pilates exercises during a one hour class each week for 6 weeks, and two 30 min sessions each week at home without any supervision. Control group: Did not participate in the Pilates exercises and continued with their normal PA levels	Visual Analog Scale. Pilates group: 18.5% significant decrease following intervention. Control group: No significant difference. No gender/age differences in results	$p < 0.05$
(Kuukkanen & Malkia, 2006) [26]	86 NSCLBP patients	Intensive training group and home exercise group completed 3-month intervention programme: 7 exercises for various parts of the body using either gym equipment, such as pulleys and bar bells (intensive training group) or without the use of extra equipment (home exercise group). Control group: Maintained their normal PA levels and did not participate in an organised exercise programme	Intensive training: 44% significant reduction post intervention. Control: 39% significant reduction post intervention. Home exercise: 32% significant reduction post intervention. No gender/age differences in results	$p < 0.05$

4.3.2. Summary

Improving the flexibility of the lumbar spine and hamstrings can significantly reduce CLBP by 18.5%–58% [25,27]. This suggests the importance of including flexibility exercises in an intervention programme for CLBP patients. However no association between hamstring flexibility and low back pain was identified in male University rowers [119].

An improvement in lumbar flexibility can increase the range of motion of the spine, which can help to reduce back pain and assist with movement [112]. Hamstring muscle shortening reduces the hip flexion range of motion which impacts upon the lumbopelvic movement [114], and a decrease in the flexibility of the hip flexor and back extensor muscles can lead to lumbar lordosis, which can result in low back pain [87]. Therefore including lumbar flexion exercises in an intervention programme for CLBP is important, as lumbar flexion exercises stretch the hip flexors and lumbar extensors [115].

5. Conclusions

Exercise intervention programmes involving either muscular strength, flexibility or aerobic fitness is beneficial for NSCLBP but not acute low back pain. Non-specific acute low back pain patients recover in 4–6 weeks with or without a treatment [5], and exercising should be avoided to reduce the swelling of the affected area [39].

NSCLBP is multi factorial in nature [110,120], and no single exercise programme is optimal for all NSCLBP patients [50]. In addition, the most appropriate specific intervention for a NSCLBP patient is often unclear [12], and NSCLBP pain should not been considered as a homogenous condition meaning all cases are identical [121]. This suggests that a specific intervention programme focusing on one area of fitness for a group of NSCLBP patients may not be appropriate. This is a limitation of this review as the NSCLBP patients in the included studies may have responded differently to the exercise interventions. Consequently, a general exercise programme which combines muscular strength, flexibility and aerobic fitness would be beneficial for rehabilitation of NSCLBP. Further research is needed into the benefits of a combined exercise intervention programme involving muscular strength, flexibility and aerobic fitness for NSCLBP patients, as the literature has supported the use of each of these fitness areas individually, but more research should be conducted combining all three.

Acknowledgments: Research funded by the University of St Mark & St John.

Author Contributions: Both authors helped to plan the review. The first author conducted the search for intervention programmes, read and reviewed the articles and completed the manuscript. The second author also read and provided improvements to the manuscript. Both authors approved the final manuscript.

References

1. Ricci, J.A.; Stewart, W.F.; Chee, E.; Leotta, C.; Foley, K.; Hochberg, M.C. Back pain exacerbations and lost productive time costs in United States workers. *Spine* **2006**, *31*, 3052–3060. [CrossRef] [PubMed]
2. Van Tulder, M.; Malmivaara, A.; Esmail, R.; Koes, B. Exercise therapy for low back pain: A systematic review within the framework of the cochrane collaboration back review group. *Spine* **2000**, *25*, 2784–2796. [CrossRef] [PubMed]
3. Chen, S.M.; Alexander, R.; Lo, S.K.; Cook, J. Effects of Functional Fascial Taping on pain and function in patients with non-specific low back pain: A pilot randomized controlled trial. *Clin. Rehabil.* **2012**, *26*, 924–933. [CrossRef] [PubMed]
4. Ebadi, S.; Ansari, N.N.; Naghdi, S.; Fallah, E.; Barzi, D.M.; Jalaei, S. A study of therapeutic ultrasound and exercise treatment for muscle fatigue in patients with chronic non specific low back pain: A preliminary report. *J. Back Musculoskelet. Rehabil.* **2013**, *26*, 221–226. [PubMed]
5. Hancock, M.J.; Maher, C.G.; Latimer, J. Spinal manipulative therapy for acute low back pain: A clinical perspective. *J. Man. Manip. Ther.* **2008**, *16*, 198–203. [CrossRef] [PubMed]
6. Kolber, M.J.; Beekhuizen, K. Lumbar stabilization: An evidence-based approach for the athlete with low back pain. *Strength Cond. J.* **2007**, *29*, 26–37. [CrossRef]
7. Lara-Palomo, I.C.; Aguilar-Ferrándiz, M.E.; Matarán-Peñarrocha, G.A.; Saavedra-Hernández, M.; Granero-Molina, J.; Fernández-Sola, C. Short-term effects of interferential current electro-massage in adults with chronic non-specific low back pain: A randomized controlled trial. *Clin. Rehabil.* **2013**, *27*, 439–450. [CrossRef] [PubMed]
8. Waddell, G.; Burton, A.K. Occupational health guidelines for the management of low back pain at work: Evidence review. *Occup. Med.* **2001**, *51*, 124–135. [CrossRef]
9. Thomas, K.J.; MacPherson, H.; Thorpe, L.; Brazier, J.; Fitter, M.; Campbell, M.J. Randomised controlled trial of a short course of traditional acupuncture compared with usual care for persistent non-specific low back pain. *Br. Med. J.* **2006**, *333*, 623–626. [CrossRef] [PubMed]
10. National Health Service (NHS). Backcare Awareness Week. Available online: http://www.nhscareers.nhs.uk/features/2012/october/ (accessed on 16 October 2014).
11. Wynne-Jones, G.; Cowen, J.; Jordan, J.; Uthman, O.; Main, C.J.; Glozier, N.; van der Windt, D. Absence from work and return to work in people with back pain: A systematic review and meta-analysis. *Occup. Environ. Med.* **2014**, *71*, 448–456. [CrossRef] [PubMed]
12. Mayer, J.; Mooney, V.; Dagenais, S. Evidence-informed management of chronic low back pain with lumbar extensor strengthening exercises. *Spine* **2008**, *8*, 96–113. [CrossRef] [PubMed]
13. Bekkering, G.E.; Hendriks, H.J.; Koes, B.W.; Oostendorp, R.A.; Ostelo, R.W.; Thomassen, J.M.; van Tulder, M.W. Dutch physiotherapy guidelines for low back pain. *Physiotherapy* **2003**, *89*, 82–96. [CrossRef]
14. National Health Service (NHS). Back Pain. Available online: http://www.nhs.uk/Conditions/Back-pain/Pages/Introduction.aspx (accessed on 16 October 2014).
15. Chan, C.W.; Mok, N.W.; Yeung, E.W. Aerobic exercise training in addition to conventional physiotherapy for chronic low back pain: A randomized controlled trial. *Arch. Phys. Med. Rehabil.* **2011**, *92*, 1681–1685. [CrossRef] [PubMed]

16. Shnayderman, I.; Katz-Leurer, M. An aerobic walking programme *versus* muscle strengthening Programme for chronic low back pain: A randomized controlled trial. *Clin. Rehabil.* **2013**, *27*, 207–214. [CrossRef] [PubMed]
17. Chatzitheodorou, D.; Kabitsis, C.; Malliou, P.; Mougios, V. A pilot study of the effects of high-intensity aerobic exercise *versus* passive interventions on pain, disability, psychological strain, and serum cortisol concentrations in people with chronic low back pain. *Phys. Ther.* **2007**, *87*, 304–312. [CrossRef] [PubMed]
18. Chatzitheodorou, D.; Mavromoustakos, S.; Milioti, S. The effect of exercise on adrenocortical responsiveness of patients with chronic low back pain, controlled for psychological strain. *Clin. Rehabil.* **2008**, *22*, 319–328. [CrossRef] [PubMed]
19. Inani, S.B.; Selkar, S.P. Effect of core stabilization exercises *versus* conventional exercises on pain and functional status in patients with non-specific low back pain: A randomized clinical trial. *J. Back Musculoskelet. Rehabil.* **2013**, *26*, 37–43. [PubMed]
20. Kim, J.D.; Oh, H.W.; Lee, J.H.; Cha, J.Y.; Ko, I.G.; Jee, Y.S. The effect of inversion traction on pain sensation, lumbar flexibility and trunk muscles strength in patients with chronic low back pain. *Isokinet. Exerc. Sci.* **2013**, *21*, 237–246.
21. Šarabon, N. Effects of trunk functional stability training in subjects suffering from chronic low back pain: A pilot study. *Kinesiol. Slov.* **2011**, *17*, 25–37.
22. Stankovic, A.; Lazovic, M.; Kocic, M.; Dimitrijevic, L.; Stankovic, I.; Zlatavovic, D. Lumbar stabilization exercises in addition to strengthening and stretching exercises reduce pain and increase function in patients with chronic low back pain: Randomized clinical open-label study. *Turk. J. Phys. Med. Rehabil.* **2012**, *58*, 177–183. [CrossRef]
23. Suni, J.; Rinne, M.; Natri, A.; Statistisian, M.P.; Parkkari, J.; Alaranta, H. Control of the lumbar neutral zone decreases low back pain and improves self-evaluated work ability: A 12-month randomized controlled study. *Spine* **2006**, *31*, 611–620. [CrossRef] [PubMed]
24. You, J.H.; Kim, S.Y.; Oh, D.W.; Chon, S.C. The effect of a novel core stabilization technique on managing patients with chronic low back pain: A randomized, controlled, experimenter-blinded study. *Clin. Rehabil.* **2014**, *28*, 460–469. [CrossRef] [PubMed]
25. Gladwell, V.; Head, S.; Haggar, M.; Beneke, R. Does a program of pilates improve chronic non-specific low Back pain? *J. Sport Rehabil.* **2006**, *15*, 338–350.
26. Kuukkanen, T.; Malkia, E. Effects of a three-month therapeutic exercise programme on flexibility in subjects with low back pain. *Physiother. Res. Int.* **2000**, *5*, 46–61. [CrossRef] [PubMed]
27. Masharawi, Y.; Nadaf, N. The effect of non-weight bearing group-exercising on females with non-specific chronic low back pain: A randomized single blind controlled pilot study. *J. Back Musculoskelet. Rehabil.* **2013**, *26*, 353–359. [PubMed]
28. Hayden, J.A.; van Tulder, M.; Tomlinson, G. Systematic review: Strategies for using exercise therapy to improve outcomes in chronic low back pain. *Ann. Intern. Med.* **2005**, *142*, 776–785. [CrossRef] [PubMed]
29. Smith, J.A.; Osborn, M. Pain as an assault on the self: An interpretative phenomenological analysis of the psychological impact of chronic benign low back pain. *Psychol. Health* **2007**, *22*, 517–534. [CrossRef]
30. Smeets, R.; Severens, J.L.; Beelen, S.; Vlaeyen, J.W.; Knottnerus, J.A. More is not always better: Cost-effectiveness analysis of combined, single behavioral and single physical rehabilitation programs for chronic low back pain. *Eur. J. Pain* **2009**, *13*, 71–81. [CrossRef] [PubMed]
31. Smith, D.; Bissell, G.; Bruce-Low, S.; Wakefield, C. The effect of lumbar extension training with and without pelvic stabilization on lumbar strength and low back pain. *J. Back Musculoskelet. Rehabil.* **2011**, *24*, 241–249. [PubMed]
32. Wai, E.K.; Rodriguez, S.; Dagenais, S.; Hall, H. Evidence informed management of chronic low back pain with physical activity, smoking cessation, and weight loss. *Spine J.* **2008**, *8*, 195–202. [CrossRef] [PubMed]
33. McCarthy, C.J.; Roberts, C.; Gittins, M.; Oldham, J.A. A process of subgroup identification in non-specific low back pain using a standard clinical examination and cluster analysis. *Physiother. Res. Int.* **2012**, *17*, 92–100. [CrossRef] [PubMed]
34. Bupa. Back Pain. Available online: http://www.bupa.co.uk/individuals/health-information/directory/b/backpain#textBlock190676 (accessed on 16 October 2014).
35. McGill, S. Designing Back Exercise: From Rehabilitation to Enhancing Performance. Available online: http://www.backfitpro.com/articles.php (accessed on 11 October 2014).

36. Del Pozo-Cruz, B.; Gusi, N.; Del Pozo-Cruz, J.; Adsuar, J.C.; Hernandez-Mocholí, M.; Parraca, J.A. Clinical effects of a nine-month web-based intervention in subacute non-specific low back pain patients: A randomized controlled trial. *Clin. Rehabil.* **2013**, *27*, 28–39. [CrossRef] [PubMed]
37. Tsauo, J.Y.; Chen, W.H.; Liang, H.W.; Jang, Y. The effectiveness of a functional training programme for patients with chronic low back pain—A pilot study. *Disabil. Rehabil.* **2009**, *31*, 1100–1106. [CrossRef] [PubMed]
38. Wells, C.; Kolt, G.S.; Marshall, P.; Bialocerkowski, A. The definition and application of pilates exercise to treat people with chronic low back pain: A delphi survey of australian physical therapists. *Phys. Ther.* **2014**, *94*, 792–805. [CrossRef] [PubMed]
39. Goertz, M.; Thorson, D.; Bonsell, J.; Bonte, B.; Campbell, R.; Haake, B. *Adult Acute and Subacute Low Back Pain*; Institute for Clinical Systems Improvement: Bloomington, MN, USA, 2012; pp. 1–91.
40. Van Tulder, M.; Becker, A.; Bekkering, T.; Breen, A.; del Real, M.; Hutchinson, A.; Koes, B.; Laerum, E.; Malmivaara, A. Chapter 3 European guidelines for the management of acute nonspecific low back pain in primary care. *Eur. Spine J.* **2006**, *15*, 169–191. [CrossRef] [PubMed]
41. Reme, S.; Shaw, W.; Steenstra, I.; Woiszwillo, M.; Pransky, G.; Linton, S. Distressed, immobilized, or lacking employer support? A sub-classification of acute work-related low back pain. *J. Occup. Rehabil.* **2012**, *22*, 541–552. [CrossRef] [PubMed]
42. Chou, R.; Qaseem, A.; Snow, V.; Casey, D.; Cross, T.; Shekelle, P. Diagnosis and treatment of low back pain: A joint clinical practice guideline from the American College of Physicians and the American Pain Society. *Ann. Intern. Med.* **2007**, *147*, 478–491. [CrossRef] [PubMed]
43. Toye, F.; Barker, K. 'I can't see any reason for stopping doing anything, but I might have to do it differently'—Restoring hope to patients with persistent non-specific low back pain—A qualitative study. *Disabil. Rehabil.* **2012**, *34*, 894–903. [CrossRef] [PubMed]
44. Savigny, P.; Watson, P.; Underwood, M. Early management of persistent non-specific low back pain: Summary of NICE guidance. *Br. Med. J.* **2009**. [CrossRef] [PubMed]
45. Ehrlich, G.E. Low back pain. *Bull. World Health Organ.* **2003**, *81*, 671–676. [PubMed]
46. Nonspecific Lower Back Pain in Adults. Available online: http://www.patient.co.uk/health/nonspecific-lower-back-pain-in-adults (accessed on 16 October 2014).
47. Josephson, I.; Hedberg, B.; Bülow, P. Problem-solving in physiotherapy—Physiotherapists' talk about encounters with patients with non-specific low back pain. *Disabil. Rehabil.* **2013**, *35*, 668–677. [CrossRef] [PubMed]
48. Benjamin, C. Low Back Pain—Acute. Available online: http://www.nlm.nih.gov/medlineplus/ency/article/007425.htm (accessed on 2 December 2014).
49. Koes, B.W.; van Tulder, M.W.; Thomas, S. Diagnosis and treatment of low back pain. *Br. Med. J.* **2006**, *332*, 1430–1434. [CrossRef] [PubMed]
50. Henchoz, Y.; Kai-Lik, S.A. Exercise and nonspecific low back pain: A literature review. *Joint Bone Spine* **2008**, *75*, 533–539. [CrossRef] [PubMed]
51. Winter, E.M.; Fowler, N. Exercise defined and quantified according to the Systeme International d'Unites. *J. Sports Sci.* **2009**, *27*, 447–460. [CrossRef] [PubMed]
52. World Health Organisation. Physical Activity. Available online: http://www.who.int/topics/physical_activity/en/ (accessed on 2 December 2014).
53. Robb, B. Exercise and Physical Activity: What's the Difference? 2009. Available online: http://www.everydayhealth.com/fitness/basics/difference-between-exercise-and-physical-activity.aspx (accessed on 18 November 2014).
54. Hayden, J.A.; van Tulder, M.W.; Malmivaara, A.; Koes, B.W. Exercise therapy for treatment of non-specific low back pain. *Cochrane Database Syst. Rev.* **2005**, *20*, 1–66.
55. Ullrich, P.F. Low Impact Aerobic Exercise. Available online: http://www.spine-health.com/wellness/exercise/low-impact-aerobic-exercise (accessed on 15 November 2014).
56. Kenny, W.L.; Wilmore, J.H.; Costill, D.L. *Physiology of Sport and Exercise*, 5th ed.; Human Kinetics: Champaign, IL, USA, 2012.
57. Stoppler, M.C.; Shiel, W.C. Endorphins: Natural Pain and Stress Fighters. 2014. Available online: http://www.medicinenet.com/script/main/art.asp?articlekey=55001 (accessed on 5 December 2014).

58. Spine-Health. Endorphins Definition. Available online: http://www.spine-health.com/glossary/endorphins (accessed on 5 December 2014).
59. Mayo, T.P.; Weissman, L. The noninvasive path to chronic back pain management. *Rehab Manag. Interdiscip. J. Rehabil.* **2011**, *24*, 18–20.
60. Duque, I.L.; Parra, J.H.; Duvallet, A. Aerobic fitness and limiting factors of maximal performance in chronic low back pain patients. *J. Back Musculoskelet. Rehabil.* **2009**, *22*, 113–119. [PubMed]
61. Lin, C.W.; McAuley, J.H.; Macedo, L.; Barnett, D.C.; Smeets, R.J.; Verbunt, J.A. Relationship between physical activity and disability in low back pain: A systematic review and meta-analysis. *Pain* **2011**, *152*, 607–613. [CrossRef] [PubMed]
62. Smeets, R.; Wittink, H.; Hidding, A.; Knottnerus, J.A. Do patients with chronic low back pain have a lower level of aerobic fitness than healthy controls? Are pain, disability, fear of injury, working status, or level of leisure time activity associated with the difference in aerobic fitness level? *Spine* **2006**, *31*, 90–97. [CrossRef] [PubMed]
63. Hoffman, M.D.; Shepanski, M.A.; Mackenzie, S.P.; Clifford, P.S. Experimentally induced pain perception is acutely reduced by aerobic exercise in people with chronic low back pain. *J. Rehabil. Res. Dev.* **2005**, *42*, 175–181. [CrossRef]
64. Jacob, T.; Baras, M.; Zeev, A.; Epstein, L. Physical activities and low back pain: a community-based study. *Med. Sci. Sports Exerc.* **2004**, *36*, 9–15. [CrossRef] [PubMed]
65. Koho, P.; Orenius, T.; Kautiainen, H.; Haanp, M.; Pohjolainen, T.; Hurri, H. Association of fear of movement and leisure-time physical activity among patients with chronic pain. *J. Rehabil. Med.* **2011**, *43*, 794–799. [CrossRef] [PubMed]
66. Swinkels-Meewisse, I.E.; Roelofs, J.; Oostendorp, R.A.; Verbeek, A.L.; Vlaeyen, J.W. Acute Low Back Pain: Pain-Related Fear and Pain Catastrophizing Influence Physical Performance and Perceived Disability. *Pain* **2006**, *120*, 36–43. [CrossRef] [PubMed]
67. Preuper, H.S.; Reneman, M.F.; Boonstra, A.M.; Dijkstra, P.U.; Versteegen, G.J.; Geertzen, J.H. Relationship between psychological factors and performance-based and self-reported disability in chronic low back pain. *Eur. Spine J.* **2008**, *17*, 1448–1456. [CrossRef] [PubMed]
68. McArthur, D.; Dumas, A.; Woodend, K.; Beach, S.; Stacey, D. Factors influencing adherence to regular exercise in middle-aged women: A qualitative study to inform clinical practice. *BMC* **2014**. [CrossRef] [PubMed]
69. Hanumanthu, V. *Assessment of an Exercise Program on Population with Chronic Medical Conditions*; ProQuest LLC: Ann Arbor, MI, USA, 2008.
70. Balint, T.; Dobrescu, T.; Rata, M.; Cristuta, A. Research regarding the assessment of a body's normal size by using the body mass index. *Gymn. J. Phys. Educ. Sports* **2010**, *11*, 14–17.
71. National Health Service (NHS). What's your BMI? Available online: http://www.nhs.uk/livewell/loseweight/pages/bodymassindex.aspx (accessed on 5 December 2014).
72. Frisco, D.J. Weight Loss for Back Pain Relief. Available online: http://www.spine-health.com/wellness/nutrition-diet-weight-loss/weight-loss-back-pain-relief (accessed on 1 December 2014).
73. Hurley, D.; O'Donoghue, G.; Tully, M.; Klaber Moffett, J.; van Mechelen, W.; Daly, L. A walking programme and a supervised exercise class *versus* usual physiotherapy for chronic low back pain: A single-blinded randomised controlled trial. *BMC Musculoskelet. Disord.* **2009**. [CrossRef] [PubMed]
74. National Institute of Arthritis and Musculoskeletal and Skin Diseases (NIAMS). Handout on Health: Back Pain. Available online: http://www.niams.nih.gov/Health_Info/Back_Pain/ (accessed on 8 December 2014).
75. Hill, E.E.; Zack, E.; Battaglini, C.; Viru, M.; Viru, A.; Hackney, A.C. Exercise and circulating cortisol levels: The intensity threshold effect. *J. Endocrinol. Investig.* **2008**, *31*, 587–591. [CrossRef] [PubMed]
76. Muhtz, C.; Rodriguez-Raecke, R.; Hinkelmann, K.; Moeller-Bertram, T.; Kiefer, F.; Wiedemann, K. Cortisol response to experimental pain in patients with chronic low back pain and patients with major depression. *Pain Med.* **2013**, *14*, 498–503. [CrossRef] [PubMed]
77. Nagarajan, M.; Nair, M.R. Importance of fear-avoidance behavior in chronic non-specific low back pain. *J. Back Musculoskelet. Rehabil.* **2010**, *23*, 87–95. [PubMed]
78. Hanney, W.J.; Kolber, M.J.; Beekhuizen, K.S. Implications for physical activity in the population with low back pain. *Am. J. Lifestyle Med.* **2009**, *3*, 63–70. [CrossRef]

79. Basler, H.D.; Luckmann, J.; Wolf, U.; Quint, S. Fear-avoidance beliefs, physical activity, and disability in elderly individuals with chronic low back pain and healthy controls. *Clin. J. Pain* **2008**, *24*, 604–610. [CrossRef] [PubMed]
80. Lante, K.; Stancliffe, R.J.; Bauman, A.; van der Ploeg, H.P.; Jan, S.; Davis, G.M. Embedding sustainable physical activities into the everyday lives of adults with intellectual disabilities: A randomised controlled trial. *BMC Public Health* **2014**. [CrossRef] [PubMed]
81. Krismer, M.; van Tulder, M. Low back pain (non-specific). *Best Pract. Res. Clin. Rheumatol.* **2007**, *21*, 77–91. [CrossRef] [PubMed]
82. Willson, J.D.; Dougherty, C.P.; Ireland, M.L.; Davis, I.M. Core stability and its relationship to lower extremity function and injury. *J. Am Acad Orthop. Surg.* **2005**, *13*, 316–325. [CrossRef] [PubMed]
83. Cho, H.Y.; Kim, E.H.; Kim, J. Effects of the CORE exercise program on pain and active range of motion in patients with chronic low back pain. *J. Phys. Ther. Sci.* **2014**, *26*, 1237–1240. [CrossRef] [PubMed]
84. Danneels, L.A.; Vanderstraeten, G.G.; Cambier, D.C.; Witvrouw, E.E.; de Cuyper, H.J. CT imaging of trunk muscles in chronic low back pain patients and healthy control subjects. *Eur. Spine J.* **2000**, *9*, 266–272. [CrossRef] [PubMed]
85. Franca, F.R.; Burke, T.N.; Hanada, E.S.; Marques, A.P. Segmental stabilisation and muscular strengthening in chronic low back pain—A comparative study. *Clinics* **2010**, *65*, 1013–1017. [CrossRef] [PubMed]
86. Amit, K.; Manish, G.; Taruna, K. Effect of trunk muscles stabilization exercises and general exercises on pain in recurrent non specific low back ache. *Int. Res. J. Med. Sci.* **2013**, *1*, 23–26.
87. Nourbakhsh, M.R.; Arabloo, A.M.; Salavati, M. The relationship between pelvic cross syndrome and chronic low back pain. *J. Back Musculoskelet. Rehabil.* **2006**, *19*, 119–128.
88. Standaert, C.J.; Weinstein, S.M.; Rumpeltes, J. Evidence-informed management of chronic low back pain with lumbar stabilisation exercises. *Spine J.* **2008**, *8*, 114–120. [CrossRef] [PubMed]
89. Hodges, P.W.; Richardson, C.A. Inefficient muscular stabilization of the lumbar spine associated with low back pain: a motor control evaluation of transversus abdominis. *Spine* **1996**, *21*, 2640–2650. [CrossRef] [PubMed]
90. Arokoski, J.P.; Valta, T.; Airaksinen, O.; Kankaanpää, M. Back and abdominal muscle function during stabilization exercises. *Arch. Phys. Med. Rehabil.* **2001**, *82*, 1089–1098. [CrossRef] [PubMed]
91. Kavcic, N.; Grenier, S.; McGill, S. Determining the stabilizing role of individual torso muscles during rehabilitation exercises. *Spine* **2004**, *29*, 1254–1265. [CrossRef] [PubMed]
92. Ferreira, P.H.; Ferreira, M.L.; Maher, C.G.; Herbert, R.D.; Refshauge, K. Specific stabilisation exercise for spinal and pelvic pain: A systematic review. *Aust. J. Physiother.* **2006**, *52*, 79–88. [CrossRef]
93. Hodges, P. Transversus abdominis: A different view of the elephant. *Br. J. Sports Med.* **2008**, *42*, 941–944. [CrossRef] [PubMed]
94. Hicks, G.E.; Fritz, J.M.; Delitto, A.; McGill, S.M. Preliminary development of a clinical prediction rule for determining which patients with low back pain will respond to a stabilization exercise program. *Arch. Phys. Med. Rehabil.* **2005**, *86*, 1753–1762. [CrossRef] [PubMed]
95. Maeo, S.; Takahashi, T.; Takai, Y.; Kanehisa, H. Trunk muscle activities during abdominal bracing: comparison among muscles and exercises. *J. Sports Sci. Med.* **2013**, *12*, 467–474. [PubMed]
96. Adler, S.; Beckers, D.; Buck, M. *PNF in Practice: An Illustrated Guide*, 3rd ed.; Springer: Berlin, Germany, 2008.
97. Shimura, K.; Kasai, T. Effects of proprioceptive neuromuscular facilitation on the initiation of voluntary movement and motor evoked potentials in upper limb muscles. *Hum. Mov. Sci.* **2002**, *21*, 101–113. [CrossRef]
98. Richardson, C.; Hodges, P.W.; Hides, J. *Therapeutic Exercise for Lumbopelvic Stabilization: A Motor Control Approach for the Treatment and Prevention of Low Back Pain*, 2nd ed.; Churchill Livingstone: Edinburgh, UK, 2004.
99. Stanton, T.; Kawchuk, G. The effect of abdominal stabilization contractions on posteroanterior spinal stiffness. *Spine* **2008**, *33*, 694–701. [CrossRef] [PubMed]
100. Chon, S.C.; Chang, K.Y.; You, J.H. Effect of the abdominal draw-in manoeuvre in combination with ankle dorsiflexion in strengthening the transverse abdominal muscle in healthy young adults: a preliminary, randomised, controlled study. *Physiotherapy* **2010**, *96*, 130–136. [CrossRef] [PubMed]
101. Katsura, Y.; Ueda, S.Y.; Yoshikawa, T.; Usui, T.; Orita, K.; Sakamoto, H.; Sotobayashi, D.; Fujimoto, S. Effects of aquatic exercise training using new water-resistance equipment on trunk muscles, abdominal circumference, and activities of daily living in elderly women. *Int. J. Sport Health Sci.* **2011**, *9*, 113–121. [CrossRef]

102. Dankaerts, W.; O'Sullivan, P.; Burnett, A.; Straker, L. Altered patterns of superficial trunk muscle activation during sitting in nonspecific chronic low back pain patients: importance of subclassification. *Spine* **2006**, *31*, 2017–2023. [CrossRef] [PubMed]
103. O'Sullivan, P.B.; Smith, A.; Beales, D.J.; Straker, L.M. Association of biopsychosocial factors with degree of slump in sitting posture and self-report of back pain in adolescents: A cross-sectional study. *Phys. Ther.* **2011**, *91*, 470–484. [CrossRef] [PubMed]
104. Spine-Health. Annulus Fibrosus Definition. Available online: http://www.spine-health.com/glossary/annulus-fibrosus (accessed on 15 December 2014).
105. Nerurkar, N.L.; Sen, S.; Huang, A.H.; Elliott, D.M.; Mauck, R.L. Engineered disk-like angle-ply structures for intervertebral disk replacement. *Spine* **2012**, *35*, 867–873. [CrossRef] [PubMed]
106. Reitmaier, S.; Shirazi-Adl, A.; Bashkuev, M.; Wilke, H.J.; Gloria, A.; Schmidt, H. *In vitro* and in silico investigations of disc nucleus replacement. *J. R. Soc.* **2012**, *9*, 1869–1879. [CrossRef] [PubMed]
107. Guerin, H.L.; Elliott, D.M. Quantifying the contributions of structure to annulus fibrosus mechanical function using a nonlinear, anisotropic, hyperelastic model. *J. Orthop. Res.* **2007**, *25*, 508–516. [CrossRef] [PubMed]
108. O'Sullivan, P.B.; Mitchell, T.; Bulich, P.; Waller, R.; Holte, J. The relationship between posture and back muscle endurance in industrial workers with flexion-related low back pain. *Man. Ther.* **2006**, *11*, 264–271. [CrossRef] [PubMed]
109. Womersley, L.; May, S. Sitting posture of subjects with postural backache. *J. Manip. Physiol. Ther.* **2006**, *29*, 213–218. [CrossRef] [PubMed]
110. Mitchell, T.; O'Sullivan, P.B.; Burnett, A.F.; Straker, L.; Smith, A. Regional differences in lumbar spinal posture and the influence of low back pain. *BMC Musculoskelet. Disord.* **2008**. [CrossRef] [PubMed]
111. Gazzi, M.L.; Maher, C.G.; Hancock, M.J.; Kamper, S.J.; McAuley, J.H.; Stanton, T.R. Predicting response to motor control exercises and graded activity for patients with low back pain: preplanned secondary analysis of a randomized controlled trial. *Phys. Ther.* **2014**, *94*, 1543–1554.
112. Ullrich, P.F. Stretching for Back Pain Relief. Available online: http://www.spine-health.com/wellness/exercise/stretching-back-pain-relief (accessed on 17 December 2014).
113. MacAuley, D.; Best, T. *Evidence-Based Sports Medicine*, 2nd ed.; Blackwell Publishing: Oxford, UK, 2007.
114. Li, Y.; McClure, P.W.; Pratt, N. The effect of hamstring muscle stretching on standing posture and on lumbar and hip motions during forward bending. *Phys. Ther.* **1996**, *76*, 836–845. [PubMed]
115. DeLisa, J.A.; Gans, B.M.; Walsh, N.E. *Physical Medicine and Rehabilitation: Principles and Practice*, 4th ed.; Lippincott Williams and Wilkins: Philadelphia, PA, USA, 2005.
116. Youdas, J.W. Lumbar lordosis and pelvic inclination in adults with chronic low back pain. *Phys. Ther.* **2000**, *80*, 261–275. [PubMed]
117. Kim, H.; Chung, S.; Kim, S.; Shin, H.; Lee, J.; Kim, S. Influences of trunk muscles on lumbar lordosis and sacral angle. *Eur. Spine J.* **2006**, *15*, 409–414. [CrossRef] [PubMed]
118. Spine-Health. Nucleus Pulposus Definition. Available online: http://www.spine-health.com/glossary/nucleus-pulposus (accessed on 19 December 2014).
119. Stutchfield, B.M.; Coleman, S. The relationships between hamstring flexibility, lumbar flexion, and low back pain in rowers. *Eur. J. Sport Sci.* **2006**, *6*, 255–260. [CrossRef]
120. O'Sullivan, P. Diagnosis and classification of chronic low back pain disorders: maladaptive movement and motor control impairments as underlying mechanism. *Man. Ther.* **2005**, *10*, 242–255. [CrossRef] [PubMed]
121. Brennan, G.P.; Fritz, J.; Hunter, S.J.; Thackeray, A.; Delitto, A.; Erhard, R. Identifying subgroups of patients with acute/subacute "nonspecific" low back pain: results of a randomized clinical trial. *Spine* **2006**, *31*, 623–631. [CrossRef] [PubMed]

Permissions

All chapters in this book were first published by MDPI; hereby published with permission under the Creative Commons Attribution License or equivalent. Every chapter published in this book has been scrutinized by our experts. Their significance has been extensively debated. The topics covered herein carry significant findings which will fuel the growth of the discipline. They may even be implemented as practical applications or may be referred to as a beginning point for another development.

The contributors of this book come from diverse backgrounds, making this book a truly international effort. This book will bring forth new frontiers with its revolutionizing research information and detailed analysis of the nascent developments around the world.

We would like to thank all the contributing authors for lending their expertise to make the book truly unique. They have played a crucial role in the development of this book. Without their invaluable contributions this book wouldn't have been possible. They have made vital efforts to compile up to date information on the varied aspects of this subject to make this book a valuable addition to the collection of many professionals and students.

This book was conceptualized with the vision of imparting up-to-date information and advanced data in this field. To ensure the same, a matchless editorial board was set up. Every individual on the board went through rigorous rounds of assessment to prove their worth. After which they invested a large part of their time researching and compiling the most relevant data for our readers.

The editorial board has been involved in producing this book since its inception. They have spent rigorous hours researching and exploring the diverse topics which have resulted in the successful publishing of this book. They have passed on their knowledge of decades through this book. To expedite this challenging task, the publisher supported the team at every step. A small team of assistant editors was also appointed to further simplify the editing procedure and attain best results for the readers.

Apart from the editorial board, the designing team has also invested a significant amount of their time in understanding the subject and creating the most relevant covers. They scrutinized every image to scout for the most suitable representation of the subject and create an appropriate cover for the book.

The publishing team has been an ardent support to the editorial, designing and production team. Their endless efforts to recruit the best for this project, has resulted in the accomplishment of this book. They are a veteran in the field of academics and their pool of knowledge is as vast as their experience in printing. Their expertise and guidance has proved useful at every step. Their uncompromising quality standards have made this book an exceptional effort. Their encouragement from time to time has been an inspiration for everyone.

The publisher and the editorial board hope that this book will prove to be a valuable piece of knowledge for researchers, students, practitioners and scholars across the globe.

List of Contributors

Agnieszka Ćwirlej-Sozańska, Agnieszka Bejer, Agnieszka Wiśniowska-Szurlej and Bernard Sozański
Institute of Health Sciences, College of Medical Sciences of the University of Rzeszow, University of Rzeszow, Rejtana16C, 35-959 Rzeszow, Poland

Anna Wilmowska-Pietruszyńska
Faculty of Medicine, Lazarski University, Świeradowska Street 43, 02-662 Warsaw, Poland

Alessandro de Sire
Physical and Rehabilitative Medicine, Department of Health Sciences, University of Eastern Piedmont, Viale Piazza D'Armi 1, 28100 Novara, Italy
Department of Geriatrics, Neurosciences, Orthopedics, Center for Geriatric Medicine (CEMI), Institute of Internal Medicine and Geriatrics, Catholic University of the Sacred Heart, L.go F.Vito 8, 00168 Rome, Italy

Renata Spalek
Department of Geriatrics, Neurosciences, Orthopedics, Center for Geriatric Medicine (CEMI), Institute of Internal Medicine and Geriatrics, Catholic University of the Sacred Heart, L.go F.Vito 8, 00168 Rome, Italy
Rehabilitation Unit, 'Mons. L. Novarese' Hospital, Str. Sotto Cerca, 13040 Vercelli, Italy

Adel Alshahrani
Rehabilitation Sciences Department, Physical Therapy Program, Najran University, Najran 55461, Saudi Arabia

Zoë C. Franklin and Paul S. Holmes
Musculoskeletal Science and Sports Medicine Research Centre, Manchester Metropolitan University, Manchester M15 6BH, UK

Neil E. Fowler
Vice Chancellor's Office, University of Salford, Salford M5 4WT, UK

Andrew Hahne
School of Allied Health, La Trobe University, Kingsbury Drive, Bundoora 3086, Australia

Jon Ford
School of Allied Health, La Trobe University, Kingsbury Drive, Bundoora 3086, Australia
Advance Healthcare, 157 Scoresby Road, Boronia 3155, Australia

Luke Surkitt, Alexander Chan and Matthew Richards
Advance Healthcare, 157 Scoresby Road, Boronia 3155, Australia

Liye Zou and Kevin W Chen
Lifestyle (Mind-Body Movement) Research Center, College of Sports Science, Shenzhen University, Shenzhen 518060, China

Yanjie Zhang
Health and Exercise Science Laboratory, Institute of Sports Science, Seoul National University, Seoul 08826, Korea

Lin Yang
Cancer Epidemiology and Prevention Research, Alberta Health Services, Calgary, AB T2S 3C3, Canada
Departments of Oncology and Community Health Sciences, Cumming School of Medicine, University of Calgary, Calgary, AB T2N 4Z6, Canada

Paul D. Loprinzi
Department of Health, Exercise Science and Recreation Management School of Applied Sciences, The University of Mississippi, Oxford, MS 36877, USA

Albert S. Yeung and Jian Kong
Department of Psychiatry, Massachusetts General Hospital, Harvard Medical School, Boston, MA 02114, USA

Wook Song
Institute on Aging, Seoul National University, Seoul 08826, Korea

Tao Xiao
College of Mathematics and Statistics, Shenzhen University, Shenzhen 518060, China

Hong Li
Shenzhen Key Laboratory of Affective and Social Cognitive Science, College of Psychology and Sociology, Shenzhen University, Shenzhen 518060, China
Shenzhen Institute of Neuroscience, Shenzhen 518057, China

Kathy Reid, Mark Simmonds and Bruce Dick
Stollery Children's Hospital, Alberta Health Services, Edmonton, AB T6G 2B7, Canada
Department of Anaesthesiology and Pain Medicine, University of Alberta, Edmonton, AB T6G 2R3, Canada

Michelle Verrier
Department of Anaesthesiology and Pain Medicine, University of Alberta, Edmonton, AB T6G 2R3, Canada

Åsa Ringqvist
Department of Neurosurgery and Pain Rehabilitation, Skåne University Hospital, SE-221 85 Lund, Sweden

Elena Dragioti, Britt Larsson and Björn Gerdle
Pain and Rehabilitation Centre, and Department of Medical and Health Sciences, Linköping University, SE-581 85 Linköping, Sweden

Mathilda Björk
Department of Social and Welfare Studies, Linköping University, SE-602 21 Norrköping, Sweden

Andrew Baird and David Sheffield
Centre for Psychological Research, Kedleston Road Campus, University of Derby, Derby DE22 1GB, UK

Arpana Jaiswal, Jeffrey F. Scherrer, Joanne Salas, Carissa van den Berk-Clark and Sheran Fernando
Department of Family and Community Medicine, Saint Louis University School of Medicine, St. Louis, MO 63104, USA

Christopher M. Herndon
Department of Family and Community Medicine, Saint Louis University School of Medicine, St. Louis, MO 63104, USA
Department of Pharmacy Practice, School of Pharmacy, Southern Illinois University Edwardsville, Edwardsville, IL 62026, USA

Stefan J. Friedrichsdorf
Children's Hospitals and Clinics of Minnesota, Minneapolis, MN 55404, USA
Department of Pediatrics, University of Minnesota Medical School, Minneapolis, MN 55455, USA

Kavita Desai Dakoji, Andrew Warmuth and Cyndee Daughtry
Children's Hospitals and Clinics of Minnesota, Minneapolis, MN 55404, USA

James Giordano
Georgetown University Medical Center, Washington, DC 20057, USA

Craig A. Schulz
Children's Hospitals and Clinics of Minnesota, Minneapolis, MN 55404, USA
Center for Spirituality & Healing, University of Minnesota, Minneapolis, MN 55455, USA

Alexander Ritter
Department of Biological and Clinical Psychology, Friedrich Schiller University of Jena, Am Steiger 3, Haus 1, Jena D-07743, Germany
Section of Neurological Rehabilitation, Hans–Berger Department of Neurology at Jena University Hospital, Erlanger Allee 101, Jena D-07747, Germany

Marcel Franz, Caroline Dietrich, Wolfgang H. R. Miltner and Thomas Weiss
Department of Biological and Clinical Psychology, Friedrich Schiller University of Jena, Am Steiger 3, Haus 1, Jena D-07743, Germany

Christian Puta
Department of Sports Medicine and Health Promotion, Friedrich Schiller University of Jena, Wöllnitzer Str. 42, Jena D-07749, Germany

Thomas Probst, Robert Jank and Christoph Pieh
Department for Psychotherapy and Biopsychosocial Health, Danube University Krems, 3500 Krems, Austria

Nele Dreyer, Stefanie Seel and Andreas Mühlberger
Institute for Psychology, Regensburg University, 93053 Regensburg, Germany

Ruth Wagner, Klaus Hanshans and Renate Reyersbach
Hospital Barmherzige Brüder, 93049 Regensburg, Germany

Claas Lahmann
Department of Psychosomatic Medicine and Psychotherapy, University Medical Center Freiburg, Faculty of Medicine, University of Freiburg, 79106 Freiburg, Germany

Jillian Vinall and Nivez Rasic
Department of Anesthesia, University of Calgary, Calgary, AB T3B 6A8, Canada

Maria Pavlova
Department of Psychology, University of Calgary, Calgary, AB T2N 1N4, Canada

Gordon J. G. Asmundson
Department of Psychology, University of Regina, Regina, SK S4S 0A2, Canada

Melanie Noel
Department of Psychology, University of Calgary, Calgary, AB T2N 1N4, Canada
Division of Behaviour and the Developing Brain, Alberta Children's Hospital Research Institute, Calgary, AB T3B 6A8, Canada

Rebecca Gordon and Saul Bloxham
Department of Sport and Health Sciences, University of St Mark and St John, Plymouth PL6 8BH, UK

Index

R

S

T

www.ingramcontent.com/pod-product-compliance
Lightning Source LLC
LaVergne TN
LVHW081029210926
848485LV00004B/979